THE Women'sHealth
BIG BOOK OF EXERCISES

RODALE

© 2010 by Rodale Inc.

First published as direct online edition/November 2009.
Special sales edition published in February 2017.

Rodale books may be purchased for business or promotional use or for special sales. For information, please write to:
Special Markets Department, Rodale Inc., 733 Third Avenue, New York, NY 10017

Women's Health is a registered trademark of Rodale Inc.

Printed in China
Rodale Inc. makes every effort to use acid-free ⊖, recycled paper ♲.

Book design by George Karabotsos with John Seeger Gilman
Cover design by Joe Heroun

Photo editor: Mark Haddad

All photography by Beth Bischoff

Cover hairstylist: Tomo Nakajima at Vivian Artists
Cover makeup artist: Lynn LaMorte at Vivian Artists
Interior hairstylist: Giovanni Giuntoli using Mac and Redken @ WT Management
Interior makeup artist: Lynn LaMorte at Vivian Artists
Styling: Thea Palad, Gail Ann Markowitz
Footwear and apparel provided by Adidas, Asics, Avia, Beyond Yoga, Brooks, Champion, Danskin,
Jockey, Lululemon Athletica, New Balance, Ryka, Splits59, and Under Armour
Anatomy illustrations by bartleby.com, except Gluteus Maximus illustration by Kurt Walters

Library of Congress Cataloging-in-Publication Data is on file with the publisher.

ISBN-13 978–1–60529–549–7   paperback
ISBN-13 978–1–62336–992–7   special sales paperback

Distributed to the book trade by Macmillan
15 17 19 20 18 16 14   paperback
2 4 6 8 10 9 7 5 3   special sales paperback

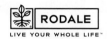

LIVE YOUR WHOLE LIFE™

We inspire and enable people to improve their lives and the world around them
For more of our products visit **rodalestore.com** or call 800-848-4735

Contents

Acknowledgments

I could never properly thank all of the people who have contributed in some way to *The Women's Health Big Book of Exercises*. But I'm particularly grateful to Steve Murphy and the Rodale family, to whom I extend my deepest appreciation for this great opportunity.

David Zinczenko: Thank you for your guidance, encouragement, and support. But most of all, thank you for the idea itself.

Michele Promaulayko and the *Women's Health* staff: I'm honored to contribute to such a great brand.

The talented and tireless George Karabotsos, who instantly shared my vision and enthusiasm for what this book should look like.

Stephen Perrine and the entire *Women's Health* Books team, with a special nod to designers John Seeger Gilman, Laura White, Elizabeth Neal, Holland Utley, and Mark Michaelson. Your efforts were heroic.

Joe Heroun: The cover is outstanding.

Karen Rinaldi, Chris Krogermeier, Marilyn Hauptly, Brooke Myers, and Jennifer Giandomenico, along with everyone else in Rodale Books who worked so hard to make this project happen.

Beth Bischoff, Michael Tedesco, and Danelle Manthey. The photography is terrific, from front to back.

Mark Haddad and Debbie McHugh: You went above and beyond.

Peter Moore, Bill Phillips, Matt Marion, Bill Stieg, Matt Goulding, Jeff Csatari, Lou Schuler, and Tom McGrath: You have influenced and inspired me beyond measure.

Bill Hartman: Your knowledge of training and anatomy is unsurpassed. I can't thank you enough for lending me your expertise.

Rachel Cosgrove: Thanks for all the coaching on exercise technique. This book is far better because of you.

Alwyn Cosgrove: I become smarter every time I talk to you. Here's hoping you never stop taking my calls.

To everyone on the *Men's Health* editorial team: I'm lucky to work with such a talented and hard-working group of people.

My friends and mentors: Craig Ballantyne, Michael Mejia, Robert dos Remedios, Joe Dowdell, Valerie Waters, Mike Boyle, Galya Talkington, Mike Wunsch, Craig Rasmussen, Alan Aragon, Stuart McGill, Ph.D., and Jeff Volek, Ph.D. Thanks for all the advice— I'm indebted to each of you.

Special thanks to Jen Ator, Adam Bornstein, Maria Masters, Kyle Western, Carolyn Kylstra, Allison Falkenberry, Charlene Lutz, Mary Rinfret, Alice Mudge, Roy Levenson, and Jaclyn Colletti. There wouldn't be a book without your behind-the-scenes work.

And, of course, to my wife, Jess: You are still my favorite.   —A.C.

Introduction:
Your New Body Starts Here

This book isn't about exercises.

It's about results.
Fast results.
The kind you want on New Year's Day.
And before your wedding.
And when summer is just 2 weeks away.

■

Of course, everyone knows you can't transform your body overnight. But if you commit to the principles and plans in these pages, you can transform it for the rest of your life. Only it won't take you a lifetime to start seeing results. It won't even take months. No, you'll notice the difference in just 14 days. And everything you need is in this book—from the workout that best fits your goals to the simple nutrition plan that you can start today.

You see, the results you want are yours for the taking. For instance, say you want to lose your gut. Using The World's Greatest 4-Week Diet and Exercise Plan, you can expect to lose 2 to 3 pounds of pure fat a week. That's an inch of belly blubber every 14 days. Those size-8 jeans? You're just a month away from a pair of 6s.

Now, these numbers aren't just made up. They're based on new scientific research from the University of Connecticut that shows you can lose up to 10 pounds of fat per month, without feeling hungry or deprived. In the study, the scientists discovered what's truly possible when you combine the right kind of diet with the right kind of exercise. The very same principles, in fact, that all the nutrition and exercise plans in this book are based on.

The benefits don't end with fat loss, though. The researchers found that people following the program reduced their risk for heart disease and diabetes, too. Results vary, of course, but the upshot is that the diet and workout plans in this book are powerful tools. Together, they make every second of every exercise you do count a little more than it ever has before. The cumulative effect of which is the fastest results of your life.

Perhaps it's not convincing you need, though; maybe you're just short on time. After all, the busy lives most of us lead leave little room for long workouts. Well, that's covered, too. You can do each of the workouts in this book in under an hour, and most take just 30 to 40 minutes. You'll also find 10 routines that can each be completed in just 15 minutes a day, 3 days a week. These aren't the kind of 15-minute workouts that are half as good as a 30-minute session. They're scientifically designed to be as effective as they are efficient. So you'll achieve the best results possible in the least amount of time. Instead of working out longer, you'll simply be working out smarter.

You'll probably be surprised at what you can accomplish in 15 minutes. University of Kansas researchers found that these short routines can double a beginner's strength. And they may be just as beneficial for your psyche: Unlike the average person, who quits a weight-training program within a month, 96 percent of the subjects stuck with the plan for the entire 6-month study. What's more, the approach also boosted participants' flab-fighting efforts beyond their workout. That's because their bodies burned more fat for the other 23 hours and 45 minutes a day—even while they were sleeping.

But these 15-minute workouts are just the start. To make this book even more useful, the world's top trainers have provided dozens of cutting-edge plans, for just about every goal, lifestyle, and experience level. All of them promise the fast results you want.

For example, if you've never even picked up a weight, you'll want to try The Get-Your-Body-Back Workout from Joe Dowdell, CSCS. Joe makes his living training models, athletes, and celebrities, and has worked with such names as Anne Hathaway, Claire Danes, Molly Sims, and Kate Hudson, as well as Victoria's Secret and *Sports Illustrated* swimsuit models. And the strategies he uses when designing workouts for his high-profile clientele are the same ones he employs to help you quickly burn fat, firm up, and improve your overall fitness.

If your goal is to look great on the beach (or naked!), The Bikini-Ready Workout will help you flatten your stomach and tighten your butt. It's designed by celebrity trainer Valerie Waters, who's perfected the body-shaping workouts you'll find here on dozens of Hollywood stars, including Jennifer Garner, Rachel Nichols, Kate Beckinsale, and Jessica Biel. Add your name to Valerie's client list to tone your total body and feel more confident than ever. And when you're ready to switch things up, you can Create Your Own Fat-Loss Workout, following the guidelines offered by Santa Clarita, California, performance coach Craig Rasmussen, CSCS. His plan allows you to choose your own flab-busting exercises for a personalized workout.

Want to look sexier in a pair of 7s? Try The Skinny Jeans Workout from Rachel Cosgrove, CSCS, author of *The Female Body Breakthrough*. In a pilot study at Rachel's gym, clients who tried the plan dropped two jeans sizes in just 8 weeks. The best part: It's perfect for any woman, whether you're a beginner or a long-time gym veteran.

In The Hard-Body Workout, fitness model and trainer Jen Heath shows you how to tone your hips, legs, and abs, and take your fitness levels to an all-time high.

But wait, there's more! You'll also find The Lose-the-Last-10-Pounds Workout, The Prenatal Workout, The Wedding Workout, The Time-Saving Couples Workout, The Best Three Exercise Workouts, and The Best Body-Weight Workouts—so you can burn fat and tone your body anywhere, anytime.

You might call *The Women's Health Big Book of Exercises* the book that keeps on giving. Giving results, that is. The fast kind.

Chapter 1:
The Genius of Weights

20 WAYS LIFTING HELPS YOU LOOK GREAT, STAY HEALTHY, AND LIVE LONGER

"You don't look like you lift weights."

I've heard this phrase more than once in my life, and it's always delivered by a burly guy in a sleeveless shirt who most certainly *does* look like he lifts weights. And who's no doubt basing his observation on the standards of a typical musclehead.

That's just it, though: Like most of you, I've never aspired to be a musclehead. Or a powerlifter. Or a strongman competitor. So do I look like any of those? Of course not.

But do I look like I lift weights? Absolutely. I'm lean and fit, and my muscles are well-defined, even if they're not busting out of my shirt.

You see, lifting weights isn't just about building 20-inch biceps. In fact, for most women, it's not about that at all, since resistance training may be the single most effective way to lose fat and look great in a swimsuit. What's more, the benefits of lifting extend into nearly every aspect of your health and well-being. So much so that after nearly 12 years of reporting in the field of health and fitness, I've come to one rock-solid conclusion: You'd have to be crazy not to lift weights—even if bigger biceps are the last thing you want.

Lifting Weights Gives You an Edge

Over belly fat.
Over stress.
Over heart disease, diabetes, and cancer.
Lifting even makes you smarter and happier.

How can the simple act of picking up a weight, putting it down, and repeating a few times bestow such a bevy of benefits? It all starts at the microscopic level of a muscle fiber.

A quick primer: When you lift weights, you cause tiny tears in your muscle fibers. This accelerates a process called muscle-protein synthesis that uses amino acids to repair and reinforce the fibers, making them resistant to future damage. So when a muscle fiber is exposed to a frequent challenge—as it is when you regularly lift weights—it makes structural adaptations in order to better handle that challenge. For example, your muscles adapt by getting bigger and stronger, or by becoming more resistant to fatigue.

These adaptations occur to reduce stress on your body, which is why you can perform everyday functions—such as walking up stairs or picking up a light object—with little effort. It's also why if you routinely lift weights, you'll find that even the hardest physical tasks become easier. In scientific circles, this is known as the training effect. Turns out, this training effect improves not only your muscles but your entire life, too. It is, in fact, what gives you the edge.

Want some proof? Here are 20 reasons you shouldn't live another day without lifting.

1. You'll Lose 40 Percent More Fat

This might be the biggest secret in fat loss. While you've no doubt been told that aerobic exercise is the key to losing your gut, weight training is actually far more valuable.

Case in point: Penn State University researchers put overweight people on a reduced-calorie diet and divided them into three groups. One group didn't exercise, another performed aerobic exercise 3 days a week, and a third did both aerobic exercise and weight training 3 days a week. Each of the groups lost nearly the same amount of weight—around 21 pounds. But the lifters shed about 6 more pounds of fat than did those who didn't pump iron. Why? Because the lifters' weight loss was almost pure fat, while the other two groups lost just 15 pounds of lard, along with several pounds of muscle. Do the math and you'll see that weights led to 40 percent greater fat loss.

This isn't a one-time finding. Research on non-lifting dieters shows that, on average, 75 percent of their weight loss is from fat, and 25 percent is from muscle. That 25 percent may reduce your scale weight, but it doesn't do a lot for your reflection in the mirror. It also makes you more likely to gain back the flab you lost. However, if you weight train as you diet, you'll protect your hard-earned muscle and burn more fat instead.

Think of it in terms of liposuction: The whole point is to simply remove unattractive flab, right? That's exactly what you should demand from your workout.

2. You'll Burn More Calories

Lifting increases the number of calories you burn while you're sitting on the couch. One reason: Your muscles need energy to repair and upgrade your muscle fibers after each resistance-training workout. For instance, a University of Wisconsin study found that when people performed a total-body workout comprising of just three big-muscle exercises, their metabolisms were elevated for 39 hours afterward. The exercisers also burned a greater percentage of calories from fat during this time, compared with those who didn't lift.

But what about during your workout? After all, many experts say jogging burns more calories than weight training. Turns out, when scientists at the University of Southern Maine used an advanced method to estimate energy expenditure, they found that lifting burns as many as 71 percent more calories than originally thought. The researchers calculated that performing just one circuit of eight exercises—which takes about 8 minutes—can expend 159 to 231 calories. That's about the same number burned by running at a 6-minute–mile pace for the same duration.

3. Your Clothes Will Fit Better

If you don't lift weights, you can say goodbye to toned arms. Research shows that between the ages of 30 and 50, you're likely to lose 10 percent of the total muscle on your body. And that percentage will double by the time you're 60.

Worse yet, it's likely that lost muscle is replaced by fat over time, according to a study in the *American Journal of Clinical Nutrition*. The scientists found that even people who maintained their body weights for up to 38 years lost 3 pounds of muscle and added 3 pounds of fat every decade. Not only does that make you look flabby, it increases your waist size. That's because 1 pound of fat takes up 18 percent more space on your body than 1 pound of muscle. Thankfully, regular resistance training can prevent this fate.

4. You'll Keep Your Body Young

It's not just the quantity of the muscle you lose that's important, it's the quality. Research shows that your fast-twitch muscle fibers are reduced by up to 50 percent as you age, while slow-twitch fibers decrease by less than 25 percent. That's important because your fast-twitch fibers are the muscles largely responsible for generating power, a combined measure of strength and speed. While this attribute is key to peak sports performance, it's also the reason you can rise from your living room chair. Ever notice how the elderly often have trouble standing up? Blame fast-twitch muscles that are underused and wasting away.

The secret to turning back the clock? Pumping iron, of course. Heavy strength training is especially effective, as is lifting light weights really fast. (Hint: Any exercise in this book with the word *explosive* or *jump* in its name is ideal for working your fast-twitch muscle fibers.)

5. You'll Build Stronger Bones

You lose bone mass as you age, which increases the likelihood that you'll one day suffer a debilitating fracture in your hips or vertebrae. That's even worse than it sounds, since UK researchers found that among older women who break a hip during a fall, more than 50 percent never walk again. In addition, significant bone loss in your spine can result in the dreaded "dowager's hump," or hunchback. The good news: A study in the *Journal of Applied Physiology* found that 16 weeks of resistance training increased hip bone density and elevated blood levels of osteocalcin—a marker of bone growth—by 19 percent.

6. You'll Be More Flexible

Over time, your flexibility can decrease by up to 50 percent. This makes it harder to squat down, bend over, and reach behind you. But in a study published in the *International Journal of Sports Medicine*, scientists found that three full-body workouts a week for 16 weeks increased flexibility of the hips and shoulders, while improving sit-and-reach

test scores by 11 percent. Not convinced that weight training won't leave you "muscle-bound"? Research shows that Olympic weight lifters rate second only to gymnasts in overall flexibility.

7. Your Heart Will Be Healthier

Pumping iron really does get your blood flowing. Researchers at the University of Michigan found that people who performed three total-body weight workouts per week for 2 months decreased diastolic blood pressure (the bottom number) by an average of eight points. That's enough to reduce the risk of a stroke by 40 percent, and the risk of a heart attack by 15 percent.

8. You'll Derail Diabetes

Call it muscle medication. In a 4-month study, Austrian scientists found that people with type 2 diabetes who started strength training significantly lowered their blood sugar levels, improving their condition. Just as important, lifting may be one of the best ways to prevent diabetes in the first place. That's because it not only fights the fat that puts you at an increased risk for the disease but also improves your sensitivity to the hormone insulin. This helps keep your blood sugar under control, reducing the likelihood that you'll develop diabetes.

9. You'll Cut Your Cancer Risk

Don't settle for an ounce of prevention; weights may offer it by the pound. A

University of Florida study found that people who performed three resistance-training workouts a week for 6 months experienced significantly less oxidative cell damage than non-lifters. That's important since damaged cells can lead to cancer and other diseases. And in a study published in *Medicine and Science in Sports and Exercise*, scientists discovered that resistance training speeds the rate at which food is moved through your large intestine by up to 56 percent, an effect that's thought to reduce the risk for colon cancer.

10. Your Diet Will Improve

Lifting weights provides a double dose of weight-loss fuel: On top of burning calories, exercise helps your brain stick to a diet. University of Pittsburgh researchers studied 169 overweight adults for 2 years and found that the participants who didn't follow a 3-hour-a-week training plan ate more than their allotted 1,500 calories per day. The reverse was also true—sneaking snacks sabotaged their workouts. The study authors say it's likely that both actions are a reminder to stay on track, reinforcing your weight-loss goal and drive.

11. You'll Handle Stress Better

Break a sweat in the weight room and you'll stay cool under pressure. Texas A&M University scientists determined that the fittest people exhibited lower levels of stress hormones than those who were the least fit. And a Medical College of Georgia study found that the blood pressure levels of the people with the most muscle returned to normal the fastest after a stressful situation, compared to those who had the least muscle.

12. You'll Shrug Off Jet Lag

Next time you travel overseas, hit the hotel gym before you unpack. When researchers at Northwestern University and the University of California at San Francisco studied muscle biopsies from people who had performed resistance exercise, they discovered changes in the proteins that regulate circadian rhythms. The researchers' conclusion? Strength training helps your body adjust faster to a change in time zones or work shifts.

13. You'll Be Happier

Yoga isn't the only exercise that's soothing. Researchers at the University of Alabama at Birmingham discovered that people who performed three weight workouts a week for 6 months significantly improved their scores on measures of anger and overall mood.

14. You'll Sleep Better

Lifting hard helps you rest easier. Australian researchers observed that patients who performed three total-body weight workouts a week for 8 weeks experienced a 23 percent improvement in sleep quality. In fact, the study participants were able to fall asleep faster and slept longer than before they started lifting weights.

15. You'll Get in Shape Faster

The term *cardio* shouldn't just describe aerobic exercise. A study at the University of Hawaii found that circuit training with weights raises your heart rate 15 beats per minute higher than does running at 60 to 70 percent of your maximum heart rate. According to the researchers, this approach not only strengthens your muscles, it provides cardiovascular benefits similar to those of aerobic exercise. So you save time without sacrificing results.

16. You'll Fight Depression

Squats may be the new Prozac. Scientists at the University of Sydney found that regularly lifting weights significantly reduces symptoms of major depression. In fact, the researchers report that a meaningful improvement was seen in 60 percent of clinically diagnosed patients, similar to the response rate from antidepressants—but without the negative side effects.

17. You'll Be More Productive

Invest in dumbbells—it could help you land a raise. UK researchers found that workers were 15 percent more productive on the days they made time to exercise compared to days they skipped their workouts. Now consider for a moment what these numbers mean to you: On days when you exercise, you can—theoretically, at least—accomplish in an 8-hour day what normally would take you 9 hours and 12 minutes. Or you'd still work 9 hours but get more done, leaving you feeling less stressed and happier with your job—another perk that the workers reported on the days they exercised.

18. You'll Add Years to Your Life

Get strong to live long. University of South Carolina researchers determined that total-body strength was linked to lower risks of death from cardiovascular disease, cancer, and all causes. Similarly, University of Hawaii scientists found that being strong at middle age was associated with "exceptional survival," defined as living until 85 years of age without developing a major disease.

19. You'll Stay Sharp

Never forget how important it is to pump iron. University of Virginia scientists discovered that men and women who lifted weights three times a week for 6 months significantly decreased their blood levels of homocysteine, a protein that's linked to the development of dementia and Alzheimer's disease.

20. You'll Even Be Smarter

Talk about a mind-muscle connection: Brazilian researchers found that 6 months of resistance training enhanced lifters' cognitive function. In fact, the workouts resulted in better short- and long-term memory, improved verbal reasoning, and a longer attention span.

Chapter 2:
All Your Lifting Questions...
Answered

THE KNOW-HOW YOU NEED TO BUILD THE BODY YOU WANT

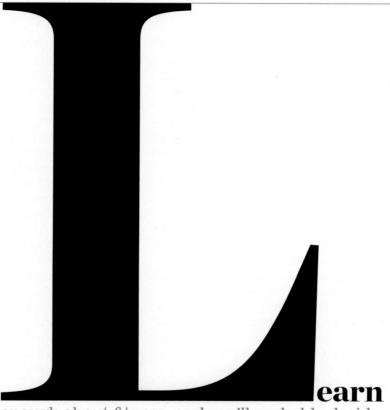

Learn enough about fitness, and you'll probably decide that the answer to just about every workout question should start with the same two words: *It depends*. After all, every person and situation is unique, and there's more than one way to achieve most goals. That's why this chapter provides you with basic principles and general guidelines, not unbreakable commandments. I've simply tackled the questions I'm asked most frequently and given you my take based on what I've learned over the years. Think of it as the Cliffs Notes for my version of Training 101. The best part: I only use the word caveat once.

"How Many Repetitions Should I Do"?

When it comes to your workout, this is always the first question you should ask. Why? Because it forces you to decide what your main goal is. For instance, do you want lose fat faster or build more muscle? The answer will determine the number of reps you do. Just make your choice, then use the guidelines that follow to find the rep range you need.

You Want to Lose Fat Faster

This one's easy: All the top trainers I know have found that doing 8 to 15 repetitions works the best for fat loss. And perhaps it's no wonder, since research shows that performing sets in that same range stimulates the greatest increase in fat-burning hormones, compared with doing a greater or fewer number of repetitions. Of course, 8 to 15 reps is a fairly broad recommendation. So you'll need to break it down further. A good approach: Use three smaller rep ranges to vary your workouts, while staying between 8 and 15 repetitions. Examples:

12 TO 15 REPS
10 TO 12 REPS
8 TO 10 REPS

All of these rep ranges are effective for burning fat. So choose one—12 to 15 reps is a great place to start, especially for beginners—and then switch to another every 2 to 4 weeks.

You Want to Build More Muscle

There's a popular gym notion that doing 8 to 12 reps is the best way to build muscle. However, the origin of this recommendation might surprise you: It's from an English surgeon and competitive bodybuilder named Ian MacQueen, MD, who published a scientific paper in which he recommended a moderately high number of reps for muscle growth. The year? 1954. Now, this approach most certainly works. But we've learned a lot about muscle science in the past half-century. And it makes more sense that using a variety of repetition ranges—low, medium, and high—will lead to even better muscle growth. (To understand why, see "There's No Such Thing as a Bad Rep" on page 14.) For the best results, you can switch up your rep ranges every 2 to 4 weeks, or even every workout.

I like this 3-day-a-week, total-body scheme from strength coach Alwyn Cosgrove, CSCS, a longtime fitness advisor to *Men's Health:*

MONDAY: 5 REPS
WEDNESDAY: 15 REPS
FRIDAY: 10 REPS

This simple approach is supported by 21st-century science. Case in point: Arizona State University researchers discovered that people who alternated their rep ranges in each of three weekly training sessions—a technique called undulating periodization—gained twice as much strength as those who did the same number of reps every workout.

"How Much Weight Should I Use"?

This question pops up a lot in my e-mail. I used to reply, "How should I know? I can't tell how strong you are over the Internet!" But I've come up with a much better answer: Choose the heaviest weight that allows you to complete all of the prescribed repetitions. That is, the lower the number of repetitions, the heavier the weight you should use. And vice versa. For instance, if you can lift a weight 15 times, it's not going to do your muscles much good to lift it only 5 times. And if you select a weight that's difficult to lift 5 times, there's no way you can pump out 15 repetitions.

So how do you figure out the right amount? Trial and error. You just have to make an educated guess and experiment. This is second nature for experienced lifters, but if you're new to training, don't stress over it; you'll catch on fast. The key is to get in there and start lifting. If you choose a weight that's too heavy or too light, just adjust it accordingly in your next set.

Of course, you'll realize pretty quickly if you're using a weight that's too heavy for your rep range. After all, you won't be able to complete all the reps. But gauging if a weight is too light is a little trickier. One simple way: Note the point at which you start to struggle.

Let's say you're doing 10 repetitions. If all 10 seem easy, then the weight you're using is too light. However, if you start to struggle on your 10th rep,

you've chosen the correct poundage. What does "start to struggle" mean? It's when the speed at which you lift the weight slows significantly. Although you can push on for another rep or two, the struggle indicates that your muscles have just about had it. This is also the point when most people start to "cheat" by changing their body posture to help them lift the weight.

Remember, the goal is to complete all the repetitions in each set with perfect form while challenging your muscles to work as hard as they can. Using the start-to-struggle approach will help you do this. Go hard, and when you start to struggle, you've completed the set. This is also a great strategy to use when you're directed to do as many repetitions as possible on body-weight exercises such as pushups, chinups, and hip raises. (You'll find this instruction in many of the workouts in Chapter 13.)

"How Many Sets of an Exercise Should I Do"?

A good rule of thumb: Do as many sets as you need to complete at least 25 repetitions for a muscle group. So if you're planning to do five reps of an exercise, you'd do five sets of that movement. If you're doing 15 reps, you'd only need to do two sets. The more reps of an exercise you do, the fewer sets you need to perform. And vice versa. This helps keep your muscles under tension for an appropriate amount of time no matter what rep range you're using.

THERE'S NO SUCH THING AS A BAD REP

Trainers don't just randomly choose the number of repetitions a person does. Well, at least the good ones don't. That's because the rep range you use dictates how your muscles adapt to your routine. In fact, by knowing the benefits of three key rep ranges, you can choose the strategy that's best for the results you want. Keep in mind that these rep ranges don't work like an on-off button; they're more like a dimmer switch. As you move up and down in reps, you're simply dialing back the benefits of one and emphasizing those of another. Here's a primer on each.

1. Low repetitions (1 to 5): This rep range allows you to use the heaviest weights, which puts your muscles under the highest amounts of tension. This increases the number of *myofibrils* in your muscle fibers. What the heck is a *myofibril*? It's the part of your muscle fiber that contains the contractile proteins. Think of it this way: When there are more of these proteins to contract, your muscles can generate greater force. That's why 1 to 5 is an ideal rep range for building strength. And, of

(continues on page 15)

If you're in good-enough shape, you can certainly do more than 25 reps per muscle group, but cap your output at 50. For example, a common bodybuilding recommendation is to do three sets of 10 of three or four different exercises for one muscle group. That's as many as 120 total reps for the working muscles. Trouble is, if you can perform even close to 100 reps for any muscle group, you're not working hard enough. Think of it this way: The harder you train, the less time you'll be able to sustain that level of effort. For example, many people can run for an hour if they jog slowly, but you'd be hard-pressed to find anyone who could do high-intensity sprints—without a major decrease in performance—for that period of time. And once performance starts to decline, you've achieved most of the benefits you can for that muscle group. So why waste your time?

"How Long Should My Workout Last"?

Only as long as it needs to, of course. The best way to gauge this is by the total number of sets you do. I first learned this years ago from famed Australian strength coach Ian King, and I find it still holds true today. The advice: Do 12 to 25 sets per workout. That is, when you add up the sets you perform for every exercise, the total should fall within this range (not including your warmup). So if you're using lengthy rest periods, your workout will take longer; and if you're using

shorter rest periods, you'll finish faster. Beginners will probably find that 12 sets are plenty, while experienced lifters may be able to handle the upper end of the range. This total-set rule isn't set in stone, of course, but it works very well for building muscle and losing fat. For most people, doing more work than this in a single workout results in rapidly diminishing returns on their time investment. It also increases the time your muscles need to recover between your bouts of exercise. If you ignore this important factor, you can wind up overstressing your body, which slows your results.

"How Long Should I Rest between Sets"?

Probably not long enough to chit-chat at the water fountain. You see, the amount of rest between sets is a crucial but often overlooked factor in most workouts. To understand why, you'll need a quick lesson in exercise science: The lower your reps—and heavier the weights—the longer you need to rest between sets; the higher your repetitions—and lighter the weights—the shorter your rest. Why? When you lift heavy weights, you're recruiting fast-twitch muscle fibers, the fibers that generate the most force but also fatigue the fastest and take the longest to recover. So giving them ample time to rest helps ensure you train them fully each set. When you use lighter weights and do more reps, you're mainly hitting your slow-twitch muscle fibers. These are not only more resistant to fatigue than fast-twitch fibers but they recover much more quickly, too. The upshot is that, even after a challenging high-rep set, they're ready for a repeat performance in a short period of time.

What does this mean in regard to your stopwatch? I use these basic guidelines:

1 TO 3 REPS: REST FOR 3 TO 5 MINUTES
4 TO 7 REPS: REST FOR 2 TO 3 MINUTES
8 TO 12 REPS: REST FOR 1 TO 2 MINUTES
13 REPS OR MORE: REST FOR 1 MINUTE

But here's the real secret: These numbers simply describe the amount of time you rest before working a muscle group again. That is, if you think strategically, you can work other muscle groups instead of waiting around while the clock ticks. The two methods I like best for this are alternating sets and circuits. They slash minutes from your workout time, without sacrificing results. That's because one muscle group rests while the other works. Here's a description of each, but you'll find them used frequently in Chapter 13.

Alternating sets: Do one set of an exercise, rest, then do a set of an exercise that works the opposite muscle group. (You can also pair an upper-body exercise with a lower-body exercise.) Rest again, and repeat until you've completed the prescribed number of sets. For instance, if you do

six reps of the bench press, you might rest for just 1 minute, instead of 2 minutes. Then you'd do a dumbbell row, and rest for 1 minute. Including the time it takes you to complete the dumbbell row, you've now rested for more than 2 minutes before repeating the bench press. The bottom line: Your rest periods can easily be cut in half.

Circuits: Do three or more (could be four, five, or even 10) exercises in succession without resting between sets. The most common approach here is to alternate between upper- and lower-body exercises. As an example, you might do the following exercises, one after another: squat, bench press, hip raise, dumbbell row, and so on. This way, your upper body rests while your lower body works. You can also add rest in between each set as well.

Ready to try these techniques? Use this chart to guide you.

PAIR THIS . . .	WITH THAT . . .
QUADRICEPS	GLUTES & HAMSTRINGS
CHEST	UPPER BACK
SHOULDERS	LATS
BICEPS	TRICEPS
UPPER BODY	LOWER BODY
UPPER BODY	CORE
LOWER BODY	CORE

course, more myofibrils increase the size of your fibers, making your muscles bigger. (Muscle trivia #1: This type of muscle growth is known as *myofibrillar hypertrophy*.)

2. High repetitions (11 or more): When you use higher reps, your muscles have to contract for long periods of time. This increases the number of mitochondria in your muscle fibers. Your mitochondria are energy-producing structures that not only burn fat (the more, the better!) but also lead to greater muscle endurance and cardiovascular fitness. What's more, these structural changes boost the fluid volume in your fibers, adding size to your muscles. (Muscle trivia #2: This type of muscle growth is called *sarcoplasmic hypertrophy*.)

3. Medium repetitions (6 to 10): With this approach, your muscles are under medium tension for a medium amount of time. Consider this just what it is: A mix of low- and high-rep lifting. So it helps you improve both muscle strength and muscle endurance. You might say it strikes a good balance between the two. However, if you use this rep range all the time, you'll miss out on the greater tension levels that come with lower reps and the longer tension time achieved by higher reps. Use them all.

"How Many Days a Week Should I Lift"?

At least 2. This number has been shown to provide many of the health benefits attributed to resistance training. So consider that the minimum. Ideally, though, you'll want to hit the weights 3 or 4 days a week, with either total-body workouts or an "upper-lower split" approach. I'll explain each.

Total-body workouts are just what they sound like. You work your entire body each workout. Then you rest a day, and repeat. There's a scientific rationale for this. In multiple studies, researchers at the University of Texas Medical Branch, in Galveston, have reported that muscle protein synthesis—a marker of muscle repair—is elevated for up to 48 hours after resistance training. So if you work out on Monday at 7 p.m., your body is in muscle-growth mode until Wednesday at 7 p.m. After 48 hours, though, the biological stimulus for your body to build new muscle returns to normal. That means it's time for another workout.

Turns out, this 48-hour period is also similar to the length of time your metabolism is elevated after you lift weights. As a result, total-body training is highly effective whether you're trying to build muscle or lose fat. In fact, I'm convinced it's the single best mode of exercise for burning blubber. That's because the more muscle you work, the more calories you burn—both during and after your workout.

The other strategy that works well is an upper-lower split. This is mainly used for adding muscle size and strength, and for improving sports performance. In this method, you work your upper body and lower body on separate days. The reason: It allows you to train the muscle groups of both halves harder than you could in a total-body routine. However, it also means that you need to give your muscles a little extra time to fully recover. For instance, you might do a 4-day-a-week plan in which you complete a lower-body workout on Monday, an upper-body workout on Tuesday, and then rest for a day or two before repeating (on Thursday and Friday perhaps). That would give you 2 to 3 full days of rest between each type of workout. Or you could alternate between lower-body and upper-body workouts every other day, 3 days a week.

Keep in mind, there's no reason to use a split routine if you're gaining muscle and strength with total-body training. But if you reach a point when you can't fit all of the sets you want to do into a total-body workout, it's likely time to make the switch. Or you may simply want to experiment with different methods, to determine what works best for your muscles and for your lifestyle. You'll find there are plenty of workouts in this book to keep you busy.

"How Many Exercises Should I Do per Muscle Group"?

One. It's an approach that's simple and effective. You actually obtain most of the benefits of weight lifting from the first exercise you do, when your muscles are fresh. For instance, let's say you complete three sets of each of the dumbbell bench press, the incline dumbbell bench press, and the dumbbell fly. By the time you reach the last exercise, the amount of weight you can handle is far lower than had you done that movement first. See for yourself by trying the routine in reverse order: You'll find that for the dumbbell bench press, you'll be able to lift far less than when you do it first—and have to use a weight you'd normally consider too light. So the benefit to your muscles will have diminished. That's why, most of the time, sticking with one exercise per muscle group makes the most sense, especially if you have a limited amount of time to work out.

Now it's okay to break the one-exercise rule if there's a good reason to do so. For example, if a muscle group has been lagging, you may want to work it a little harder for a 4-week period by doubling the total number of sets you do for that area. This is called prioritizing a muscle group. So instead of doing all of your sets with one exercise, you might use two or three different exercises, as in the example of the dumbbell bench press, incline dumbbell bench press, and dumbbell fly. (See "Build the Perfect Chest" in Chapter 4 for a ready-made plan.) While you won't be able to use as much weight in the second two exercises as you would if you had done them when your muscles were fresh, you will increase the total amount of work the muscle group has to perform.

This can help you break through plateaus and spark new muscle growth.

One *caveat*: If you try this method and find you're getting weaker, the workload is too high for you. Dial it back so that your muscles can better recover between workouts. What's more, prioritizing one muscle group may mean you have to cut back a little on other muscle groups. That's because the total-set-per-workout recommendation still applies. (See "How Long Should My Workout Last"? on page 14.)

"How Fast Should I Lift"?

Do this: Lower slowly, lift fast. Research shows that taking longer to lower the weight helps you build strength faster, and quickly lifting the weight activates the greatest number of muscle fibers. For most exercises, take 2 or 3 seconds to lower the weight, pause for a second in the "down" position, and then lift the weight as quickly as you can while maintaining control over it at all times. One big exception: If an exercise is to be performed explosively, perform the entire lift quickly, from start to finish.

Keep in mind that on some exercises, like the lat pulldown, it will seem like the lowering portion is the part of the lift in which your muscles are contracting. But realize that as you pull the bar down, the weight stack is actually rising.

"Do I Need a Spotter"?

The politically correct answer is yes. After all, a barbell might fall on your neck. This is no joke, because this very kind of accident happens every year. It kills people. But there's a bigger lesson here: Don't try to lift a weight that's too heavy for you, especially if that weight is attached to a bar. For instance, like many people, I work out by myself at home. So a spotter isn't an option. However, there's zero chance that I'll be pinned helplessly underneath a barbell. That's because I do my heavy pressing with dumbbells, which I can just drop to the floor if needed.

I also use the start-to-struggle strategy with every exercise. (See "How Much Weight Should I Use"? on page 13.) If I choose a weight that's too heavy for six reps, I'll know it before I ever reach the point of complete failure and I'll be able to simply end the set before trouble starts. How then, do I figure out my one-rep max? I don't. It's not really important to me. But if it is to you, my advice is simple: Anytime you test your limits, make sure you have a spotter.

"What Equipment Do I Need"?

You already have enough to get started: your body. In fact, check out "The Best Body-Weight Workouts" in Chapter 13 for a workout you can do today. But if you want to build your own home gym, here's a rundown of everything worth having—from the essentials to the extras.

The Essentials

Dumbbells. If I could have only one training tool, the dumbbell would be my pick. It's simple, versatile, and durable. If you have the space, any type of dumbbell will do. The least expensive kind is a basic cast-iron hex dumbbell. (At the time of this printing, 1 dollar a pound was a competitive price.) Shop around; you may be able to find a special on an entire set. If you're strapped for space, consider buying a pair of PowerBlocks (www.powerblock. com). This all-in-one dumbbell set allows you to quickly change the weight you want to use, and it requires little storage room.

Bench. A basic flat bench is fairly inexpensive, but if you're going to invest the money, consider an adjustable bench so that you can perform exercises on both an incline and a decline. (The Web site www.fitnessfactory.com has several options.) This can instantly give you dozens of more exercise variations.

Chinup bar. If you're handy, you can create and install your own using a piece of 1-inch diameter pipe. Or purchase a pre-made joist-, wall-, or ceiling-mount chinup bar, like one of those at www.newyorkbarbells.com. You can also buy the kind that hangs on a door. I like a product called the Perfect Pullup (www.perfectpullup. com) because you can lower the bar's height to perform inverted rows. This is a unique feature that really improves its usefulness. The downsides: You have to use screws to attach the bar to the inside of a doorframe; and at $100, it's relatively expensive.

Swiss ball. This is also called a stability ball, a physio ball, and an exercise ball. (Why did I go with Swiss ball? Habit.) The Swiss ball is great for core exercises, but it also doubles as an inexpensive substitute for the bench. In fact, a set of dumbbells, a Swiss ball, and a chinup bar will give you a complete home gym. You can pick up a basic Swiss ball just about anywhere—including Target and Wal-Mart—but heavier-duty balls such as those from Sissel and Duraball are available at www.performbetter.com.

Barbell and weight plates. Two options here: a standard barbell or an Olympic barbell. A standard bar weighs 20 pounds and is less expensive, but the Olympic bar—which weighs about 45 pounds—is the kind you'll find in most gyms. The Olympic bar is also heavier duty. My advice: If you already have a standard bar, your muscles won't know the difference. But opt for a 7-foot Olympic barbell if you're starting your home gym or upgrading. Shop around and you can find an Olympic barbell with a 300-pound Olympic weight set for $300.

Power rack. You absolutely need a power or squat rack if you want to do barbell squats. But a good rack can also vastly expand your home gym. That's because you can buy one equipped with a chinup bar and high and low pulley systems for doing lat pulldowns, cable rows, and just about

any other cable exercise. I recommend the EFS Multi High/Low Pulley Rack at www.elitefts.com.

The Extras

Cable station. This gives you hundreds more exercise variations. The most economical—in terms of both money and space—is a cable pulley system that's attached to a power rack. But if you have the space and the cash, the Free Motion EXT Dual Cable Cross is state of the art. The arms swivel into 108 different positions, allowing you to work every muscle from every conceivable angle. See for yourself at www.freemotionfitness.com.

EZ-curl bar. When you do curls, this angled bar is easier on your wrists than a straight bar. It's also shorter than a barbell, making it easier to move to an open spot in the gym.

Kettlebells. These Russian imports—which look like bowling balls with handles—have been around for years but are just now taking hold in gyms and exercise routines across the United States. You can use them like dumbbells, but you'll find that they make the same exercises more challenging. That's because the weight is off-center, which forces your stabilizer muscles to work even harder. Check out the single-arm kettlebell swing on page 268, and feel free to substitute a kettlebell for almost any movement in this book that requires a dumbbell.

Medicine ball. Some equipment never goes out of style. Use medicine balls for core exercises, sports-specific training, and even as a way to make pushups harder (place each hand on a ball). For the most versatile version, buy a ball that bounces—such as a First Place Elite Medicine Ball—so that you can throw it against a wall, catch, and repeat. (Go to www.performbetter.com for a great selection.)

Valslides. These foam-topped plastic sliders transform hard floors and carpets into ice rinks, intensifying old standbys like lunges by decreasing your stability and keeping your muscles under tension for the entire movement. What's more, Valslides are perhaps most useful for core exercises, because they provide an all-new way to work your abs, as you'll see in Chapter 10. Find them at www.valslide.com.

TRX Suspension Trainer. This set of nylon straps allows you take your workout anywhere. You can lock these lightweight straps onto any elevated fixture—a pullup bar, door, or tree branch—and you'll instantly be equipped to do hundreds of lower-body, upper-body, and core exercises that can be adjusted for any fitness level. (An accompanying DVD provides the complete instructions for different goals.) So it's perfect for anyone who travels or wants to add an effective new training tool to their workout arsenal. The fitness industry is plagued with plenty of gimmicky products, but TRX fully delivers on its promises. Check it out at www.fitnessanywhere.com.

Blast straps. Just loop these straps over any sturdy bar—at the gym, in your house, or even at the park—adjust the strap length, and you can do suspended pushups, chinups, and inverted rows. Because the straps aren't stabilized, they allow you to challenge your body in all three planes of movement: forward and backward, up and down, and side to side. This literally adds an all-new dimension to these exercises, helping to eliminate weak spots and correct muscle imbalances. Blast straps are available at www.elitefts.com.

Step or box. You can do stepups on a bench, but a box or step works better because you can adjust the height. A Reebok step or generic aerobic step with risers will do the trick, but I really like the box squat box at www.elitefts.com. It provides a stable, no-slip surface to lift from, and you can quickly raise and lower the height of this box for stepups, single-leg squats, box lunges, split squats, depth jumps, and elevated pushups.

Large bands. These are oversized rubber bands that allow you to perform assisted chinups without a special machine. (For details on how to do the band-assisted chinup, see Chapter 5.) The wider the bands, the more they'll assist in the movement. Look for Superbands at www.ihpfit.com and flex bands at www.elitefts.com.

Mini bands. Also known as thera-bands (available at www.performbetter.com), these small elastic bands are especially useful for working your glutes and your inner thighs. You'll find that they're utilized throughout this book in exercises such as band walks, band hip abduction, and body-weight squats with knee press-out.

Bosu ball. Bosu stands for "both sides utilized." This training tool allows you to make pushups and hip raises more difficult. You can find it at just about any fitness outlet, or order it online at any number of Internet fitness stores.

Sandbag. The sand shifts as you lift the bag, changing your center of gravity. This forces your core to work harder to keep you from falling over. You might say these bags are awkward, but in a way that's great for your body. Plus, a sandbag is odd-sized compared to a barbell or dumbbell, so it more closely mimics the objects—such as a baby carrier, TV, or suitcase—that you have to pick up in real life. One problem: The sand leaks out of the bags you buy at Home Depot or Lowe's. But you can solve that problem with a Woody Bag (www.ironwoodyfitness. com), which houses the sand in a rugged PVC shell.

Airex Balance Pad. Doing lower-body exercises while standing on this soft foam pad forces the muscles that stabilize your ankle, knee, and hip joints to work harder. So that's one use. But you'll also see that, in this book, I've used the pad in other ways—for example, as a pad to press your knees against in the hip raise with knee squeeze (Chapter 9). You can pick one up at www.performbetter.com.

Chapter 3:
The World's Greatest 4-Week Diet and Exercise Plan

THE FAST WAY TO A LEAN BODY

If you want fast

results, and you want to start today, there's no easier way than this 4-week diet and exercise plan. It's based on the scientific research of Jeff Volek, PhD, RD, one of the world's top nutrition scientists.

In a recent study at the University of Connecticut, Volek and his colleagues found that the combination of a low-carb diet, workout nutrition, and weight training is an incredibly potent formula for shedding fat and quickly improving health. Study participants lost up to 10 pounds of pure fat per month, and many reported that, after just a week or two on the plan, they had higher energy levels and slept better.

More important, the study subjects slashed their risks of heart disease and diabetes—even more so than those who followed a low-fat diet. Case in point: The low-carb lifters dropped their total cholesterol by 12 percent, reduced triglycerides by 32 percent, decreased insulin by 32 percent, and lowered C-reactive protein (CRP)—a marker of inflammation—by 21 percent. And they did all of this simply by following a diet and exercise plan like the one in this chapter.

Consider this your 4-week quick-start guide to losing your gut and getting healthy for life.

The Diet Plan

The way this diet works is simple: Cutting back on carbs reduces your calorie intake, causing weight loss. But it also triggers your body to use its fat stores—instead of sugar—as its primary source of energy. Research shows this helps people better control blood sugar, hunger, and cravings. So you'll eat less without feeling deprived. The end result is that you'll lose fat faster and more easily than ever before.

What to Eat

Eat any combination of the foods from the three categories listed in the chart on page 25, until you feel satisfied but not stuffed. It's likely that this simple approach will regulate your appetite. The upshot: You'll automatically eat less and lose fat—without having to count calories.

The Guidelines

Consume high-quality protein at every meal. Eating protein ensures that your body always has the raw material to build and maintain your muscle, even while you lose fat. It also helps you feel fuller, faster.

Go ahead, eat fat. Dietary fat is a crucial factor in helping you control the total number of calories your body craves. That's because it's very effective at keeping you feeling satisfied after you've eaten. So know this: As long as you're losing fat, you're not eating too much of it.

Indulge in vegetables. When researchers at SUNY Downstate Medical Center in New York City polled more than 2,000 low-carbohydrate dieters, they found that, on average, those who were most successful consumed at least four servings of low-starch vegetables each day.

Avoid foods that contain sugar and starch. These are the foods that are high in carbohydrates. The list includes bread, pasta, potatoes, rice, beans, candy, regular soda, and baked goods—as well any other foods that contain grains, flour, or sugar. An easy way to gauge: Read the ingredients label. If a food contains more than 5 grams of carbohydrate per serving, skip it. And don't obsess either. When ordering food at a restaurant, just worry about the main components of the meal. Sure, there could be hidden sugar or starch in a dish, but if the recommended foods are the major players, you'll be fine. Just use your best judgment.

Limit your fruit and milk intake. In the study, participants were told to avoid these two foods as well, in order to keep their total carbohydrate intake below 50 to 75 grams a day without having to count carbs. However, you can consume milk as well as low-calorie fruits, particularly berries and melons, if you don't overdo it and you monitor your overall carb consumption.

As a general rule, limit yourself to two total servings of fruit and milk combined. A serving of fruit is ½ cup; a serving of milk is 1 cup (8 ounces). Each contains about 10 grams of carbohydrate. So in a day, you might have ½ cup of berries and a cup of milk, or just 1 cup of berries.

A Meal-by-Meal Guide

Don't complicate your eating plan. Just think of it as a meat-and-vegetables diet. Here's a sampling of what you might eat throughout your day.

Breakfast: Any type of eggs, whether scrambled, fried, boiled, poached, or made into an omelet (with all the fixings). You can add cheese, of course, and serve with any type of meat—even bacon and sausage.

Snacks: Just about any type of cheese makes a great snack, as do nuts and seeds—almonds, peanuts, sunflower

About the Expert
Jeff Volek, PhD, RD, is an associate professor at the University of Connecticut and has published more than 185 scientific papers on diet and exercise. In 2007, Dr. Volek and I teamed up to write the *Men's Health TNT Diet*, a book that details all of the science behind the plan you see here, complete with step-by-step instructions, recipes, and even more workouts.

HIGH-QUALITY PROTEINS	LOW-STARCH VEGETABLES*		NATURAL FATS
BEEF	ARTICHOKES	MUSHROOMS	AVOCADOS
CHEESE	ASPARAGUS	ONIONS	BUTTER
EGGS	BROCCOLI	PEPPERS	COCONUT
FISH	BRUSSELS SPROUTS	SPINACH	CREAM
PORK	CAULIFLOWER	TOMATOES	NUTS AND SEEDS**
POULTRY	CELERY	TURNIPS	OLIVES, OLIVE OIL, AND CANOLA OIL
WHEY AND CASEIN PROTEINS	CUCUMBERS	ZUCCHINI	FULL-FAT SOUR CREAM AND SALAD DRESSINGS

* These are just a few common examples of low-starch vegetables, but you can consider any vegetable besides potatoes, peas, and corn to be fair game.

** Limit yourself to two servings a day (a serving is about a handful).

seeds, and pumpkin seeds are ideal. So are fresh vegetables dipped in ranch dressing. And, of course, a protein shake works at any time of day.

Lunch: A great choice is a big salad that includes chicken, turkey, or tuna—for example, a chicken Caesar or a Cobb salad. But you could also eat a burger without a bun, or you could have left-overs from the previous night's dinner.

Dinner: This should be your easiest meal of the day. Just pair any meat with any approved vegetable and you're sticking to the plan. A great meal might be a sirloin with a Caprese salad of tomatoes and mozzarella, or roast chicken with steamed broccoli.

What to Drink

You can consume any beverage that has 5 or fewer calories per serving. What's on the list? Water, of course. But also unsweetened coffee or tea (you can use cream), and no-calorie beverages such as diet soda and Crystal Light.

As for alcohol, it's fine in moderation. Limit yourself to two drinks per day of wine, light beer, or hard liquor. Just make sure any liquor you down isn't combined with a mixer that contains calories, such as juice or regular soda.

Workout Nutrition

Use these guidelines, as study partici-pants did, anytime you perform the workout. Here's what to do: Consume at least 20 grams of protein anywhere from an hour before to 30 minutes after your workout. A protein shake is ideal at this time. Use a product that's mostly protein, with only small amounts of carbs and fat. For instance, At Large Nutrition Nitrean (www.atlargenutrition. com) is an excellent choice. One serving has 24 grams of protein, 2 grams of carbs, and 1 gram of fat. So use that for comparison shopping. You can also eat regular food, of course. Here are some easy options:

- A small can (*3.5 ounces*) of tuna
- 3 to 4 ounces (*three to four slices*) of deli meat, such as turkey or chicken
- A serving of any kind of lean meat that's about the size of a deck of cards
- 3 eggs: hard-boiled, scrambled, fried

Troubleshooting

1. If you're not achieving the results you want, monitor your calorie intake. Simply multiply your target body weight by 10 to 12. The total is the number of daily calories you should shoot for.

2. Don't be surprised if you're irritable or tired for the first 3 to 4 days. Your body typically needs a few days to adjust. If it's been 5 or more days and you still feel tired, make sure you're getting adequate salt and drinking enough water. A good rule of thumb: Consume 8 to 12 ounces of water for every 2 hours that you're awake. And don't avoid fat. This diet increases your body's use of fat for energy, so you absolutely need to eat fat.

3. If you're having GI discomfort, try taking a fiber supplement—such as Metamucil or Benefiber—once a day.

The Exercise Plan

Now you can lose fat your way, thanks to Craig Rasmussen, CSCS, who has designed a cutting-edge flab-busting workout that allows you to choose the exercises. Think of it as DIY fat loss: Just plug and play—and watch your gut melt away.

How to Do This Workout

• Select your exercises using the guidelines provided. Then refer to the charts on pages 28 and 29 for the prescribed sets, reps, and rest.

• Three days a week, alternate between Workout A and Workout B, resting for at least a day after each session. So if you plan to lift on Monday, Wednesday, and Friday, you'd do Workout A on Monday, Workout B on Wednesday, and Workout A again on Friday. The next week, you'd do Workout B on Monday and Friday, and Workout A on Wednesday.

• Do the exercises in the order shown. For each exercise, use the heaviest weight that allows you to complete all of the prescribed repetitions. (See "How Much Weight Should I Use"? in Chapter 2, for more detailed instructions.)

• Perform Exercise 1 as a straight set. That is, complete all of your sets of that movement before moving on to Exercise 2A. Rest for 1 minute after each set.

• Perform Exercises 2A and 2B as a pair. Do one set of Exercise 2A, rest for 1 minute, then do one set of Exercise 2B. Rest

for 1 minute again, then repeat until you've completed all three sets of both exercises. Then move on to Exercise 3A.

• Perform Exercises 3A and 3B as a pair. Do one set of exercise 3A, rest for 1 minute, then do one set of Exercise 3B. Rest for 1 minute again, then repeat until you've completed all three sets of both exercises. Then move on to your Cardio Workout.

• Do the Cardio Workout immediately after each Weight Workout.

• Prior to each workout, complete a 5- to 10-minute warmup. Use the "Create Your Own Warmup" guide in Chapter 12 to design a routine you enjoy.

About the Expert
Craig Rasmussen, CSCS, is a performance coach at Results Fitness in Santa Clarita, California. He's been helping clients lose fat and improve athletic performance for more than 8 years.

Workout A

EXERCISES	SETS	REPS	REST
1. Core (Chapter 10)	3	12	1 min
2A. Glutes and hamstrings (Chapter 9)	3	12	1 min
2B. Upper back (Chapter 5)	3	12	1 min
3A. Quadriceps (Chapter 8)	3	12	1 min
3B. Chest (Chapter 4)	3	12	1 min

- **Exercise 1: Core** Choose any core exercise (Chapter 10) from the section labeled "Stability Exercises" (page 278). The plank (page 278), side plank (page 284), mountain climber (page 288), and Swiss-ball jackknife (page 290) are all great choices. *Note:* If the exercise—such as a plank or side plank—is done for "time" instead of "reps," simply hold it for the amount of time suggested in the exercise instructions. That's one set.
- **Exercise 2A: Glutes and Hamstrings** Choose any glutes/hamstrings exercise (Chapter 9) in which you work one leg at a time. This might be a single-leg barbell straight-leg deadlift (page 254), a single-leg hip raise (page 240), or a dumbbell stepup (page 262).
- **Exercise 2B: Upper Back** Choose any back exercise (Chapter 5) from the section labeled "Upper Back" (pages 72 to 95). So that's any variation of the dumbbell row (pages 78 to 82), barbell row (pages 76 to 77), or cable row (pages 92 to 95).
- **Exercise 3A: Quadriceps** Choose any quadriceps exercise (Chapter 8) in which you work both legs at the same time. This will be a version of the squat, such as the dumbbell squat (page 203), goblet squat (page 204), or barbell front squat (page 199).
- **Exercise 3B. Chest** Choose any chest exercise (Chapter 4). For example, you might choose a variation of the pushup (pages 34 to 43), a dumbbell bench press (pages 52 to 53), or a Swiss-ball dumbbell chest press (pages 56 to 57).

CARDIO

- Choose any "Finishers" from "The Fastest Cardio Workouts of All Time" (Chapter 14) or any of the cardio workouts that accompany other routines in this chapter.

Workout B

EXERCISES	SETS	REPS	REST
1. Core (Chapter 10)	3	12	1 min
2A. Quadriceps (Chapter 8)	3	12	1 min
2B. Lats (Chapter 5)	3	12	1 min
3A. Glutes and Hamstrings (Chapter 9)	3	12	1 min
3B. Shoulders (Chapter 6)	3	12	1 min

- **Exercise 1: Core** Choose any core exercise (Chapter 10) from the section labeled "Stability Exercises" (page 278). The plank (page 278), side plank (page 284), mountain climber (page 288), and Swiss-ball jackknife (page 290) are all great choices. *Note:* If the exercise—such as a plank or side plank—is done for "time" instead of "reps," simply hold it for the amount of time suggested in the exercise instructions. That's one set.
- **Exercise 2A: Quadriceps** Choose any quadriceps exercise (Chapter 8) in which you work one leg at a time. This will be any version of the barbell or dumbbell lunge (pages 206 to 211), barbell or dumbbell split squat (pages 212 to 221), dumbbell lunge (pages 216 to 217), or a single-leg squat (pages 196 to 197).
- **Exercise 2B: Lats** Choose any back exercise (Chapter 5) from the section labeled "Lats" (pages 96 to 107). For example, you could choose any version of the chinup (pages 96 to 100), lat pulldown (pages 102 to 105), or pullover (pages 106 to 107).
- **Exercise 3A: Glutes and Hamstrings** Choose any glutes/hamstrings exercise (Chapter 9) in which you work both legs at the same time. This might be a barbell deadlift (page 248), a dumbbell straight-leg deadlift (page 256), or a Swiss-ball hip raise and leg curl (page 243).
- **Exercise 3B: Shoulders** Choose any shoulder exercise (Chapter 6), such as the dumbbell shoulder press (page 120), lateral raise (page 126), or scaption and shrug (page 143).

CARDIO

- Choose any "Finishers" from "The Fastest Cardio Workouts of All Time" (Chapter 14) or any of the cardio workouts that accompany other routines in this chapter.

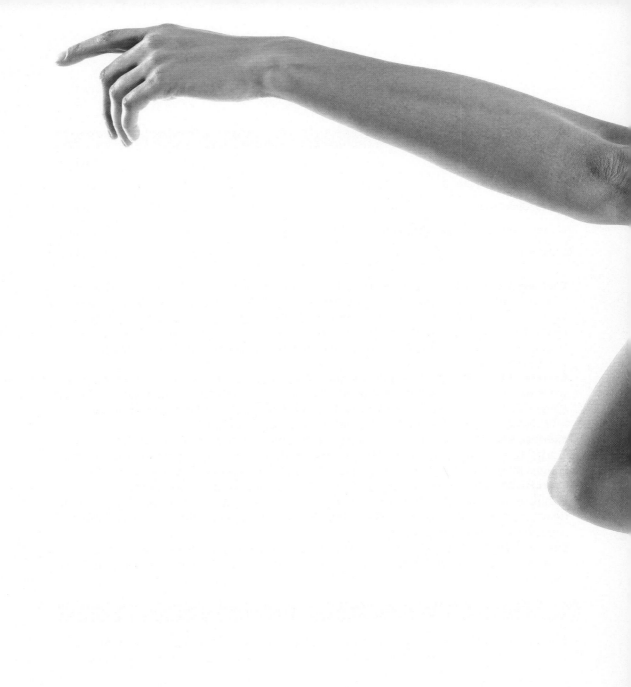

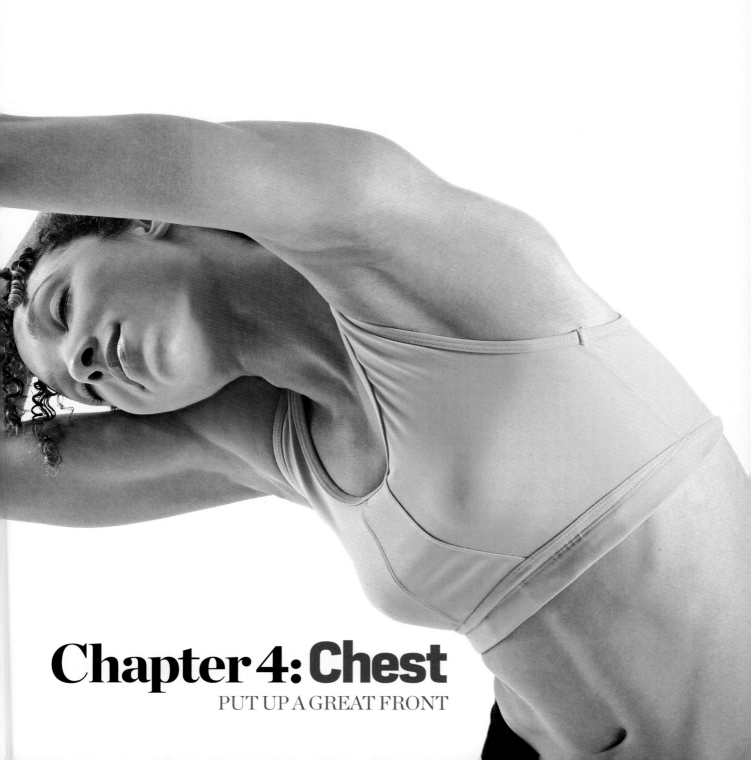

Chapter 4: Chest
PUT UP A GREAT FRONT

Chest

It's true: Most women aren't looking to make their pecs pop. But there are still plenty of reasons to work your chest. After all, the best exercises for targeting your pectoral muscles also help shape and firm your deltoids and triceps. So consider the movements in this chapter to be sculpting tools for your shoulders and arms as well as your chest. And that makes these exercises among the best ways to improve your upper-body strength. (Hey, who says you can't be skinny and strong?)

What's more, working all those muscles burns lots of calories. Or perhaps you should think of it this way: Skip your chest, and you'll be missing out on that burn. The take-home message: Regularly training your chest also helps you fight belly fat.

Bonus Benefits

Perkier breasts! When combined with perfect posture, regularly working your chest muscles may even give your bosom a lift. Hint: Always keep your chest raised high, as if there's a string pulling it toward the ceiling.

A stronger swing: Forehand strokes in tennis and other racquet sports rely on your chest muscles for velocity, in addition to your core musculature.

A stronger core: Pushups aren't just a chest exercise; they're great for your abs, too.

Meet Your Muscles

Pectoralis Major

Your main chest muscle is the pectoralis major [1]. Its job: to pull your upper arms toward the middle of your body. Think about that in terms of a bench press. As you push the bar away from your torso, your upper arms move closer to your chest as they straighten. This is because your pectoralis major attaches to the inside of your upper arm bone. So when your pectorals contract, the muscle fibers shorten, pulling your upper arms toward the muscles' origin, your mid-chest.

This is why exercises such as pushups and bench presses are the best way to make your pecs pop. By holding a weight in your hands when you do a bench press, for instance, you increase the weight of your upper arms, which forces your pectoral muscles to contract harder. The end result: a bigger, stronger chest.

The muscle fibers that make up the clavicular portion form what many call the upper chest.

The fibers of your pectoralis major originate at three places on your chest: your collar bone [2], your breast bone [3], and your ribs [4], just below your breast bone.

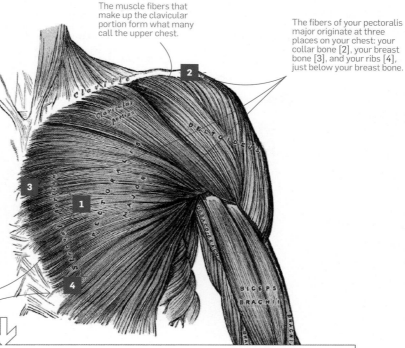

The sternal portion of the muscle is collectively considered to be your lower chest.

Pectoralis Minor

The pectoralis minor [5] is a thin, triangular muscle that lies beneath your pectoralis major. It starts at your third, fourth, and fifth ribs, and attaches near your shoulder joint. Although this muscle is technically a "chest muscle," its main duty is to assist in pulling your shoulders forward—an action that occurs in back exercises such as the dumbbell pullover.

Chest | PUSHUPS

In this chapter, you'll find 63 exercises that target the muscles of your chest. Throughout, you'll notice that certain exercises have been designated as a Main Move. Master this basic version of a movement, and you'll be able to do all of its variations with flawless form.

PUSHUPS AND DIPS

These exercises target your pectoralis major. However, they also hit your front deltoids and triceps, since these muscles assist in just about every version of the movements. What's more, your rotator, trapezius, serratus anterior, and abdominals all contract to keep your shoulders, core, and hips stable as you perform the moves.

MAIN MOVE
Pushup

A

- Get down on all fours and place your hands on the floor so that they're slightly wider than and in line with your shoulders.

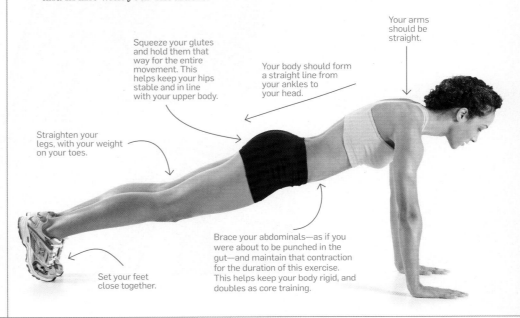

Your arms should be straight.

Squeeze your glutes and hold them that way for the entire movement. This helps keep your hips stable and in line with your upper body.

Your body should form a straight line from your ankles to your head.

Straighten your legs, with your weight on your toes.

Set your feet close together.

Brace your abdominals—as if you were about to be punched in the gut—and maintain that contraction for the duration of this exercise. This helps keep your body rigid, and doubles as core training.

75

Percent of your body weight you lift when you do a standard pushup, according to research by the National Strength and Conditioning Association.

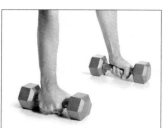

SPARE YOUR WRISTS
If it hurts your wrists to put your hands directly on the floor, place a pair of hex dumbbells at the spots where you position your hands. Then grasp the dumbbells' handles and keep your wrists straight as you perform the exercise.

 B

- Lower your body until your chest nearly touches the floor.
- Pause at the bottom, and then push yourself back to the starting position as quickly as possible.
- If your hips sag at any point during the exercise, your form has broken down. When this happens, consider that your last repetition and end the set.

Why the Pushup Is King

While exercises like the pushup and the bench press both work your chest, shoulders, and triceps, the pushup also trains your abs, lower back, upper back, and glutes. So it bestows a bevy of total-body benefits. What's more, unlike the bench press, performing pushups with perfect form actually helps make your shoulders healthier. The bottom line: Pushups not only work the front of your body, but just about everywhere else, too.

Tuck your elbows as you lower your body so that your upper arms form a 45-degree angle with your body in the bottom position of the movement.

Don't drop your hips.

Your head should stay in the same position from start to finish.

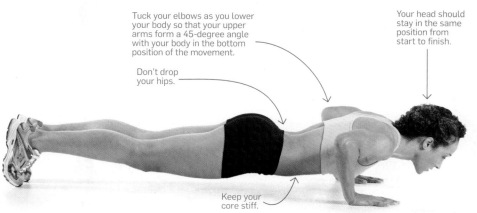

Keep your core stiff.

Chest | PUSHUPS

VARIATION #1
Incline Pushup

- Place your hands on a box, bench, or step instead of the floor. This reduces the amount of your body weight you have to lift, making the exercise easier.

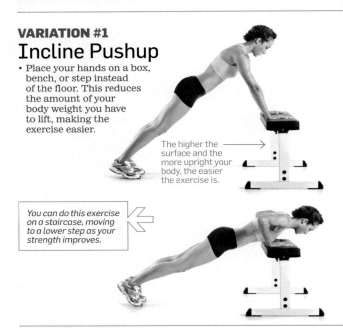

The higher the surface and the more upright your body, the easier the exercise is.

You can do this exercise on a staircase, moving to a lower step as your strength improves.

VARIATION #2
Modified Pushup

- Instead of performing the exercise with your legs straight, bend your knees and cross your ankles behind you. This is another way to make the classic pushup easier.

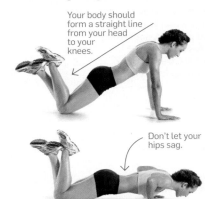

Your body should form a straight line from your head to your knees.

Don't let your hips sag.

65

Percent of your body weight you lift when you do a modified pushup.

VARIATION #3
Decline Pushup

- Place your feet on a box or bench as you perform a pushup. This increases the amount of your body weight you have to lift, making the exercise harder.

STRENGTHEN YOUR SHOULDERS
Researchers in Texas found that the decline pushup works the muscles that stabilize your shoulders better than a traditional pushup.

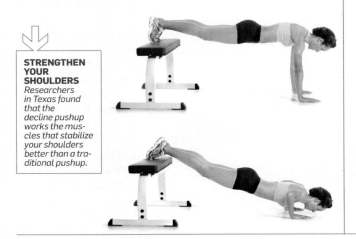

VARIATION #4
Single-Leg Decline Pushup

- Place one foot on a box or bench and hold the other in the air.

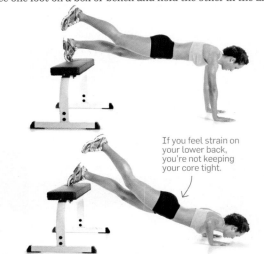

If you feel strain on your lower back, you're not keeping your core tight.

VARIATION #5
Pushup with Feet on Swiss Ball

 A

- Perform the movement with your feet placed on Swiss ball.

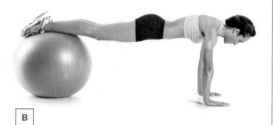

B

- Lower your body as far as you can, without allowing your hips to sag.

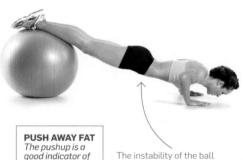

PUSH AWAY FAT
The pushup is a good indicator of whether or not you're exercising enough now to avoid fat later, according to a Canadian study. The researchers found that people who perform poorly in a pushup test are 78 percent more likely to gain 20 pounds of flab over the next two decades.

The instability of the ball forces your core to work harder, increasing the difficulty of the exercise.

VARIATION #6
Stacked-Feet Pushup
- Place one foot on top of the other so that only the lower one supports your body.

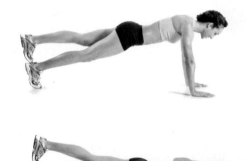

VARIATION #7
Weighted Pushup
- Have a workout partner place a weight plate on your back, at the level of your shoulder blades.

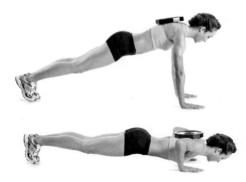

You can also increase the amount you're lifting by wearing a weighted vest or placing a heavy chain on your back.

The Pushup Spectrum

HARDEST

9. SWISS-BALL PUSHUP

8. BOSU PUSHUP

7. SINGLE-LEG DECLINE PUSHUP

6. PUSHUP WITH FEET ON SWISS BALL

5. DECLINE PUSHUP

4. STACKED-FEET PUSHUP

3. PUSHUP

2. INCLINE PUSHUP

1. MODIFIED PUSHUP

EASIEST

Chest | PUSHUPS

VARIATION #8
Triple-Stop Pushup

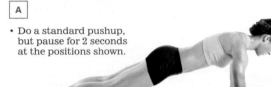

A

- Do a standard pushup, but pause for 2 seconds at the positions shown.

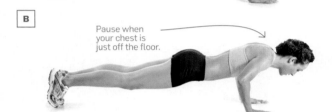

B

Pause when your chest is just off the floor.

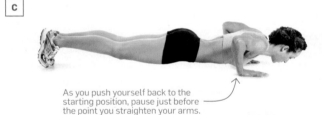

C

As you push yourself back to the starting position, pause just before the point you straighten your arms.

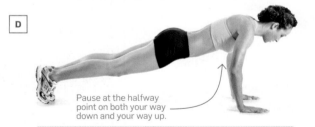

D

Pause at the halfway point on both your way down and your way up.

MAKE TIME FOR THIS MOVE
Pausing briefly at each point increases strength at that joint angle and 10 degrees in either direction. So this method eliminates any weak point you might have. It also increases the time your muscles are under tension, stimulating growth.

VARIATION #9
Wide-Hands Pushup

- Place your hands about twice shoulder-width apart.

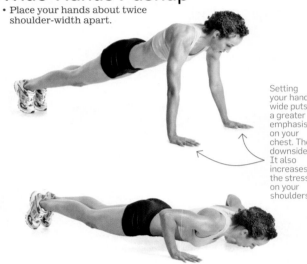

Setting your hands wide puts a greater emphasis on your chest. The downside: It also increases the stress on your shoulders.

VARIATION #10
Close-Hands Pushup

- Place your hands directly under your shoulders.

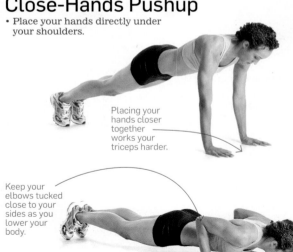

Placing your hands closer together works your triceps harder.

Keep your elbows tucked close to your sides as you lower your body.

VARIATION #11
Staggered-Hands Pushup
• Place one hand in standard pushup position and your other hand a few inches farther forward.

Staggering your hands increases the challenge to your core and shoulder muscles.

Alternate which hand is placed forward each set.

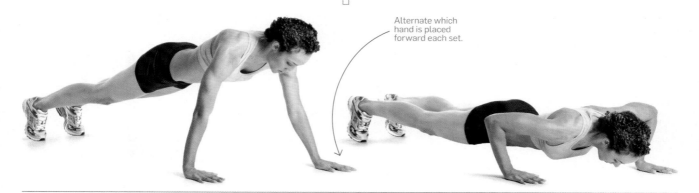

VARIATION #12
Spiderman Pushup

A

• Assume the standard pushup position.

B

• As you lower your body toward the floor, lift your right foot off the floor, swing your right leg out sideways, and try to touch your knee to your elbow.

• Reverse the movement, then push your body back to the starting position. Repeat, but on your next repetition, touch your left knee to your left elbow. Continue to alternate back and forth.

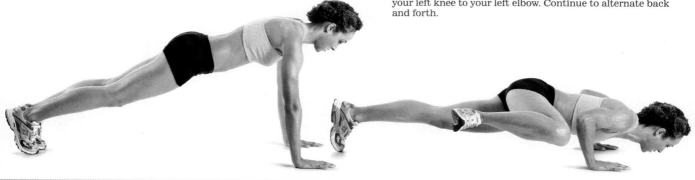

Chest | PUSHUPS

VARIATION #13
Swiss-Ball Pushup
- Place your hands on a Swiss ball instead of the floor.

TARGET YOUR TRICEPS
This exercise trains your triceps 30 percent harder than a standard pushup. The reason: The Swiss ball forces your triceps to stabilize your elbow and shoulder joints, which results in the recruitment of more muscle fibers.

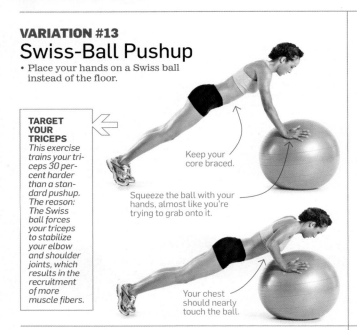

Keep your core braced.

Squeeze the ball with your hands, almost like you're trying to grab onto it.

Your chest should nearly touch the ball.

VARIATION #14
Medicine-Ball Pushup
- Place both hands on a medicine ball.

CHISEL YOUR ABS
When you place your hands on a Swiss ball or a medicine ball, the instability causes your core muscles to work 20 percent harder than when you do pushups on the floor, report New Zealand researchers.

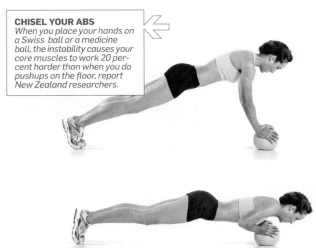

VARIATION #15
Single-Arm Medicine-Ball Pushup
- Place one hand on a medicine ball.

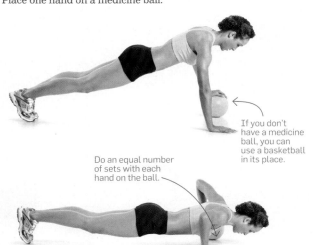

If you don't have a medicine ball, you can use a basketball in its place.

Do an equal number of sets with each hand on the ball.

VARIATION #16
Two-Arm Medicine-Ball Pushup
- Place each hand on a medicine ball.

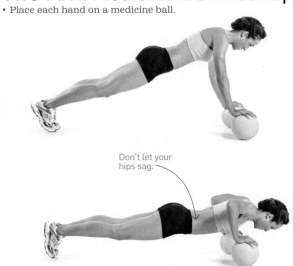

Don't let your hips sag.

VARIATION #17
T-Pushup

- Place a pair of hex dumbbells at the spot where you position your hands.
- Grasp the dumbbell handles and set yourself in pushup position.

Set your feet hip-width apart.

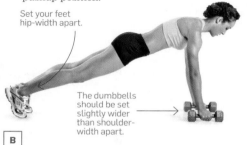

The dumbbells should be set slightly wider than shoulder-width apart.

B

- Lower your body to the floor.

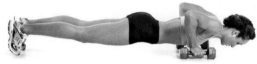

C

- As you push yourself back up, rotate the right side of your body upward as you bend your right arm and pull the right dumbbell to your torso. Then straighten your arm so that the dumbbell is above your right shoulder.
- Lower the dumbbell back down, and repeat, this time performing the move to your left.

Raise the dumbbell and rotate your body in one fluid motion.

As you rotate your body, pivot on your toes and then lower your heels to the floor.

Your arms should form a T with your body.

VARIATION #18
Judo Pushup

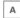

- Begin in standard pushup position, but move your feet forward and raise your hips so your body almost forms an upside-down "V."

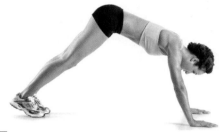

B

- Keeping your hips elevated, lower your body until your chin nearly touches the floor.

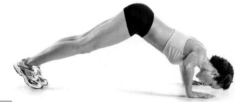

C

- Lower your hips until they almost touch the floor, as you simultaneously raise your head and shoulders toward the ceiling. Reverse the movement back to the starting position and repeat.

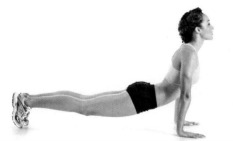

Pump Up Your Pushups

If you struggle to do standard pushups, use variation #1, the incline pushup. Perform as shown, but if that's still too hard, use this trick. Set a barbell in a power rack at about chest height. Now place your hands on the bar and get into pushup position—your body will be more vertical than horizontal. Try to do 12 pushups with perfect form. If you can do more, lower the bar one notch and repeat until you're challenged. If you can't complete 12 reps, raise the bar one notch and test yourself again.

Chest | PUSHUPS

VARIATION #19
Explosive Pushup

- After you lower your body, press yourself up so forcefully that your hands leave the floor.

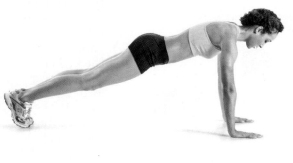

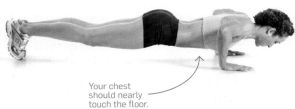

Your chest should nearly touch the floor.

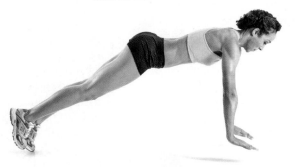

VARIATION #20
Iso-Explosive Pushup

- Do this movement just like the explosive pushup, but first pause 5 seconds in the down position. This pause technique eliminates all the elasticity in your muscles, which allows you to activate a maximum number of fast-twitch muscle fibers. These are the muscle fibers with greatest potential for size and strength gains.

VARIATION #21
Explosive Crossover Pushup

A

- Place your left hand on the floor and your right hand on the smooth side of a weight plate.

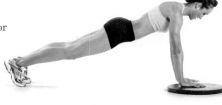

B

- Lower your body to the floor.

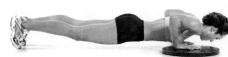

C

- Explosively push up and to the right so your hands leave the floor.

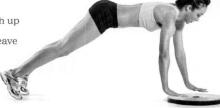

D

- Land with your left hand on the plate and your right hand on the floor.

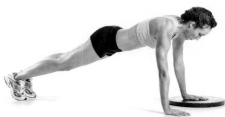

E

- Then lower and repeat, alternating back and forth each repetition.

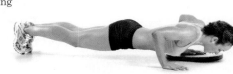

The crossover portion of this movement forces your upper arms toward the center of your body, which is the main function of the pectoralis major, your largest chest muscle.

VARIATION #22
Bosu Pushup

- Turn a Bosu ball over, so that the half-ball portion is on floor, and position your hands on the sides of the platform.

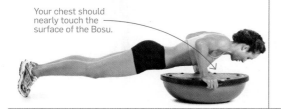

Brace your core and glutes.

Your chest should nearly touch the surface of the Bosu.

VARIATION #23
Suspended Pushup

A
- Attach a pair of straps with handles to a secure bar, so that the handles are a foot or so off the floor.

Keep your body in a straight line from your ankles to your head.

B
- Lower your body until your upper arms dip below your elbows.

One option for suspended pushups: Blast Straps, which can be found at elitefts.com.

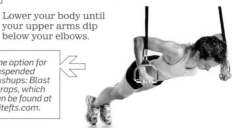

VARIATION #24
Pushup and Row

A
- Place a pair of hex dumbbells at the spot where you position your hands.
- Grasp the dumbbell handles and set yourself in pushup position.

B
- Lower your body to the floor, pause, then push yourself back up.

C
- Once you're back in the starting position, row the dumbbell in your right hand to the side of your chest, by pulling it upward and bending your arm.
- Pause, then lower the dumbbell back down, and repeat the same movement with your left arm. That's one repetition.

THE ALL-IN-ONE UPPER BODY EXERCISE
The pushup and row works your middle and upper back as hard as it does your chest.

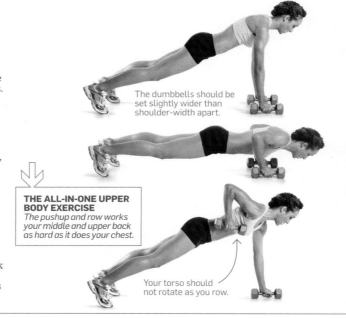

The dumbbells should be set slightly wider than shoulder-width apart.

Your torso should not rotate as you row.

Hang On for More Strength

Performing pushups while suspended from straps increases muscle activation in your abs and upper back, according to a study by Canadian researchers. One caution: This exercise can also place more stress on your lower back. To protect your spine, make sure to keep your core and glutes tight, as you should when you do any variation of the pushup. Simply brace your abs forcefully and squeeze your glutes, and hold those contractions as you lower and raise your body.

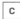

Chest | DIPS

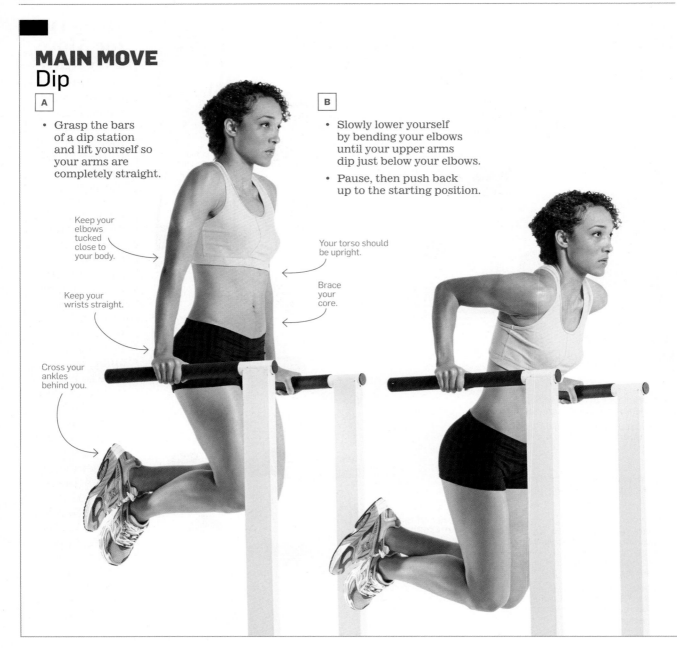

MAIN MOVE
Dip

A

- Grasp the bars of a dip station and lift yourself so your arms are completely straight.

Keep your elbows tucked close to your body.

Keep your wrists straight.

Cross your ankles behind you.

B

- Slowly lower yourself by bending your elbows until your upper arms dip just below your elbows.

- Pause, then push back up to the starting position.

Your torso should be upright.

Brace your core.

VARIATION #1
Incline Dip

SAVE YOUR SHOULDERS
This version of the dip redistributes your weight so that your torso leans forward as you lower your body, placing more of the stress on your chest instead of your shoulders. It's particularly useful if you find the standard dip causes shoulder pain, but since it places less strain on your shoulder joint regardless, most people would be better off sticking with this variation all the time.

VARIATION #2
Weighted Dip

• Perform the exercise with a dipping belt attached to your waist.

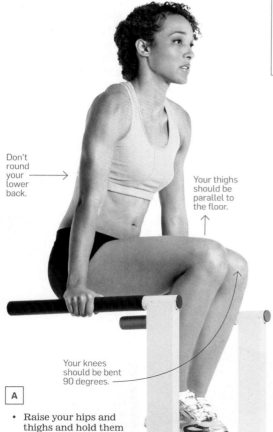

Don't round your lower back.

Your thighs should be parallel to the floor.

Your knees should be bent 90 degrees.

A

• Raise your hips and thighs and hold them that way for the entire movement.

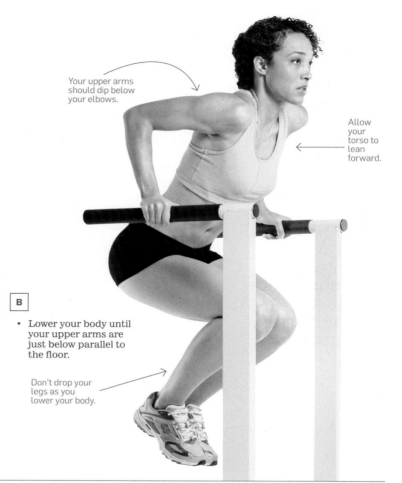

Your upper arms should dip below your elbows.

Allow your torso to lean forward.

B

• Lower your body until your upper arms are just below parallel to the floor.

Don't drop your legs as you lower your body.

Chest | PRESSES

These exercises target your pectoralis major, the largest muscle of your chest. Most of the movements also hit your front deltoids and triceps, since these muscles assist in just about every version of the exercise. Your rotator cuff and trapezius also contract to help keep your shoulders stable as you perform the moves.

MAIN MOVE
Barbell Bench Press

A

- Grasp a barbell with an overhand grip that's just wider than shoulder-width, and hold it above your sternum with arms completely straight.

TRAINER'S TIP
Imagine that you're pushing your body away from the bar, instead of pushing the bar away from your body. This simple mind trick automatically encourages your body to use good form.

As you push the bar off your chest, squeeze and press the bar outward, as if you were trying to tear it apart. This forces more muscle fibers into play.

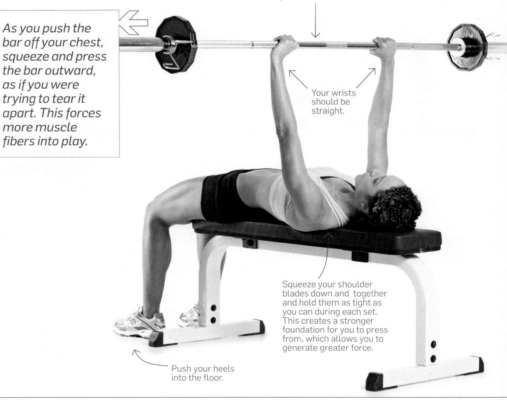

Hold the bar above your sternum.

Your wrists should be straight.

Squeeze your shoulder blades down and together and hold them as tight as you can during each set. This creates a stronger foundation for you to press from, which allows you to generate greater force.

Push your heels into the floor.

WHY FORM MATTERS

Pay closer attention to your exercise technique and you may notice something: People who review proper lifting form before bench-pressing may increase barbell velocity by 183 percent, report researchers at Barry University. The benefit: Faster bar speed helps you blast through sticking points, allowing you to lift heavier loads.

B

- Lower the bar straight down, pause, then press the bar in a straight line back up to the starting position.
- Keep your elbows tucked in, so that your upper arms form a 45-degree angle with your body in the down position. This reduces stress on your shoulder joints.

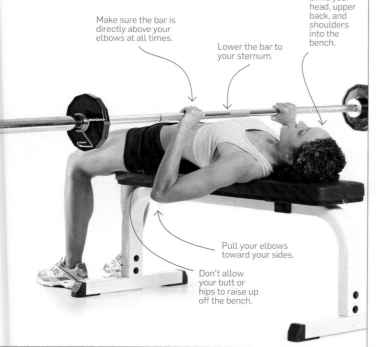

Make sure the bar is directly above your elbows at all times.

Lower the bar to your sternum.

Drive your head, upper back, and shoulders into the bench.

Pull your elbows toward your sides.

Don't allow your butt or hips to raise up off the bench.

VARIATION #1
Close-Grip Barbell Bench Press

- Use an overhand grip that's shoulder-width apart.

MORE TRICEPS!
Using a close grip forces your triceps to work harder. In fact, the close-grip bench press is one of the best exercises for building size and strength in your triceps.

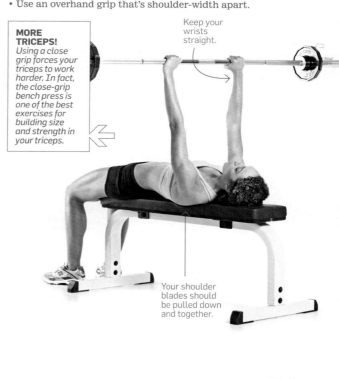

Keep your wrists straight.

Your shoulder blades should be pulled down and together.

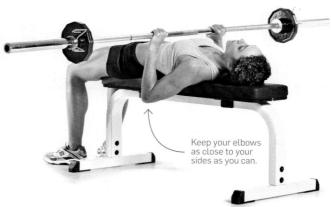

Keep your elbows as close to your sides as you can.

Chest | PRESSES

VARIATION #2
Reverse-Grip Barbell Bench Press
• Use an underhand grip that's about shoulder-width apart.

BUILD YOUR UPPER CHEST
Canadian researchers found that the reverse-grip bench press activates your upper-chest muscles better than other versions of the flat bench press.

Your palms should be facing behind you.

Your arms should be completely straight.

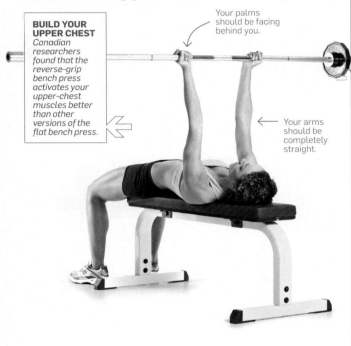

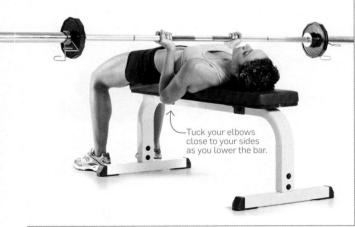

Tuck your elbows close to your sides as you lower the bar.

VARIATION #3
Barbell Towel Press
• Roll a towel and place it long ways in the middle of your chest. Now perform a bench press, lowering the bar to the towel instead of to your chest.

Use a thick towel for this exercise.

Rest the bar on the towel momentarily before you push it back to the starting position.

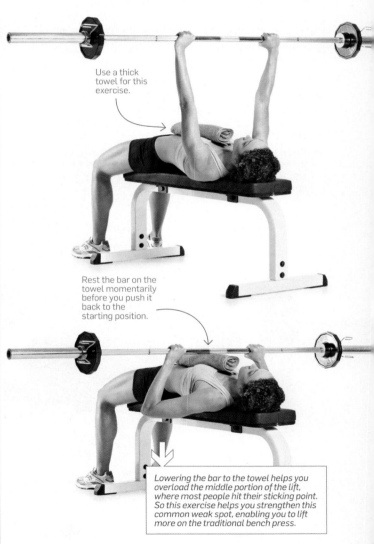

Lowering the bar to the towel helps you overload the middle portion of the lift, where most people hit their sticking point. So this exercise helps you strengthen this common weak spot, enabling you to lift more on the traditional bench press.

VARIATION #4
Triple-Stop Barbell Bench Press

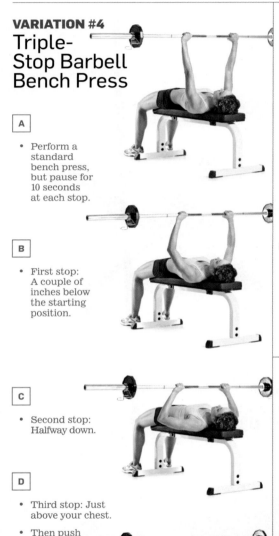

A

- Perform a standard bench press, but pause for 10 seconds at each stop.

B

- First stop: A couple of inches below the starting position.

C

- Second stop: Halfway down.

D

- Third stop: Just above your chest.

- Then push the bar back to the starting position. That's one set.

VARIATION #5
Isometric Barbell Bench Press

- Lift the bar off the uprights and lower it until it's about 4 inches off your chest. Hold that position for 40 seconds to build more muscle; hold the position for 6 to 8 seconds for greater gains in strength. That's one set.

- Warning: Never perform the isometric barbell bench press without an experienced spotter.

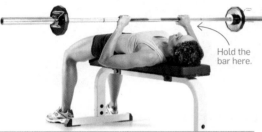

Hold the bar here.

HOW MUCH WEIGHT?
Choose the heaviest weight that allows you to maintain the isometric hold for the length of time that matches your goal. So if you're building strength, you'll use a heavier weight than if you're focusing on faster muscle growth.

VARIATION #6
Barbell Pin Press

- Place a bench inside a power rack. Then set the safety pins just below where you think your sticking point is. Rest the bar on the pins. Lie on the bench, press the bar up, and then slowly lower it back onto the pins. Pause for a second and repeat.

VARIATION #7
Barbell Board Press

- Perform this the same way as the towel press, but instead of the towel, use a pair of stacked 12-inch-long two-by-fours. Just make sure they're secured together with a screw or a tight band.

FIND YOUR STICKING POINT
Your sticking point is the position of the bar at which your muscles give out and you can't complete the rep. You don't have to completely fail to find this spot; it's also the first place you start to struggle as you become fatigued.

Strong Chest, Healthy Eyes?

Researchers at Mississippi State University report that you can slash your risk of glaucoma with bench presses. In the study, 30 people who performed three sets of bench presses reduced the pressure within their eyes by 15 percent. This results in decreased pressure on the optic nerve, thus reducing the likelihood of nerve damage and glaucoma, say the scientists. Exercises that recruit a lot of muscle mass, such as the bench press or squat, provide the most benefit.

Chest | PRESSES

Incline Barbell Bench Press

A

- Set an adjustable bench to its lowest incline, about 15 to 30 degrees.
- Lie faceup on the bench and grab the barbell with an overhand grip that's slightly beyond shoulder width.

Hold the bar above your shoulders.

Your arms should be completely straight.

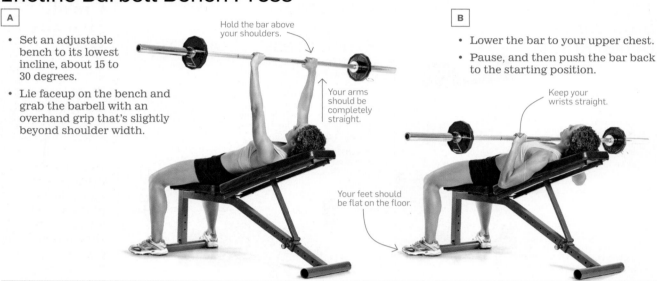

Your feet should be flat on the floor.

B

- Lower the bar to your upper chest.
- Pause, and then push the bar back to the starting position.

Keep your wrists straight.

Decline Barbell Bench Press

A

- Lie faceup on a decline bench and grab the barbell with an overhand grip that's slightly beyond shoulder width.
- Hold the bar above your chest with your arms straight.

Your palms should face forward.

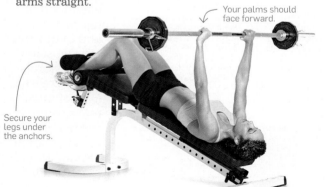

Secure your legs under the anchors.

B

- Lower the bar to your lower chest.
- Pause, and then push the bar back to the starting position.

The bar should nearly touch your lower chest.

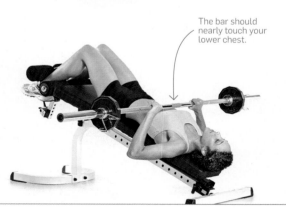

Barbell Floor Press

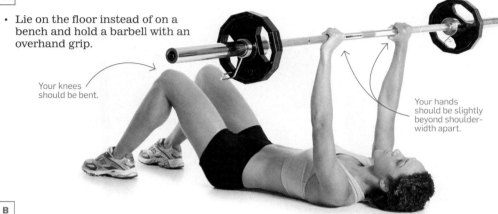

- Lie on the floor instead of on a bench and hold a barbell with an overhand grip.

Your knees should be bent.

Your hands should be slightly beyond shoulder-width apart.

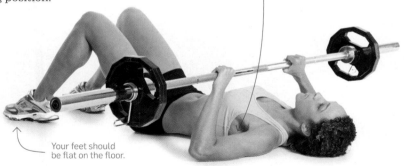

- Lower the barbell until your upper arms touch the floor.
- Keep your elbows pulled in toward your sides as you lower the bar.
- Pause, then push the bar back to the starting position.

Your upper arms should form a 45-degree angle with the sides of your torso.

Your feet should be flat on the floor.

MORE ON THE FLOOR!
The floor keeps your upper arms from descending below parallel, which limits your range of motion and concentrates the work on the muscles used during the last (and toughest) part of the bench press.

The Secret of Your Soreness

All of the chest exercises in this chapter work your entire pectoralis major. But you'll notice that when you perform an incline bench press, the upper portion of your chest is the area that's the most sore the next day. For decline bench presses, it's the lower portion. That's because changing the angle of your body puts more tension on a specific segment of your pecs. This causes a greater amount of muscle damage to those fibers, resulting in greater soreness.

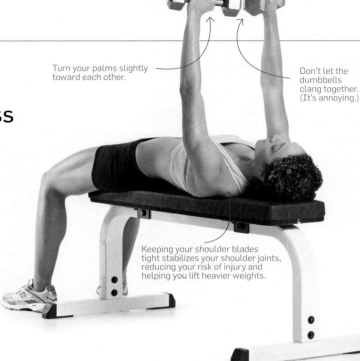

Turn your palms slightly toward each other.

Don't let the dumbbells clang together. (It's annoying.)

MAIN MOVE
Dumbbell Bench Press

A

- Grab a pair of dumbbells and lie on your back on a flat bench, holding the dumbbells over your chest so that they're nearly touching.

- Your palms should be facing out, but turned slightly inward.

- Before you begin, pull your shoulder blades down and together, and hold them as tight as you can throughout the entire exercise.

Keeping your shoulder blades tight stabilizes your shoulder joints, reducing your risk of injury and helping you lift heavier weights.

B

- Without changing the angle of your hands, lower the dumbbells to the sides of your chest.

- Pause, then press the weights back up to the starting position as quickly as you can.

- Straighten your arms completely at the top of each repetition.

In the down position, both your upper arms and the dumbbells should form a 45-degree angle to your body.

Your wrists should be straight.

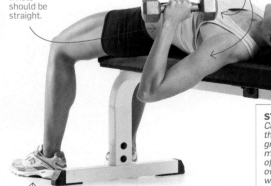

LIFT MORE—TODAY!
UK researchers found that people bench-press 12 percent more weight when they psych themselves up before a lift than when they're distracted. In the study, the scientists gave experienced weight lifters 20 seconds to mentally prepare. The take-home message: Before you approach the bench, skip the small talk and focus on the task at hand.

Keep your feet flat on the floor at all times.

STAY GROUNDED
Canadian researchers found that raising your feet off the ground while benching shifts as much as 30 percent of the load off your upper body and onto an overmatched core, significantly weakening your lift.

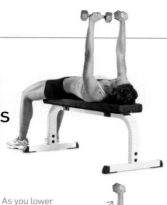

VARIATION #1
Alternating Dumbbell Bench Press

• Instead of pressing both dumbbells up at once, lift them one at a time, in an alternating fashion.

As you lower one dumbbell, press the other up.

VARIATION #2
Alternating Neutral-Grip Dumbbell Bench Press

The dumbbells should almost touch.

• Instead of pressing both dumbbells up at once, lift them one at a time, in an alternating fashion. So as you lower one dumbbell, press the other one up.

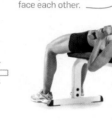

Your palms should face each other.

Alternating dumbbell presses increase your core activation because you're continually changing the weight distribution on each side of your body.

VARIATION #3
Neutral-Grip Dumbbell Bench Press

• Hold the dumbbells so that your palms face each other.

HIT YOUR CHEST HIGHER
Like the incline press, the neutral-grip bench press puts more of the emphasis on your upper chest. So if you don't have an adjustable bench, it's an effective way to target that part of your pectoralis major.

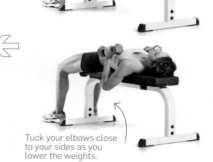

Tuck your elbows close to your sides as you lower the weights.

VARIATION #4
Single-Arm Dumbbell Bench Press

• For this exercise, simply use the same form as for a dumbbell chest press but complete the prescribed number of repetitions with one arm before immediately doing the same number with your other arm.

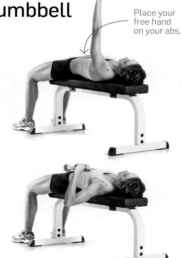

Place your free hand on your abs.

BENCH FOR ABS
Doing any exercise with one dumbbell at a time forces your core to work harder.

Chest | PRESSES

MAIN MOVE
Incline Dumbbell Bench Press

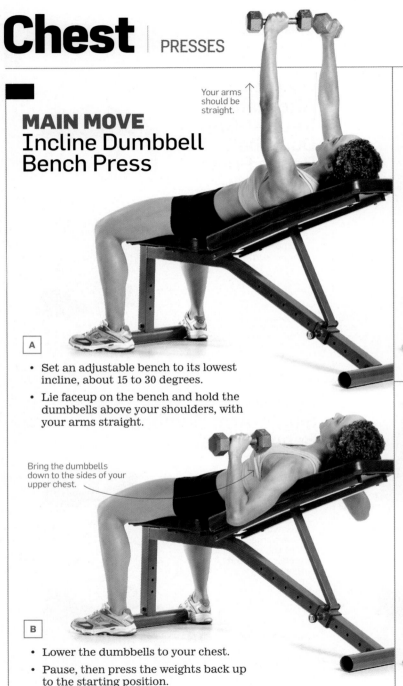

Your arms should be straight. ↑

A

- Set an adjustable bench to its lowest incline, about 15 to 30 degrees.
- Lie faceup on the bench and hold the dumbbells above your shoulders, with your arms straight.

Bring the dumbbells down to the sides of your upper chest.

B

- Lower the dumbbells to your chest.
- Pause, then press the weights back up to the starting position.

Neutral-Grip Incline Dumbbell Bench Press
- Hold the dumbbells so that your palms face each other.

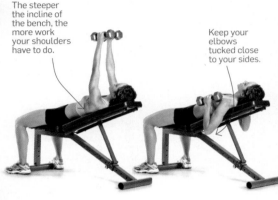

The steeper the incline of the bench, the more work your shoulders have to do.

Keep your elbows tucked close to your sides.

VARIATION #2
Alternating Incline Dumbbell Bench Press
- Instead of pressing both dumbbells up at once, lift them one at a time, in an alternating fashion.

As you lower one dumbbell, press the other one up.

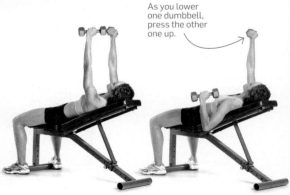

Decline Dumbbell Bench Press

A

- Grab a pair of dumbbells and lie faceup on a decline bench.
- Hold the dumbbells above your chest.

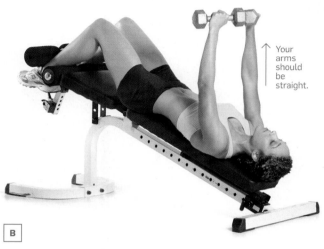

Your arms should be straight.

B

- Lower the dumbbells to the sides of your lower chest.
- Pause, then press the weights back up to the starting position.

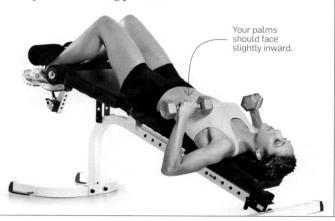

Your palms should face slightly inward.

Dumbbell Floor Press

A

- Grab a pair of dumbbells and lie faceup on the floor.
- Hold the dumbbells above your chest with your arms straight.

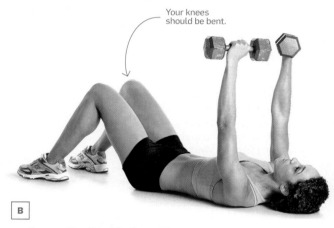

Your knees should be bent.

B

- Lower the dumbbells until your upper arms touch the floor.
- Pause, then press the weights back up to the starting position.

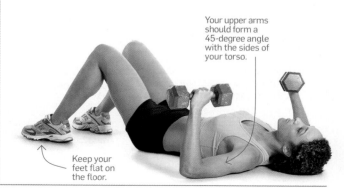

Your upper arms should form a 45-degree angle with the sides of your torso.

Keep your feet flat on the floor.

Chest | PRESSES

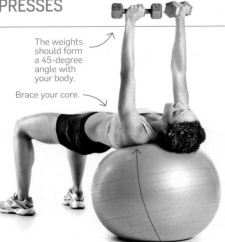

MAIN MOVE
Swiss-Ball Dumbbell Chest Press

The weights should form a 45-degree angle with your body.

Brace your core.

A

- Grab a pair of dumbbells and lie on your back on a Swiss ball.
- Raise your hips so that your body forms a straight line from your knees to your shoulders.
- Your palms should be facing out, but turned slightly inward.

Your upper and middle back should be placed firmly on the ball.

Keep your wrists as straight as you can.

Don't drop your hips.

Your feet should be flat on the floor at all times.

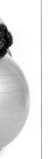

B

- Without changing the angle of your hands, lower the dumbbells to the sides of your chest.
- Pause, then press the weights back up to the starting position as quickly as you can.
- Straighten your arms completely at the top of each repetition.

A HARD CORE CHEST EXERCISE
Performing the chest press on a Swiss ball makes your core work 54 percent harder than when you do the exercise on a bench, according to an Australian study. However, it also reduces the amount of weight you can press, decreasing the demand on your chest muscles.

Alternating Swiss-Ball Dumbbell Chest Press

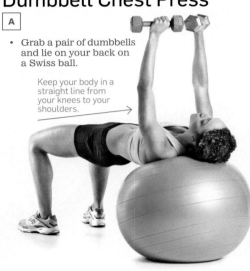

A

- Grab a pair of dumbbells and lie on your back on a Swiss ball.

Keep your body in a straight line from your knees to your shoulders.

B

- Instead of pressing both dumbbells up at once, lift them one at a time, in an alternating fashion.

As you lower one dumbbell, press the other one up.

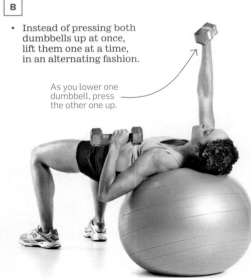

MAIN MOVE
Incline Swiss-Ball Dumbbell Chest Press

- Position yourself on your back on a Swiss ball so your torso is at a 45-degree angle to the floor.
- Hold the dumbbells straight above your chin, with your arms straight.

Keep your core braced.

Your feet should be flat on the floor.

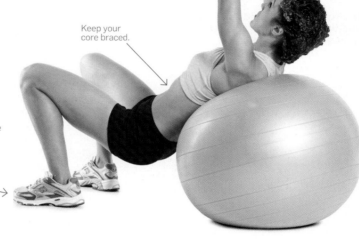

- Lower the dumbbells so that they end up just outside your upper chest.
- Pause, then press the weights back up to the starting position.

Don't let your hips drop.

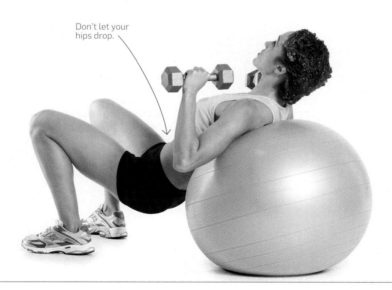

Single-Arm Cable Chest Press

A

- With your right hand, grab the high-pulley handle of a cable station and face away from the weight stack.

- Stagger your feet and hold the handle at shoulder height, with your right arm bent and parallel to the floor.

B

- Push the handle forward and straighten your right arm in front of you.

- Then slowly bend your right elbow to return to the starting position.

- Complete the prescribed number of reps with your right arm, then switch hands and do the same number with your left.

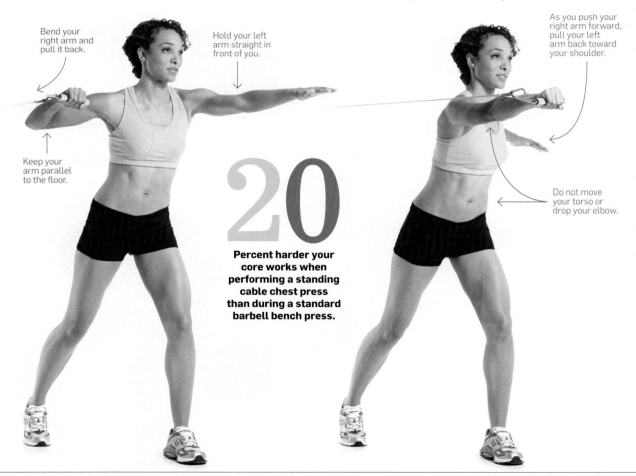

Bend your right arm and pull it back.

Hold your left arm straight in front of you.

Keep your arm parallel to the floor.

As you push your right arm forward, pull your left arm back toward your shoulder.

Do not move your torso or drop your elbow.

20

Percent harder your core works when performing a standing cable chest press than during a standard barbell bench press.

Medicine-Ball Chest Pass

A

- Grab a medicine ball and stand about 3 feet in front of a concrete wall.
- Hold the ball with both hands next to your chest.
- Set your feet shoulder-width apart.

B

- Throw the ball at the wall with both hands, as if you were throwing a chest pass in basketball.
- Catch the ball as it rebounds off the wall, and repeat.

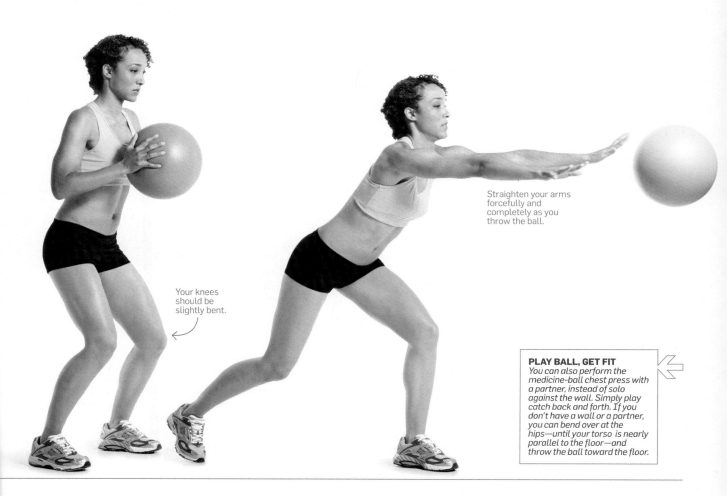

Your knees should be slightly bent.

Straighten your arms forcefully and completely as you throw the ball.

PLAY BALL, GET FIT
You can also perform the medicine-ball chest press with a partner, instead of solo against the wall. Simply play catch back and forth. If you don't have a wall or a partner, you can bend over at the hips—until your torso is nearly parallel to the floor—and throw the ball toward the floor.

Chest | FLYS

These exercises target your pectoralis major. Your front deltoids assist in the movements.

MAIN MOVE
Dumbbell Fly

- Grab a pair of dumbbells and lie faceup on a flat bench.
- Hold the dumbbells over your chest with your elbows slightly bent and your palms facing out.

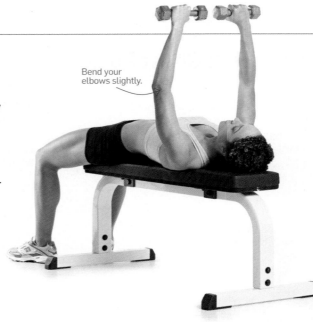

Bend your elbows slightly.

B

- Without changing the bend in your elbows, slowly lower the dumbbells down and slightly back until your upper arms are parallel to the floor.
- Pause, then lift the dumbbells back to the starting position.

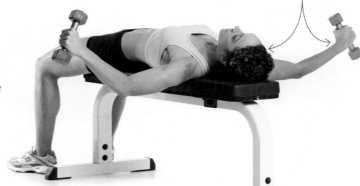

In the down position, the dumbbells should be in line with your ears.

A PECKING ORDER FOR PEC EXERCISES
The chest fly is best placed at the end of your workout. Researchers at Truman State University found that pectoral muscles are activated for 23 percent less time during the chest fly than during the bench press. As a result, the scientists say that dumbbell and barbell chest presses can be used interchangeably but that the fly shouldn't be your primary lift for working your chest.

VARIATION #1
Incline Dumbbell Fly
• Lie faceup on a bench set to a low incline.

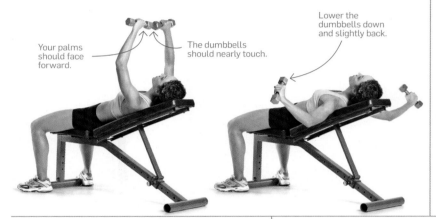

Your palms should face forward.

The dumbbells should nearly touch.

Lower the dumbbells down and slightly back.

VARIATION #2
Incline Dumbbell Fly to Press

• This exercise combines the incline fly with an incline press. Start by doing the incline fly, performing as many repetitions as you can until you start to struggle. Then immediately switch to incline dumbbell presses and complete as many repetitions as you can with perfect form.

MUSCLE MISTAKE
You Still Use the Chest Fly Machine

The chest fly machine, also known as the pec deck, can overstretch the front of your shoulder and cause the muscles around the rear of your shoulder to stiffen. The result is a higher risk for a painful injury called shoulder impingement syndrome. So skip the fly machine, and stick with the exercises in this chapter instead. For any exercise, perform it only if you can complete it pain-free for the full range of motion.

VARIATION #3
Decline Dumbbell Fly
• Lie faceup on a decline bench.

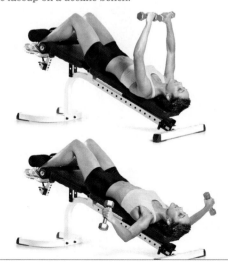

VARIATION #4
Swiss-Ball Dumbbell Fly

• Lie with your middle and upper back placed firmly on a Swiss ball.

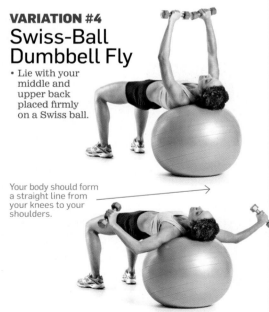

Your body should form a straight line from your knees to your shoulders.

Chest | FLYS

Standing Cable Fly

A

- Attach two stirrup handles to the high-pulley cables of a cable-crossover station.
- Grab a handle with each hand, and stand in a staggered stance in the middle of the station.

B

- Without changing the angle of your elbows, pull the handles down and together, until they cross in front of your body.
- Pause, then return to the starting position.

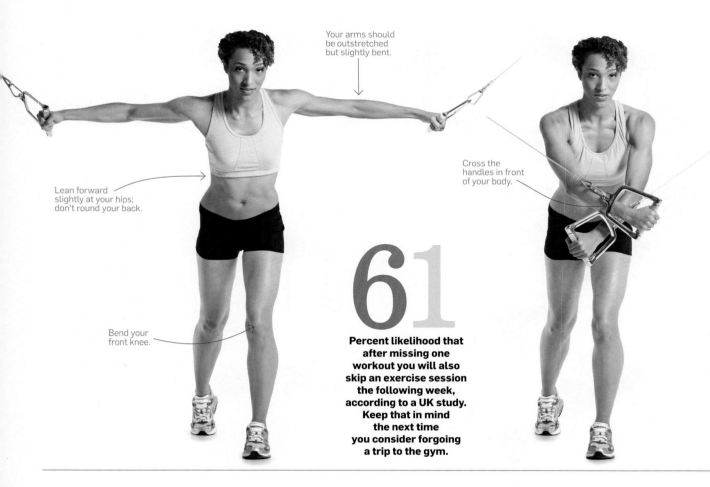

Your arms should be outstretched but slightly bent.

Lean forward slightly at your hips; don't round your back.

Bend your front knee.

Cross the handles in front of your body.

61

Percent likelihood that after missing one workout you will also skip an exercise session the following week, according to a UK study. Keep that in mind the next time you consider forgoing a trip to the gym.

Turn the page to see
THE BEST CHEST EXERCISE YOU'VE NEVER DONE

Chest

THE BEST CHEST EXERCISE YOU'VE NEVER DONE
Pushup Plus

Besides working your chest, this exercise is highly effective at engaging your serratus anterior, a small but important muscle that helps move your shoulder blades. Neglect this muscle, as most people do, and it becomes weak. That puts you at high risk for shoulder impingement—a painful injury in which a muscle tendon becomes entrapped in your shoulder joint. What's more, serratus anterior weakness often causes your shoulder blades to tilt forward and down, resulting in rounded shoulders—giving you a permanent slump.

Now, the classic pushup does work your serratus anterior. But adding the "plus"—pushing your upper back toward the ceiling at the end of the movement—makes the exercise even more effective. In fact, University of Minnesota researchers found that the pushup plus activates your serratus anterior 38 percent more than the standard pushup does.

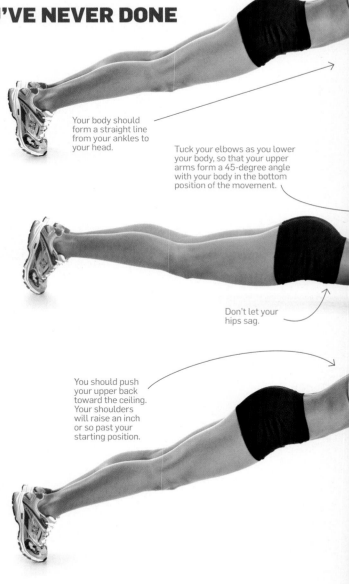

Your body should form a straight line from your ankles to your head.

Tuck your elbows as you lower your body, so that your upper arms form a 45-degree angle with your body in the bottom position of the movement.

Don't let your hips sag.

You should push your upper back toward the ceiling. Your shoulders will raise an inch or so past your starting position.

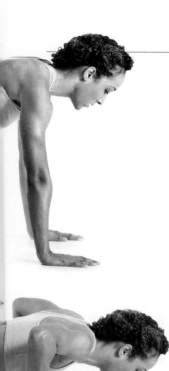

A

- Get down on all fours and place your hands on the floor so that they're slightly wider than and in line with your shoulders.
- Brace your abdominals—as if you were about to be punched in the gut—and hold them that way for the duration of this exercise.

B

- Lower your body until your chest nearly touches the floor.

C

- Pause, and then push yourself back to the starting position as quickly as possible.
- Once your arms are straight again, push your upper back toward the ceiling. The movement is very slight; it's hard to see, but you'll feel the difference.
- Pause for a count of one, then do another pushup and repeat.

BONUS EXERCISE!
Swiss-Ball Pushup Plus

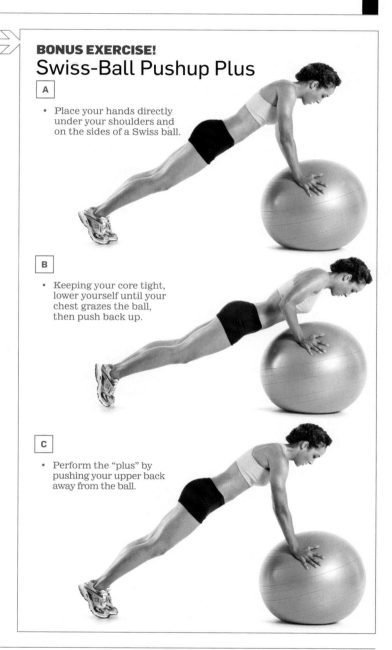

A

- Place your hands directly under your shoulders and on the sides of a Swiss ball.

B

- Keeping your core tight, lower yourself until your chest grazes the ball, then push back up.

C

- Perform the "plus" by pushing your upper back away from the ball.

Chest

THE BEST STRETCH FOR YOUR CHEST
Doorway Stretch

Why it's good:
This stretch loosens your pectoralis minor. When these muscles are stiff—as they are in almost anyone who works a desk job—they yank your shoulder blades forward, making you appear hunched instead of tall and straight.

Make the most of it: Hold this stretch for 30 seconds on each side, then repeat twice for a total of three sets. Do this routine daily, and up to three times a day if you're really tight.

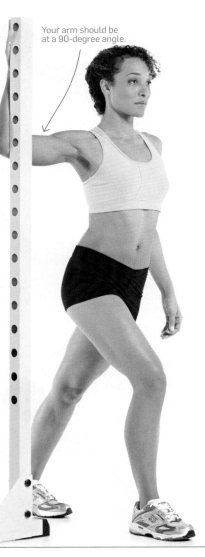

Your arm should be at a 90-degree angle.

A

- Bend your right arm 90 degrees (the "high-five" position) and place your forearm against a door frame.

B

- Step through the doorway with your right foot until you feel a comfortable stretch in your chest and the front of your shoulder. Switch arms and legs and repeat for your other side.

SCULPT THE PERFECT CHEST

Pick your plan: Here are three routines for the results you want.

The Chest-Chiseling Complex

The premise behind this workout is simple: Don't allow your muscles time to fully recover and they'll learn to withstand fatigue better. As a result, over time you'll improve your ability to churn out more repetitions of any chest exercise. And that means better results.

What to do: Do eight dips and eight pushups without pausing between exercises. Continue alternating between moves, reducing the number of reps you do by one each time. So you'll do seven dips and seven pushups next, six and six, and so on, until you're down to one rep. Rest for 90 seconds, then try to repeat the complex. As your strength improves, add one rep to your starting number of reps. Do this workout once every 5 days, maximum.

The Super-Strength Workout

Research shows that people who vary their repetition ranges in a wavelike fashion—known by scientists as undulating periodization—gain twice as much strength as those who do the same routine every workout.

What to do: Do three workouts a week, resting for at least a day between sessions.

- On Monday (Workout 1), perform four sets of the barbell bench press, followed by four sets of the incline barbell bench press. Do four to six repetitions of each exercise, resting for 90 seconds between sets.

- On Wednesday (Workout 2), do three sets of the single-arm cable chest press, followed by three sets of the incline dumbbell bench press; perform 10 to 12 repetitions of each exercise, resting for 60 seconds between sets.

- On Friday (Workout 3), do two sets of dips followed by two sets of pushups. Perform 15 to 20 repetitions of each exercise, resting for 45 seconds between sets.

The Time-Saving Trifecta

Sure, performing three consecutive chest exercises without resting saves you time. But organizing your workout this way also keeps your muscles under tension longer, which is an effective means of conditioning your muscles.

What to do: Perform one set each of three different exercises in succession, without resting—a routine known as a triset. Mix and match movements as you like, choosing one from each of the exercise groups below (A, B, and C). Simply do four to six reps of Exercise A, 10 to 12 reps of Exercise B, and then 15 to 20 reps of Exercise C. Rest for 60 seconds, then repeat three times for a total of four rounds. Perform this workout 2 days a week, resting for at least 3 days between sessions.

EXERCISE GROUP A
Dumbbell bench press (page 52)

Alternating dumbbell bench press (page 53)

Neutral-grip dumbbell bench press (page 53)

Alternating neutral-grip dumbbell bench press (page 53)

Swiss-ball dumbbell chest press (page 56)

Alternating Swiss-ball dumbbell chest press (page 56)

Barbell bench press (page 46)

EXERCISE GROUP B
Incline dumbbell bench press (page 54)

Alternating incline dumbbell bench press (page 54)

Neutral-grip incline dumbbell bench press (page 54)

Incline Swiss-ball dumbbell chest press (page 57)

Reverse-grip barbell bench press (page 48)

Incline barbell bench press (page 50)

EXERCISE GROUP C
Any variation of the pushup or dip (pages 34–45)

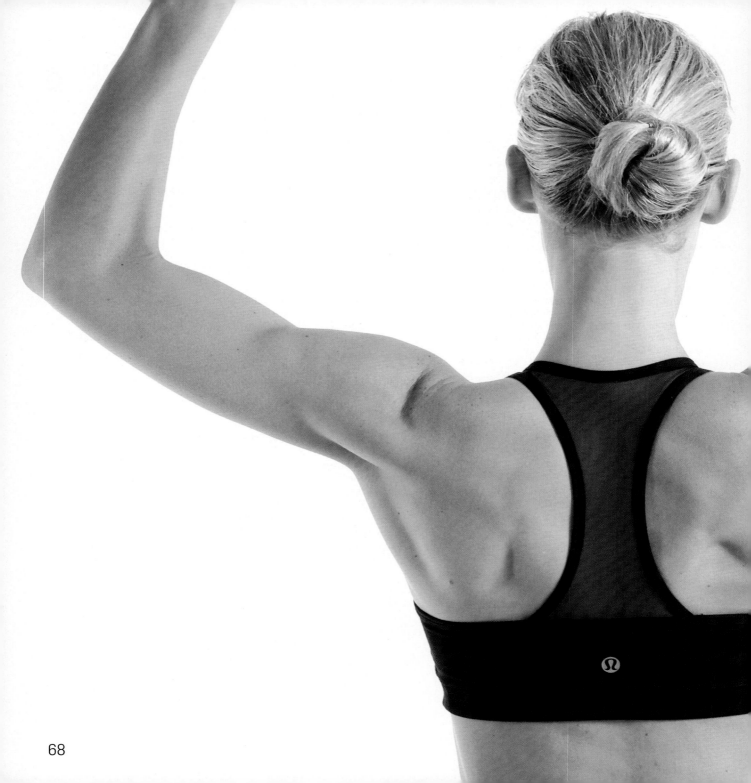

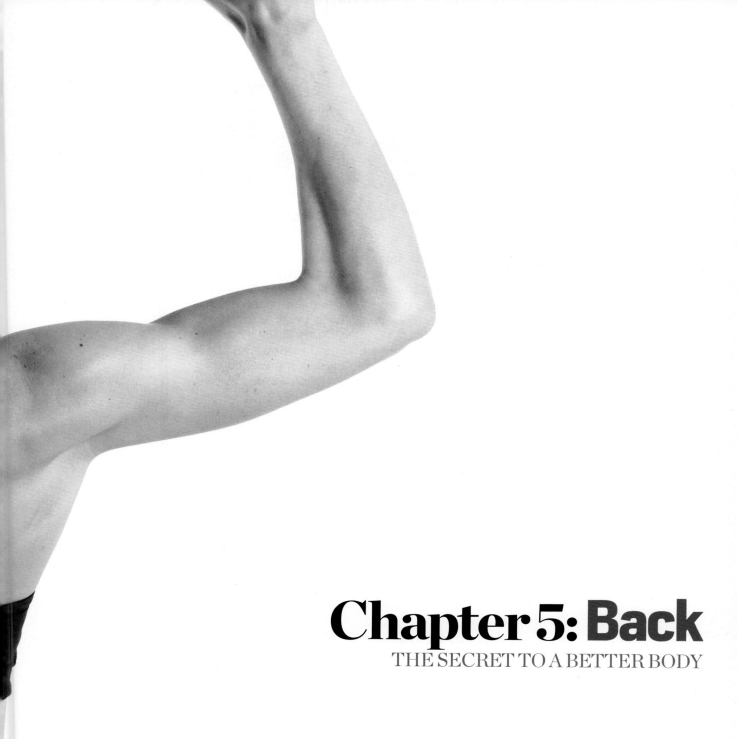

Chapter 5: Back
THE SECRET TO A BETTER BODY

Back

When it comes to sex appeal, a nicely toned back may be your most underrated asset. That's because it not only allows you to look your best in the most revealing of dresses—the backless ones, naturally— but it's also a key to perfect posture. You see, the muscles of your upper back help pull your shoulders down and back, so that you stand tall and staight, instead of hunched over. The added benefit, of course, is that this lifts your front up, too. (Think perky, not saggy.)

So use the back exercises in this chapter to sculpt a top half that has heads turning as fast when you're walking away as they do on your approach.

Bonus Benefits

Sexier arms! Exercises that work your back are also great for targeting your arms. That's because any time that you have to bend your elbows to lift a weight, you're training your biceps—whether you're doing an arm curl, or a classic "back" exercise such as a row or chinup. Think about it: How would your arms know the difference?

A tighter tummy! Working your back can torch belly fat. It's metabolism 101: The more muscles you train, the more calories you burn.

A strong upper body! The muscles of your upper- and mid-back are key for stabilizing your shoulder joints. And strong, stable shoulders allow you to lift heavier weights in just about every upper-body exercise, from the bench press to the arm curl.

Meet Your Muscles

Rear Deltoid
While your rear deltoid [1] is typically thought of as a shoulder muscle (and you'll learn more about it in Chapter 6), it's actually emphasized by many of the exercises that work your upper back. That's because its job is to pull your upper arm backward, a movement that you perform whenever you do a rowing exercise.

Teres Major
The teres major [2] starts on the outer edge of your shoulder blade, or scapula, and—like your lats—attaches to the inside of your upper arm. So it assists your lats in pulling your upper arm down to the side of your torso.

Latissimus Dorsi
Your latissimus dorsi [3] originates on the lower half of your back, along your spine and hip, and attaches to the inside of your upper arm. The primary job of your two lats is to pull your upper arms from a raised position down to the sides of your torso, as when you grab an object off a high shelf. That's why exercises that require this movement, such as chinups, pullups, lat pulldowns, and pullovers, are such popular back builders.

Trapezius
Your trapezius [4] is a long, triangle-shaped muscle located on the upper half of your back. Because of the way its muscle fibers are arranged, your traps have several jobs.

The upper portion of your traps [A] are responsible for lifting your shoulder blades. This allows you to shrug your shoulders. It's worth noting that the best movements for working these fibers—lateral raises, and shrugs—are classified as shoulder exercises and are found in Chapter 6.

The middle portion of your traps [B], with fibers running perpendicular to your spine, are responsible for pulling your shoulder blades closer together, toward the middle of your back. Rowing exercises emphasize these muscle fibers.

The lower portion of your traps [C], with fibers ascending to your shoulder blades, pull your shoulder blades down. Rowing movements work these fibers as well.

Rhomboids
Beneath your trapezius lie your rhomboids, specifically the rhomboid major [5] and rhomboid minor. [6] These are small muscles that start at your spine and attach to your shoulder blades. They assist your traps with pulling your shoulder blades together.

Upper Back | ROWS & RAISES

In this chapter, you'll find 103 exercises that target the muscles of your back. These exercises are divided into two major sections: Upper-Back Exercises and Lat Exercises. Within each section, you'll notice that certain exercises have been given the designation Main Move. Master this basic version of a movement, and you'll be able to do all of its variations with flawless form.

ROWS & RAISES

These exercises target your middle and lower traps, your rhomboid major, and your rhomboid minor. They also hit your upper traps, rear deltoids, and rotator cuff muscles, which assist in the rowing movement or act as stabilizers in every version of these exercises.

MAIN MOVE
Inverted Row

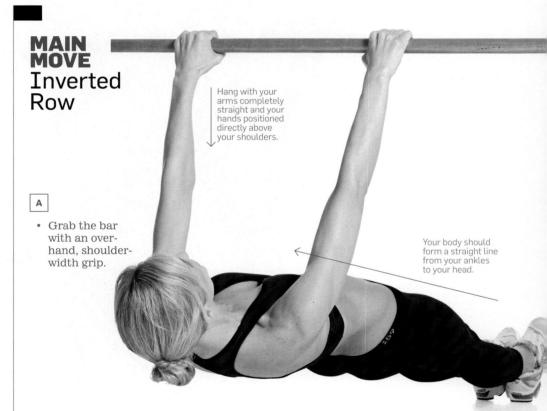

Hang with your arms completely straight and your hands positioned directly above your shoulders.

Your body should form a straight line from your ankles to your head.

A

- Grab the bar with an over-hand, shoulder-width grip.

Why Rows Matter

Rowing exercises train your trapezius and rhomboids, muscles that help keep your shoulder blades from moving as you lift a weight. That's important because unstable shoulders can limit your strength in exercises for your chest and arms. For instance, your chest muscles might be capable of bench-pressing 115 pounds, but if your shoulders can't support that weight, you won't be able to complete one rep. So boost your strength on rows to boost your strength all over.

THE REVERSE PUSHUP?
The inverted row is to your back as the pushup is to your chest. Not only is it great for working the muscles of your middle and upper back but it also challenges your core.

If your wrists start to "curl" as you perform the movement—that is, if you have trouble keeping them straight, it's a sign that your upper back and/or your biceps are weak.

Try to keep your wrists straight.

Keep your body rigid for the entire movement.

B

• Initiate the movement by pulling your shoulder blades back, then continue the pull with your arms to lift your chest to the bar.

• Pause, then slowly lower your body back to the starting position.

Upper Back | ROWS & RAISES

VARIATION #1
Modified Inverted Row
• Instead of performing an inverted row with your legs straight, start with your knees bent 90 degrees.

Bending your knees reduces the amount of your body weight that you have to lift.

VARIATION #2
Underhand-Grip Inverted Row
• Use a shoulder-width, underhand grip.

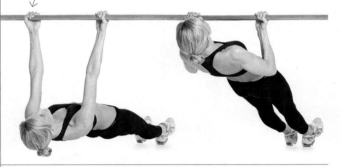

An underhand grip forces your biceps to work harder.

VARIATION #3
Elevated-Feet Inverted Row
• Place your heels on a bench or box, instead of on the floor.

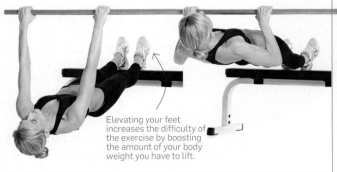

Elevating your feet increases the difficulty of the exercise by boosting the amount of your body weight you have to lift.

VARIATION #4
Inverted Row with Feet on Swiss Ball
• Instead of placing your heels on the floor, position them on a Swiss ball.

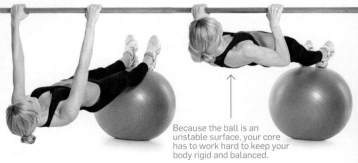

Because the ball is an unstable surface, your core has to work hard to keep your body rigid and balanced.

VARIATION #5
Weighted Inverted Row

- To make the inverted row even harder, perform the movement with a weight plate positioned on your chest.

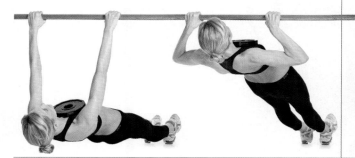

VARIATION #6
Single-Arm Inverted Row

- Grab the bar overhand with your left hand, but keep your right hand free and hold it in the air, with your elbow bent 90 degrees.

- Pull your body up with your left arm, as you straighten your right arm and reach high with your right hand.

- Complete the prescribed number of repetitions with your left arm, then immediately switch arms, grabbing the bar with your right hand to do the same number of reps.

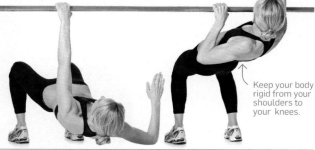

Keep your body rigid from your shoulders to your knees.

VARIATION #7
Suspended Inverted Row

- Attach a pair of straps with handles to a secure bar so that the handles are about 3 feet off the floor.

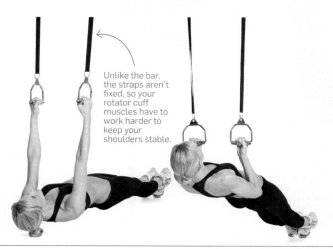

Unlike the bar, the straps aren't fixed, so your rotator cuff muscles have to work harder to keep your shoulders stable.

VARIATION #8
Towel-Grip Inverted Row

- Find your hand positions for an inverted row, then drape a towel over each of those spots on the bar.

- Grab the ends of each towel so that your palms are facing each other.

- Pull your chest as high as you can.

Grasping the towels increases the demand on your forearm muscles, helping improve grip strength as you build your back.

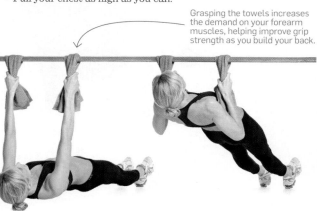

Upper Back | ROWS & RAISES

MAIN MOVE
Barbell Row

A

- Grab the barbell with an overhand grip that's just beyond shoulder width, and hold it at arm's length.

- Bend at your hips and knees and lower your torso until it's almost parallel to the floor.

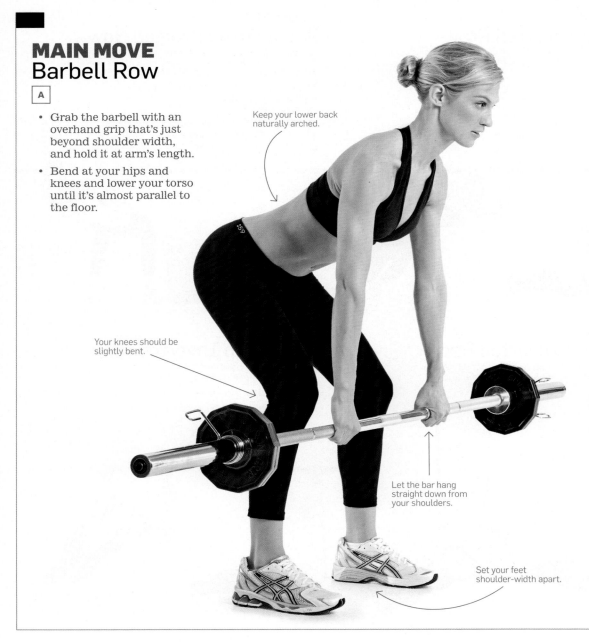

Keep your lower back naturally arched.

Your knees should be slightly bent.

Let the bar hang straight down from your shoulders.

Set your feet shoulder-width apart.

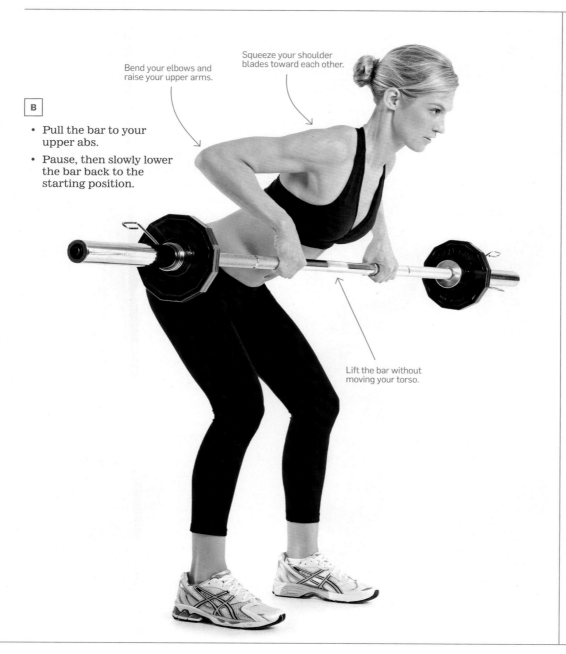

Bend your elbows and raise your upper arms.

Squeeze your shoulder blades toward each other.

B

- Pull the bar to your upper abs.
- Pause, then slowly lower the bar back to the starting position.

Lift the bar without moving your torso.

MUSCLE MISTAKE
You Round Your Lower Back When You Row

This mistake can lead to injuries such as herniated disks. Here's how to avoid it: Pick up the weight and stand tall— with your lower back naturally arched. Keeping your upper body rigid, bend your knees slightly as you push your hips backward as far as possible. Then without changing the posture of your torso, lower your upper body until it's nearly parallel to the floor. Now check your form in the mirror.

Upper Back | ROWS & RAISES

Mix and match one of four grip positions—overhand, neutral, underhand, elbows-out—with any of the eight versions of the dumbbell row that follow. All of the grips are interchangeable with each type of row, giving you 32 back-building options from this one classic move.

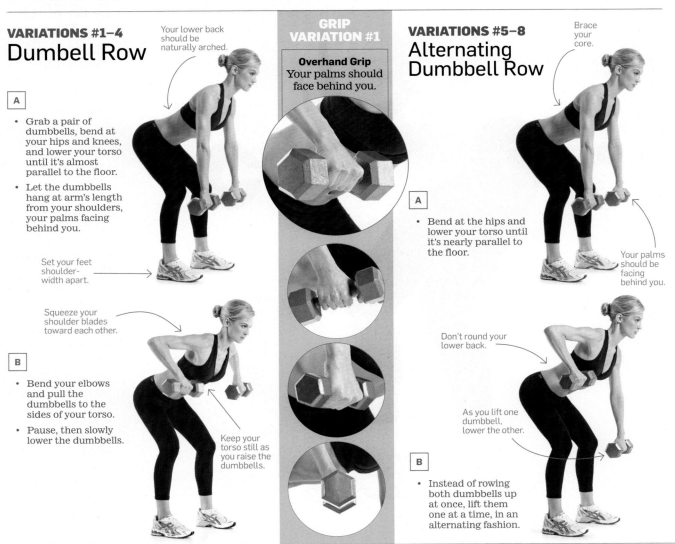

VARIATIONS #1–4
Dumbell Row

A

- Grab a pair of dumbbells, bend at your hips and knees, and lower your torso until it's almost parallel to the floor.
- Let the dumbbells hang at arm's length from your shoulders, your palms facing behind you.

Set your feet shoulder-width apart.

Your lower back should be naturally arched.

Squeeze your shoulder blades toward each other.

B

- Bend your elbows and pull the dumbbells to the sides of your torso.
- Pause, then slowly lower the dumbbells.

Keep your torso still as you raise the dumbbells.

GRIP VARIATION #1

Overhand Grip
Your palms should face behind you.

VARIATIONS #5–8
Alternating Dumbbell Row

Brace your core.

A

- Bend at the hips and lower your torso until it's nearly parallel to the floor.

Your palms should be facing behind you.

Don't round your lower back.

As you lift one dumbbell, lower the other.

B

- Instead of rowing both dumbbells up at once, lift them one at a time, in an alternating fashion.

VARIATIONS #9–12
Single-Leg Neutral-Grip Dumbbell Row

A

- Bend at the hips and lower your torso until it's nearly parallel to the floor.
- Raise one leg and hold it in the air.

Your lower back should be naturally arched.

Your palms should be facing each other.

B

- Row the dumbbells to the sides of your torso.
- Each set, switch the leg you balance on.

Tuck your elbows close to your sides.

Keep your leg elevated as your row.

GRIP VARIATION #2

Neutral Grip
Your palms should face each other. When you row the weight, keep your elbows close to your sides.

VARIATIONS #13–16
Single-Arm Neutral-Grip Dumbbell Row

Brace your core.

Place your free hand behind your back, palm facing up.

Use a neutral grip, so that your right palm is facing left.

A

- Grab a dumbbell in your right hand, bend at your hips and knees, and lower your torso until it's almost parallel to the floor.
- Let the dumbbell hang at arm's length from your shoulders.

The single-arm row allows you to work each side of your body separately, helping to shore up muscle imbalances while increasing the challenge to your core.

B

- Pull the dumbell to the side of your torso, keeping your elbow tucked close to your side.

Don't rotate or lift your torso as you row the weight.

Bend your knees slightly.

Upper Back | ROWS & RAISES

VARIATIONS #17–20
Lying Supported Elbows-Out Dumbbell Row

A

- Instead of standing, perform the exercise while lying chest down on a bench set to its lowest incline.
- Let the dumbbells hang at arm's length from your shoulders.

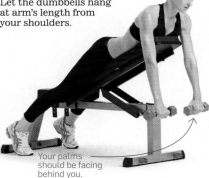

Your palms should be facing behind you.

B

- Keeping your elbows flared out, row the dumbbells toward the sides of your chest.

Keep your lower back naturally arched as you perform the movement, instead of allowing your upper body to "collapse" against the bench.

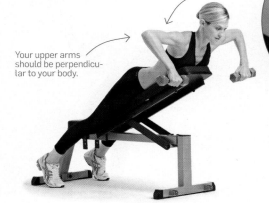

Your upper arms should be perpendicular to your body.

GRIP VARIATION #3

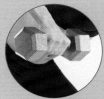
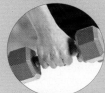

Elbows-Out Overhand Grip
Your palms should face behind you. As you row, keep your elbows flared so upper arm is perpendicular to your torso.

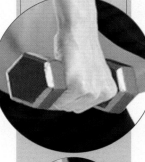

VARIATIONS #21–24
Kneeling Supported Elbows-Out Single-Arm Dumbbell Row

A

- Place your left hand and left knee on a flat bench.
- Your lower back should be naturally arched and your torso parallel to the floor.

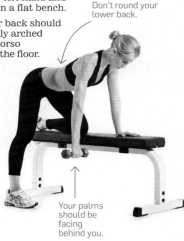

Don't round your lower back.

Your palms should be facing behind you.

B

- Keeping your upper arm perpendicular to your body, row the weight toward the side of your chest.

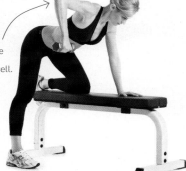

Flare your elbow out to your side as you lift the dumbbell.

VARIATIONS #25–28
Single-Arm, Single-Leg Underhand-Grip Dumbbell Row

Your lower back should be naturally arched.

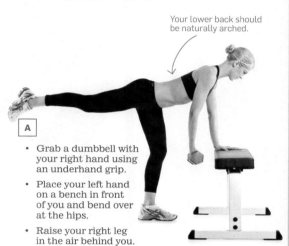

A

- Grab a dumbbell with your right hand using an underhand grip.
- Place your left hand on a bench in front of you and bend over at the hips.
- Raise your right leg in the air behind you.

Your palm should be facing forward.

Your raised leg should be in line with your upper body.

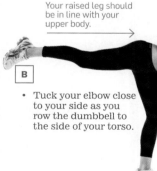

B

- Tuck your elbow close to your side as you row the dumbbell to the side of your torso.

Bend your knee slightly.

GRIP VARIATION #4

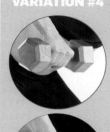

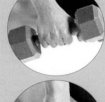

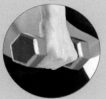

Underhand Grip
Your palms should face forward. Like the neutral grip, keep your elbows close to your sides as you row.

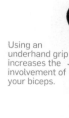

VARIATIONS #29–32
Standing Supported, Single-Arm Underhand-Grip Dumbbell Row

A

- Grab a dumbbell in your right hand.
- Place your left hand on a bench in front of you and bend over at the hips.
- Let the dumbbell hang at arm's length, your palm facing forward.

Your torso should be nearly parallel to the floor.

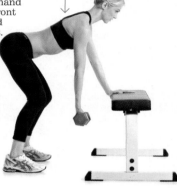

B

- Keep your elbow next to your side as you row the weight to the side of your torso.

Using an underhand grip increases the involvement of your biceps.

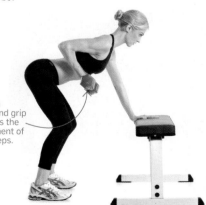

Upper Back | ROWS & RAISES

VARIATION #33
Dumbbell Face Pull with External Rotation

- Grab a pair of dumbbells and lie chest down on a bench set to a low incline.

- Let your arms hang straight down from your shoulders, with your palms facing each other.

- In one movement, bend your arms and pull the dumbbells toward the sides of your face as you simultaneously raise your upper arms as high as you can.

- Pause, then reverse the movement to the start.

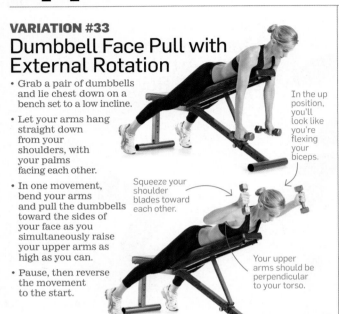

In the up position, you'll look like you're flexing your biceps.

Squeeze your shoulder blades toward each other.

Your upper arms should be perpendicular to your torso.

VARIATION #34
Single-Arm, Neutral-Grip Dumbbell Row and Rotation

- Instead of using two dumbbells, work one arm at a time.

- As you row the dumbbell, rotate the same side of your torso upward.

- Pause, then lower your body and the weight back to the start.

- Complete the prescribed number of reps with one arm, then do the same number with your other arm.

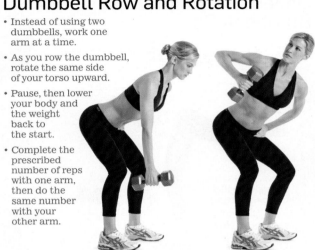

VARIATION #35
Single-Leg, Single-Arm Rotational Dumbbell Row

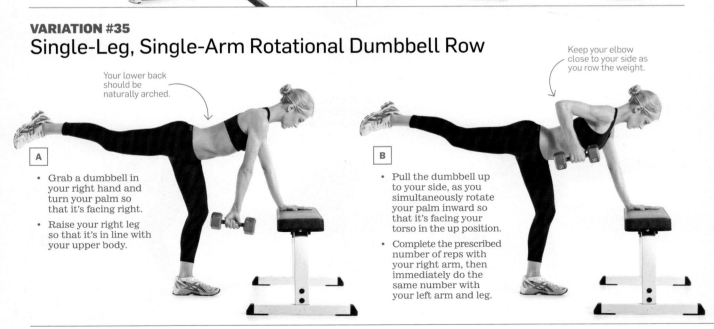

Your lower back should be naturally arched.

Keep your elbow close to your side as you row the weight.

A

- Grab a dumbbell in your right hand and turn your palm so that it's facing right.

- Raise your right leg so that it's in line with your upper body.

B

- Pull the dumbbell up to your side, as you simultaneously rotate your palm inward so that it's facing your torso in the up position.

- Complete the prescribed number of reps with your right arm, then immediately do the same number with your left arm and leg.

MAIN MOVE
Rear Lateral Raise

A

- Grab a pair of dumbbells and bend forward at your hips until your torso is nearly parallel to the floor.
- Let the dumbbells hang straight down from your shoulders, your palms facing each other.

B

- Without moving your torso, raise your arms straight out to your sides until they're in line with your body.
- Pause, then slowly return to the starting position.

The Most Surprising Back Exercise?

Most people think of the rear lateral raise as strictly a shoulder exercise, since it targets your rear deltoid. But consider: It's actually the same movement as a row, only you're not bending your elbows as you lift the weight. So it's also highly effective at working the muscles of your middle and upper back, which is why it's included in this chapter. For best results, focus on squeezing your shoulder blades together as you do the exercise.

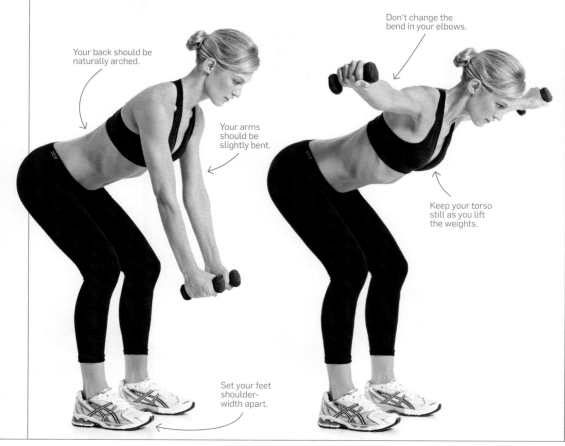

Your back should be naturally arched.

Your arms should be slightly bent.

Set your feet shoulder-width apart.

Don't change the bend in your elbows.

Keep your torso still as you lift the weights.

Upper Back | ROWS & RAISES

VARIATION #1
Underhand-Grip Rear Lateral Raise
- Perform the movement with an underhand grip. Your palms should be facing forward, instead of facing each other.

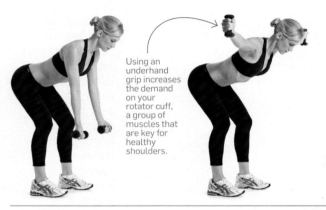

Using an underhand grip increases the demand on your rotator cuff, a group of muscles that are key for healthy shoulders.

VARIATION #2
Overhand-Grip Rear Lateral Raise
- Perform the movement while holding the dumbbells with an overhand grip. Your palms should be facing behind you, instead of facing each other.

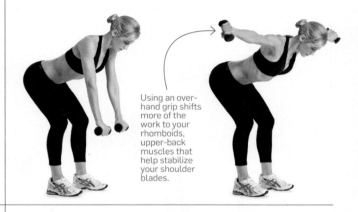

Using an overhand grip shifts more of the work to your rhomboids, upper-back muscles that help stabilize your shoulder blades.

VARIATION #3
Seated Rear Lateral Raise
- Grab a pair of dumbbells and sit at the end of a bench, instead of standing.

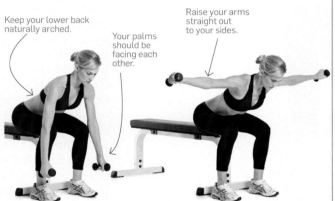

Keep your lower back naturally arched.

Your palms should be facing each other.

Raise your arms straight out to your sides.

VARIATION #4
Lying Dumbbell Raise
- Grab a dumbbell in your right hand and lie on your left side on a flat bench.
- Prop yourself up with your left elbow.
- Let your right arm hang straight down so that it's perpendicular to the floor, with your palm facing behind you and your elbow slightly bent.
- Without changing the bend in your elbow, raise your arm straight above your shoulder, while rotating your arm so that your palm is facing your head.
- Slowly return to the starting position.

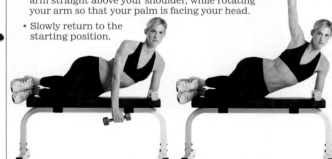

VARIATION #5

Crossover Rear Lateral Raise

- Attach two stirrup handles to the low cables of a cable-crossover station.
- Grab the left handle with your right hand and the right handle with your left, and stand in the middle of the station.
- Bend at your hips and knees and lower your torso until it's nearly parallel to the floor.

- Without changing the bend in your elbows, raise your arms until they're parallel to the floor.
- Pause, then slowly return to the starting position.

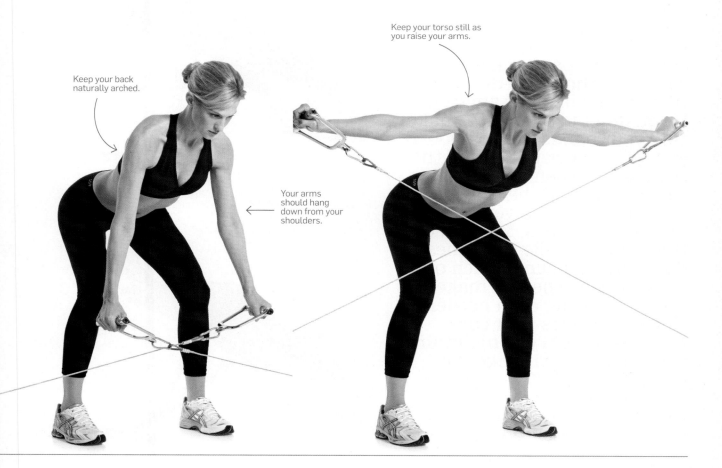

Keep your torso still as you raise your arms.

Keep your back naturally arched.

Your arms should hang down from your shoulders.

Upper Back | ROWS & RAISES

Y-T-L-W-I RAISE

This is a fantastic, multi-part exercise that targets the muscles of your upper back that stabilize your shoulder blades—particularly your trapezius. It also strengthens your shoulder muscles in every direction, emphasizing your rotator cuff and deltoids.

You can perform all parts of the Y-T-L-W-I raise as a *complete* upper-back workout, with or without the dumbbells (depending on your ability). If you don't use weights, make sure your hands are positioned just as if you were holding the dumbbells. When using weights, you'll likely find that all you'll need is, at most, a very light pair of dumbbells. You can do the exercise while lying chest down on an incline bench or a Swiss ball. The ball makes the movements even harder, since it engages your core muscles to help you maintain your position. Three of the movements—Y-T-I—can also be effectively performed on the floor, which can come in handy in a hotel room.

Incline Y Raise

A

- Set an adjustable bench to a low incline and lie with your chest against the pad.

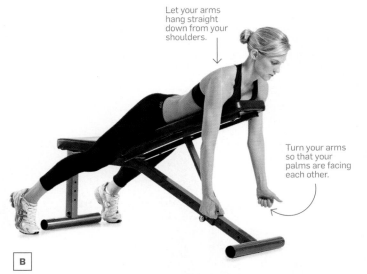

Let your arms hang straight down from your shoulders.

Turn your arms so that your palms are facing each other.

B

- Raise your arms at a 30-degree angle to your body (so that they form a Y) until they're in line with your body.
- Pause, then slowly lower back to the starting position.

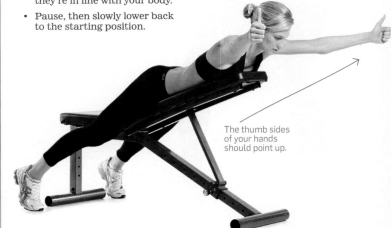

The thumb sides of your hands should point up.

Floor Y Raise

 A

- Lie facedown on the floor. Allow your arms to rest on the floor, completely straight and at a 30-degree angle to your body, your palms facing each other.

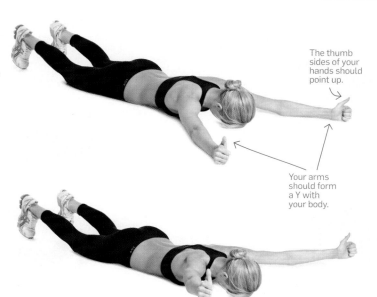

The thumb sides of your hands should point up.

Your arms should form a Y with your body.

 B

- Raise your arms as high as you can.
- Pause, then slowly lower back to the starting position.

Swiss-Ball Y Raise

A

- Lie facedown on top of a Swiss ball so that your back is flat and your chest is off the ball.

B

- Raise your arms at a 30-degree angle to your body (so that they form a Y) until they're in line with your body.
- Pause, then slowly lower back to the starting position.

Let your arms hang straight down from your shoulders.

Turn your arms so that your palms are facing each other.

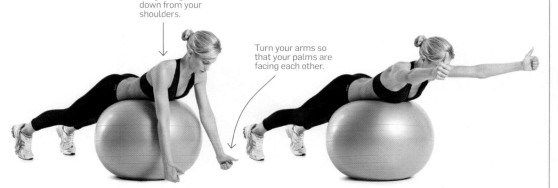

The Complete Upper-Back Workout

Do 10 reps of the Y raise, then immediately do 10 reps of the T raise. Continue on until you've done all five movements of the Y-T-L-W-I raise. Rest for 2 minutes and repeat one time.

The No-Equipment Back Workout

Do 12 repetitions each of Y-T-I while lying facedown on the floor, without resting between movements.

Five More Exercises!

Besides performing Y-T-L-W-I raises on an incline bench, a Swiss ball, and the floor, you can do each of the movements in the same bent-over position in which you do barbell and dumbbell rows. Just make sure to keep your lower back naturally arched as you perform the exercises.

Upper Back | ROWS & RAISES

Incline T Raise

- Lie chest down on an adjustable bench set to a low incline.

- Raise your arms straight out to your sides until they're in line with your body.

- Pause, then slowly lower back to the starting position.

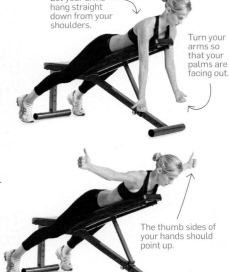

Let your arms hang straight down from your shoulders.

Turn your arms so that your palms are facing out.

The thumb sides of your hands should point up.

Floor T Raise

- Move your arms so that they're out to your sides—perpendicular to your body with the thumb sides of your hands pointing up—and raise them as high as you comfortably can.

- Pause, then slowly lower back to the starting position.

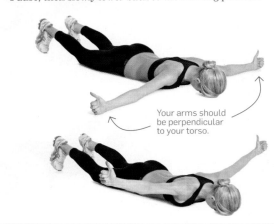

Your arms should be perpendicular to your torso.

Swiss Ball T Raise

A

- Lie facedown on top of a Swiss ball so that your back is flat and your chest is off the ball.

B

- Raise your arms straight out to your sides until they're in line with your body.

- Pause, then slowly lower back to the starting position.

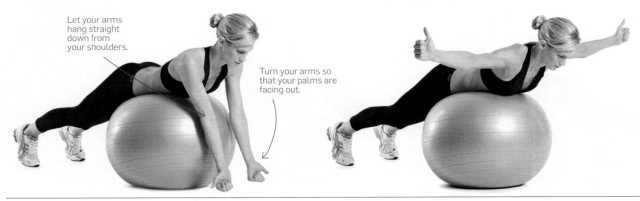

Let your arms hang straight down from your shoulders.

Turn your arms so that your palms are facing out.

Incline L Raise

A

- Lie chest down on an adjustable bench set to a low incline.
- Let your arms hang straight down from your shoulders, your palms facing behind you.

B

- Keeping your elbows flared out, lift your upper arms as high as you can by bending your elbows and squeezing your shoulder blades together.

Your upper arms should be perpendicular to your torso.

C

- Without changing your elbow position, rotate your upper arms up and back as far as you can.
- Pause, then slowly lower back to the starting position.

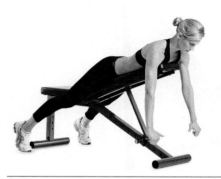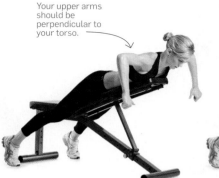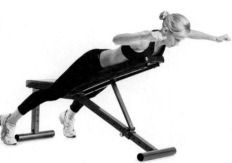

Swiss-Ball L Raise

A

- Lie facedown on top of a Swiss ball so that your back is flat and your chest is off the ball.

Let your arms hang straight down from your shoulders, your palms facing behind you.

B

- Keeping your elbows flared out, lift your upper arms as high as you can by bending your elbows and squeezing your shoulder blades together.
- Your upper arms should be perpendicular to your torso at the top of the move.

C

- Without changing your elbow position, rotate your upper arms up and back as far as you can.
- Pause, then slowly lower back to the starting position.

Keep your chest up.

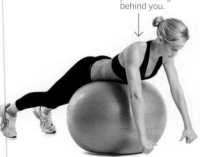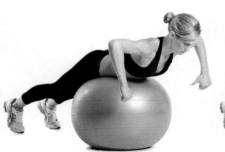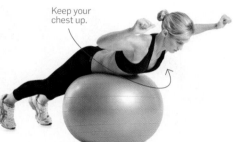

Upper Back | ROWS & RAISES

Incline W Raise

A

- Lie chest down on an adjustable bench set to a low incline.
- Bend your elbows more than 90 degrees and hold them close to your sides with your palms facing up, the thumb side of your hands pointing out.

B

- Without changing the bend in your elbows, squeeze your shoulder blades together as you raise your upper arms.
- At the top of the movement, your arms should form a W.
- Pause, then slowly lower back to the starting position.

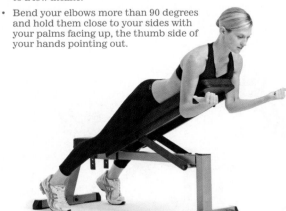
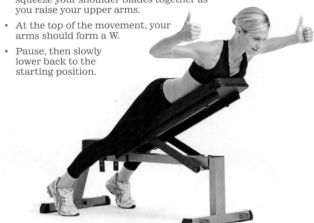

Swiss-Ball W Raise

A

- Lie facedown on top of a Swiss ball so that your back is flat and your chest is off the ball.
- Bend your elbows more than 90 degrees with your palms facing up, the thumb side of your hands pointing out.

B

- Without changing the bend in your elbows, squeeze your shoulder blades together as your raise your upper arms.
- At the top of the movement, your arms should form a W.
- Pause, then slowly lower back to the starting position.

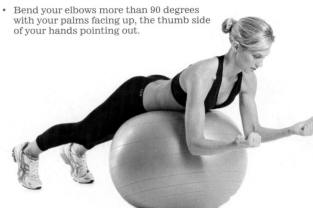

Keep your chest up.

Incline I Raise

- Lie chest down on an adjustable bench set to a low incline.

- Let your arms hang straight down from your shoulders, your palms facing each other.

- Raise your arms straight up, so that they're in line with your body and form an I.

- Pause, then slowly lower back to the starting position.

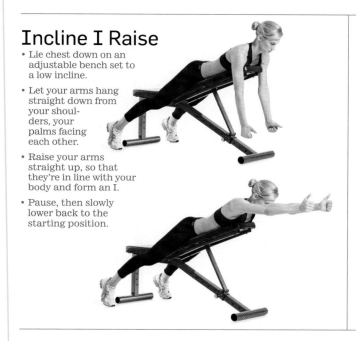

Floor I Raise

- Position your arms straight above your shoulders so your body forms a straight line from your feet to your fingertips.

- Raise your arms as high as you comfortably can.

- Pause, then slowly lower back to the starting position.

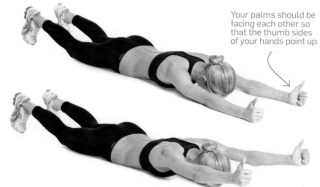

Your palms should be facing each other so that the thumb sides of your hands point up.

Swiss-Ball I Raise

A

- Lie facedown on top of a Swiss ball so that your back is flat and your chest is off the ball.

B

- Raise your arms straight up, so that they're in line with your body and form an I.

- Pause, then slowly lower back to the starting position.

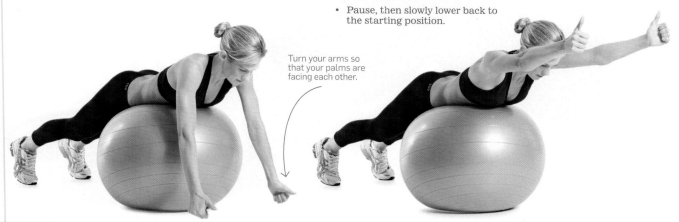

Turn your arms so that your palms are facing each other.

Upper Back | ROWS & RAISES

MAIN MOVE
Cable Row

- Attach a straight bar to the cable and position yourself with your feet braced.
- Grab the bar with an overhand grip that's just beyond shoulder width.

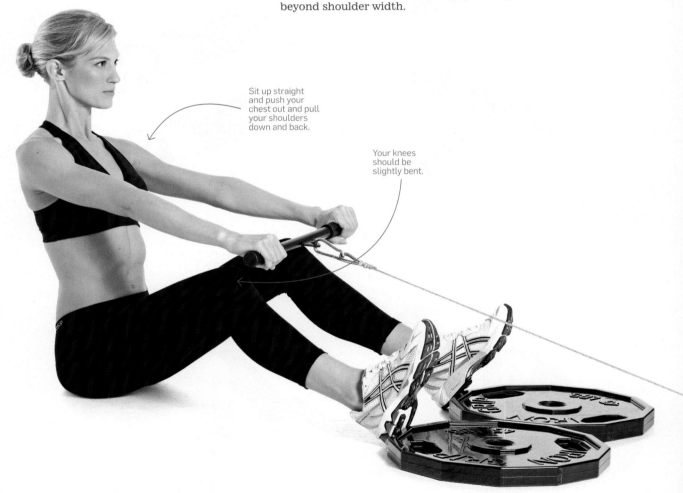

Sit up straight and push your chest out and pull your shoulders down and back.

Your knees should be slightly bent.

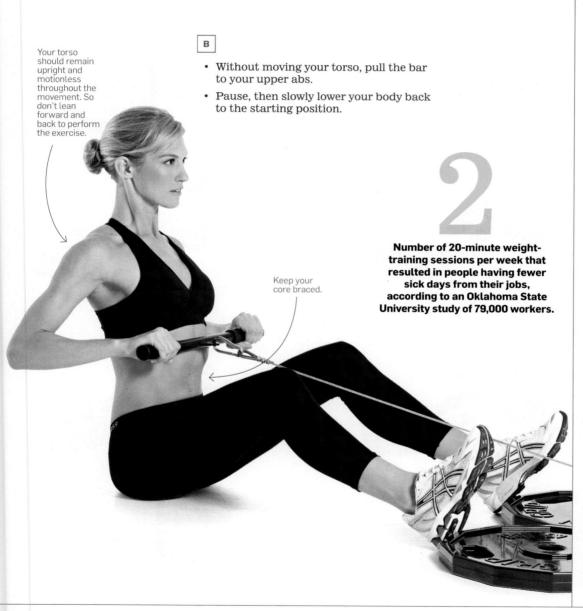

Your torso should remain upright and motionless throughout the movement. So don't lean forward and back to perform the exercise.

B

- Without moving your torso, pull the bar to your upper abs.
- Pause, then slowly lower your body back to the starting position.

Keep your core braced.

2

Number of 20-minute weight-training sessions per week that resulted in people having fewer sick days from their jobs, according to an Oklahoma State University study of 79,000 workers.

MUSCLE MISTAKE
You Row with High Shoulders

When you do any type of row, start the movement by pulling your shoulders back and down. Why? Because otherwise, you'll tend to keep your shoulders elevated, which allows you to hyperextend them as you row your elbows back. This stresses both the front of your shoulder and a rotator cuff muscle called the *subscapularis*. Over time, this can cause your shoulder joint to become unstable, which often leads to injuries.

Upper Back | ROWS & RAISES

VARIATION #1
Wide-Grip Cable Row
- Position your hands about 1½ times shoulder-width apart, and pull the bar to your lower chest.

The wider grip increases the involvement of your rear deltoids.

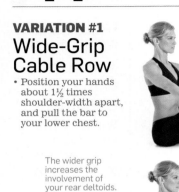

VARIATION #2
Underhand-Grip Cable Row
- Grasp the bar with a shoulder-width, underhand grip and pull the bar to your lower abs.

The underhand grip allows your biceps to work harder.

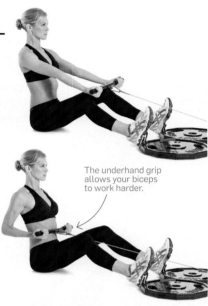

VARIATION #3
Rope-Handle Cable Row
- Attach a rope handle to the cable, grab an end with each hand, and perform a cable row.

Pull toward your upper abs.

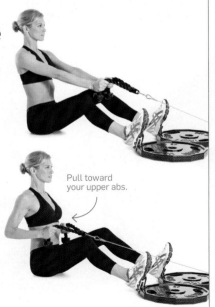

VARIATION #4
V-Grip Cable Row
- Attach a V-grip to the cable, grasp it with both hands, and pull it toward your midsection.

Keep your torso upright; don't lean forward or back.

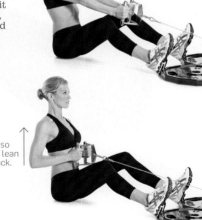

VARIATION #5
Single-Arm Cable Row

- Attach a stirrup handle to the cable and perform the movement with one arm at a time. Without moving your torso, pull the handle to your side.

- Complete the prescribed number of repetitions to your right side, then immediately do the same number to your left side.

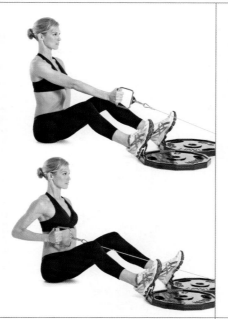

VARIATION #6
Single-Arm Cable Row and Rotation

- Attach a stirrup handle to the cable and grasp it with your right hand.

- Pull the handle toward your right side as you rotate your torso to the right.

- Pause, then reverse the movement back to the starting position.

Sit tall and keep your torso upright.

Keep your core tight as you perform this exercise.

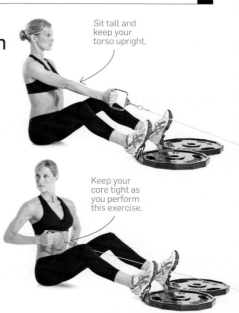

VARIATION #7
Cable Row to Neck with External Rotation

- Attach a rope handle to the cable and position yourself in front of the machine.

- Pull the middle of the rope toward your face, as you squeeze your shoulder blades together and rotate your upper arms and forearms up and back.

- Pause, then slowly return to the starting position.

Grab the bottom of the rope with each hand, your palms facing each other.

Rotating your upper arms backward strengthens your rotator cuff, muscles that help stabilize your shoulder joints.

Sit up straight.

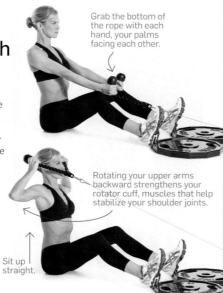

VARIATION #8
Standing Single-Arm Cable Row

- Attach a stirrup handle to the low pulley of a cable station, grab it with your right hand, and stand in a staggered stance.

- Pull the handle toward your right side as you rotate your torso to the right.

- Pause, then reverse the movement back to the starting position.

- Complete the prescribed number of repetitions to your right side, then immediately do the same number to your left side.

Keep your lower back naturally arched.

Your arm should be straight, your palm facing your left.

Lean forward at your hips.

Set your left foot in front of your right.

Brace your core.

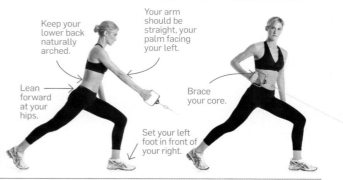

Lats | CHINUPS & PULLUPS

CHINUPS & PULLUPS

These exercises target your lats. They also hit your teres major and biceps. What's more, your core and middle and upper back muscles are involved, assisting in the movement or acting as stabilizers in most versions of this exercise.

MAIN MOVE
Chinup

A

- Grab the chinup bar with a shoulder-width, underhand grip.

- Hang at arm's length. You should return to this position—known as a dead hang—each time you lower your body back down.

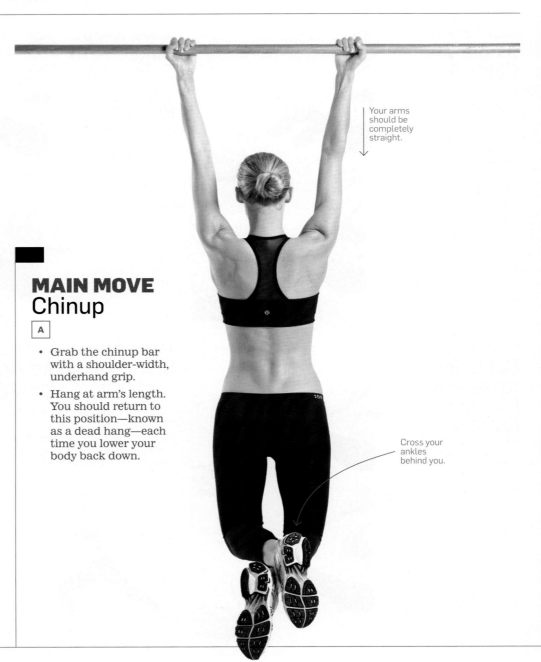

Your arms should be completely straight.

Cross your ankles behind you.

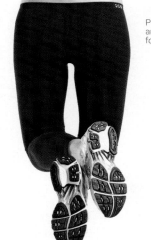

TRAINER'S TIP
Imagine that you're pulling the bar to your chest, instead of your chest to the bar.

Squeeze your shoulder blades together.

Pull your upper arms down forcefully.

B

- Pull your chest to the bar.
- Once the top of your chest touches the bar, pause, then slowly lower your body back to a dead hang.

LIFT YOURSELF HIGHER
Perhaps a better name for the chinup and pullup would be the chest-up. That's because to attain the most benefit from this exercise, you should actually pull your chest to the bar. This increases the range of motion for the exercise, engaging more of the muscles that surround your shoulder blades.

The Chinup vs the Pullup

In case you're wondering about the difference between a chinup and a pullup, it's simple: For a chinup, you use an underhand grip; for the pullup, you use an overhand grip. Of course, you'll quickly discover that the chinup is a little easier. (Or perhaps "less hard" would be more accurate.) This is because an underhand grip allows your biceps to be more involved with the exercise, providing more total muscle power to pull you up.

Lats | CHINUPS & PULLUPS

VARIATION #1
Negative Chinup

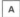

- Set a bench under a chinup bar, step up on the bench, and grasp the bar using a shoulder-width, underhand grip.
- From the bench, jump up so that your chest is next to your hands, then cross your ankles behind you.

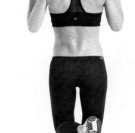

- Try to take 5 seconds to lower your body until your arms are straight. If that's too hard, lower yourself as slowly as you can.
- Jump up to the starting position and repeat.

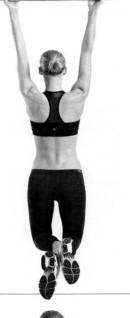

Lower your body at the same rate of speed from the top position of the negative chinup to the bottom. If you notice that you speed up at a specific point, make a mental note. Then, on your next set, pause for a second or two just above that point as you lower your body. This will help you improve your performance faster. A good way to gauge your progress: Once you can complete a 30-second negative chinup, you can probably perform one full standard chinup.

VARIATION #2
Band-Assisted Chinup

- Loop one end of a large rubber band around a chinup bar and then pull it through the other end of the band, cinching the band tightly to the bar.
- Grab the bar with a shoulder-width, underhand grip, place your knees in the loop of the band, and hang at arm's length.

- Perform a chinup by pulling your chest to the bar.
- Once the top of your chest touches the bar, pause, then slowly lower your body back to a dead hang.

The band-assisted method will allow you to do full chinups, and it more accurately mimics the movement than does the assisted-chinup machine you find in commercial gyms. Try a SuperBand (available at www.ihpfit.com) or a Jump Stretch Mini Flex Band (which you can find at www.elitefts.com).

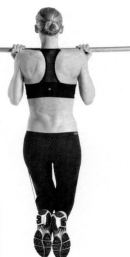

VARIATION #3
Close-Grip Chinup
• Use an underhand grip with your hands placed 6 to 8 inches apart.

When you place your hands closer together, your biceps become even more involved in the exercise. This makes the exercise easier than the classic chinup.

VARIATION #4
Neutral-Grip Chinup
• Grab the parallel handles of a chinup station, so that your palms are facing each other. Now pull your chest to the level of the bars.

VARIATION #5
Pullup
• This is the same movement as a chinup except that you grab the bar with an overhand grip that's slightly wider than shoulder width.

THE BICEPS TONER
When West Point researchers measured muscle activity during the pullup, they found that the exercise targets your biceps just as much as your lats.

VARIATION #6
Wide-Grip Pullup
• Use an overhand grip that's about 1½ times shoulder width.

You can position your hands even wider, but as you do, the strain on your shoulder joint will increase.

The Chinup Spectrum

HARDEST

8. WIDE-GRIP PULLUP

7. PULLUP

6. MIXED-GRIP CHINUP

5. NEUTRAL-GRIP CHINUP

4. CHINUP

3. CLOSE-GRIP CHINUP

2. BAND-ASSISTED CHINUP

1. NEGATIVE CHINUP

EASIEST

Lats | CHINUPS & PULLUPS

VARIATION #7
Mixed-Grip Chinup
- Placing your hands shoulder-width apart, use an underhand grip with one hand and an overhand grip with the other.

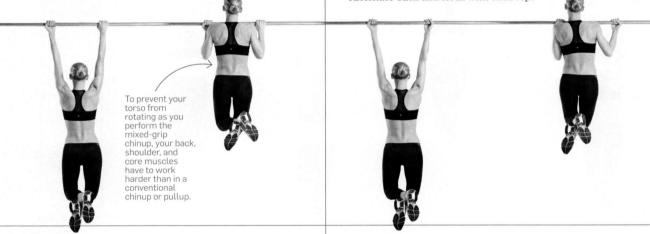

To prevent your torso from rotating as you perform the mixed-grip chinup, your back, shoulder, and core muscles have to work harder than in a conventional chinup or pullup.

VARIATION #8
Crossover Chinup
- Instead of pulling your chest straight to the bar, pull toward your right hand. Pause, then lower back to the start. On your next repetition, aim for your left hand. Alternate back and forth with each rep.

VARIATION #9
Suspended Chinup
- Attach a pair of straps with handles to a chinup bar, grasp the handles, and hang at arm's length. Then perform a chinup, allowing your arms to rotate naturally as you pull yourself up.

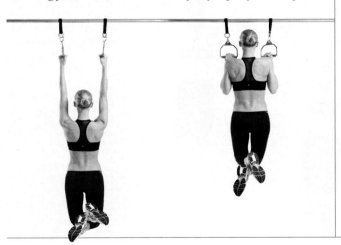

VARIATION #10
Towel Pullup
- Find your hand positions for a chinup, then drape a towel over each of those spots on the bar.
- Grab the ends of the towels so that your palms are facing each other, cross your ankles behind you, and hang at arm's length.
- Pull your chest as high as you can.
- Pause, then slowly lower your body back to a dead hang.

Grasping the towels engages more of your forearm muscles, improving grip strength and endurance.

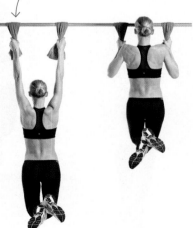

Scapular Retraction

A

- Grab a chinup bar with an overhand grip and hang at arm's length.

B

- Without moving your arms, pull your shoulder blades down and together. Hold this position for 5 seconds, breathing steadily. That's one repetition.

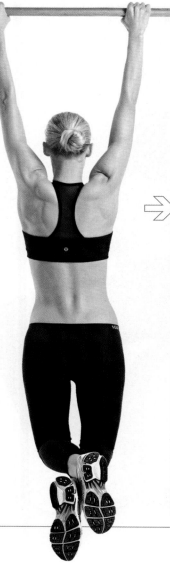

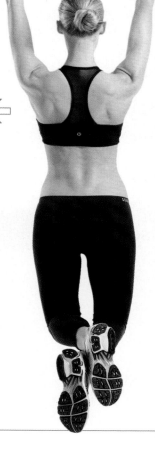

TEST YOUR UPPER BACK
Try to hold the hanging scapular retraction for as long as you can. If you don't last at least 10 seconds, you have an upper back weakness, and this exercise should instantly become a part of your workout. This move also trains you to hold your shoulders down and back, which promotes good posture.

Lats

PULLDOWNS & PULLOVERS

These exercises target your lats. They also hit your teres major and biceps. What's more, your middle and upper back muscles are involved to varying degrees, assisting in the movement or acting as stabilizers in most versions of the exercises.

MAIN MOVE
Lat Pulldown

A

- Sit down in a lat pulldown station and grab the bar with an overhand grip that's just beyond shoulder width.

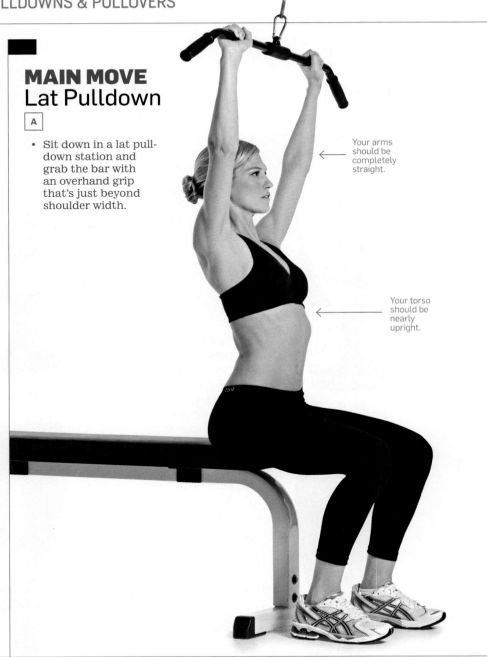

Your arms should be completely straight.

Your torso should be nearly upright.

B

- Without moving your torso, pull the bar down to your chest as you continue to squeeze your shoulder blades.
- Pause, then slowly return to the starting position.

THE CHINUP ALTERNATIVE
Walk into any gym and look around: Of all the exercises in this chapter, you'll find that the lat pulldown is probably the most popular. That's because it's the most logical substitute for a classic chinup (other than a negative chinup or a band-assisted chinup).

Initiate the movement by pulling your shoulders back and down.

Don't lean back to pull the bar to your chest; your upper body should remain in nearly the same position from start to finish.

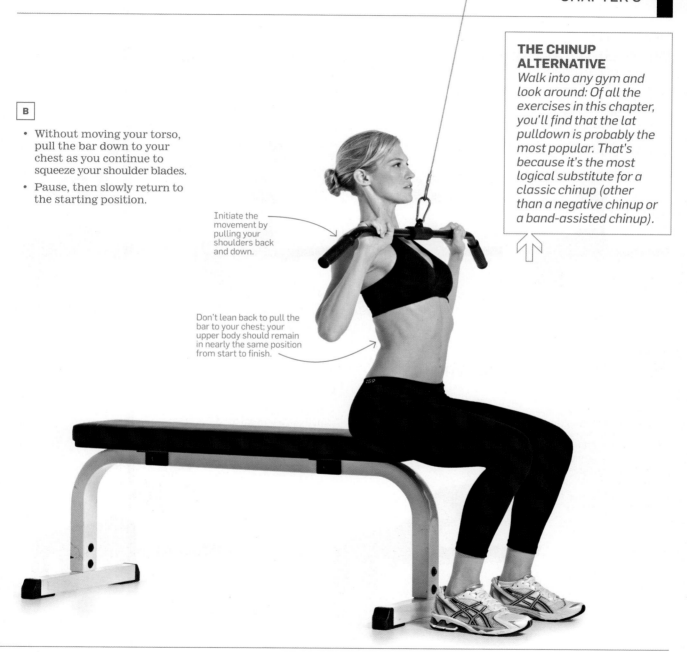

Lats | PULLDOWNS & PULLOVERS

VARIATION #1
Wide-Grip Lat Pulldown
• Use an overhand grip that's about 1½ times shoulder width.

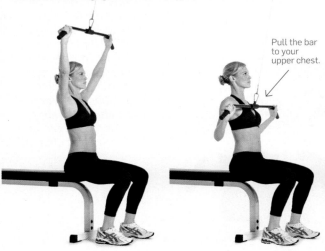

Pull the bar to your upper chest.

VARIATION #2
Underhand-Grip Lat Pulldown
• Use a shoulder-width, underhand grip.

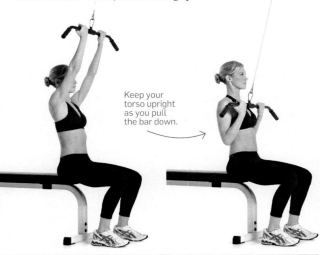

Keep your torso upright as you pull the bar down.

VARIATION #3
30-Degree Lat Pulldown

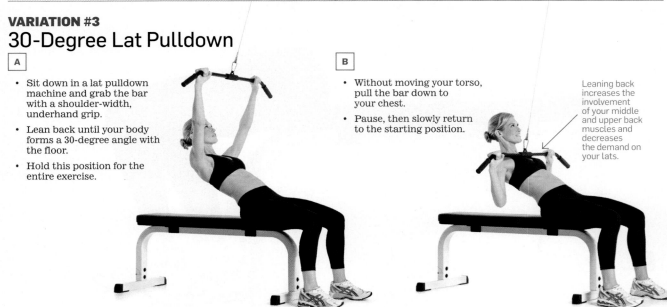

A

• Sit down in a lat pulldown machine and grab the bar with a shoulder-width, underhand grip.

• Lean back until your body forms a 30-degree angle with the floor.

• Hold this position for the entire exercise.

B

• Without moving your torso, pull the bar down to your chest.

• Pause, then slowly return to the starting position.

Leaning back increases the involvement of your middle and upper back muscles and decreases the demand on your lats.

VARIATION #4
Close-Grip Lat Pulldown
• Use an underhand grip with your hands placed 6 to 8 inches apart.

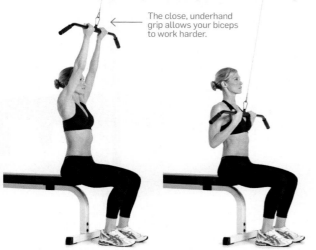

The close, underhand grip allows your biceps to work harder.

VARIATION #5
Kneeling Lat Pulldown
• Instead of sitting in the machine, position yourself on your knees in front of it, your body forming a straight line from your shoulders to your knees.

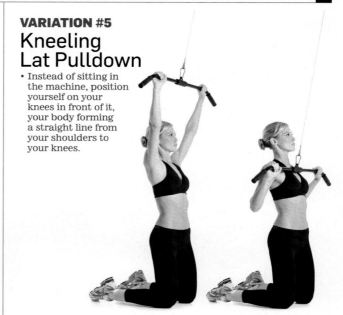

VARIATION #6
Kneeling Underhand-Grip Lat Pulldown

A

• Grab a lat pulldown bar with a shoulder-width, underhand grip.

• Instead of sitting in the machine, position yourself on your knees in front of it, your body forming a straight line from your shoulders to your knees.

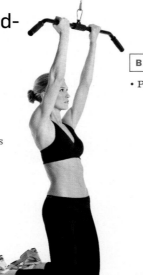

B

• Pull the bar to your upper chest.

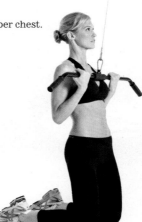

WHY KNEEL?
Because in real life, your lats work with your glutes, or butt muscles. However, when you sit, your glutes are "turned off." So kneeling keeps your glutes switched on, as they would be when you're walking or, say, doing a chinup. You won't be able to use as heavy of a weight, but that doesn't mean that your lats aren't working hard.

Lats | PULLDOWNS & PULLOVERS

MAIN MOVE
EZ-Bar Pullover

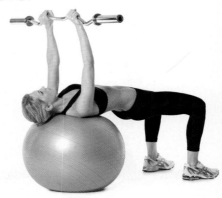

Bend your arms slightly.

A

- Grab an EZ-curl bar with an overhand grip, your hands a little less than shoulder-width apart.

- Lie faceup on a flat bench and hold the bar straight over your chin.

B

- Without changing the angle of your elbows, slowly lower the bar back beyond your head until your upper arms are in line with your body or parallel to the floor.

- Pause, then slowly raise the bar back to the starting position.

Keep your feet flat on the floor at all times.

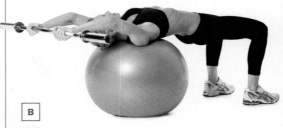

A

- Instead of lying on a bench, perform the movement on a Swiss ball. Place your middle and upper back firmly on the ball. Raise your hips so that your body forms a straight line from your knees to your shoulders.

B

- Without changing the bend in your elbows, lower the bar until it's in line with your body.

If you don't have access to a chinup bar or a lat pulldown machine, the pullover gives you another great option for working your lats. The reason: Even though you perform the movement lying down, it requires that you pull your upper arms from above your head down toward your torso, utilizing one of the main functions of your lats.

Standing Cable Pullover

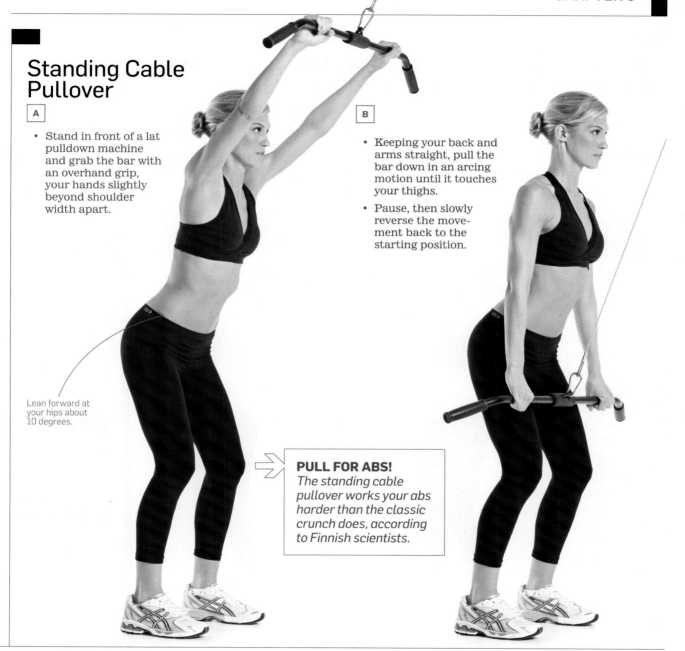

A

- Stand in front of a lat pulldown machine and grab the bar with an overhand grip, your hands slightly beyond shoulder width apart.

Lean forward at your hips about 10 degrees.

B

- Keeping your back and arms straight, pull the bar down in an arcing motion until it touches your thighs.

- Pause, then slowly reverse the movement back to the starting position.

PULL FOR ABS!
The standing cable pullover works your abs harder than the classic crunch does, according to Finnish scientists.

Back

THE BEST BACK EXERCISE YOU'VE NEVER DONE
Cable Face Pull with External Rotation

This unique movement simultaneously targets your upper back's scapular muscles and the rotator cuff muscles of your shoulders. Collectively, these muscles, which tend to be a weak spot in most people, are the key to stable, healthy shoulders. As a result, the face pull with external rotation will help you avoid injuries and improve your upper-body strength. In fact, according to a survey of top *Women's Health* fitness advisors, this exercise is one of the best you can do.

A

- Attach a rope to the high pulley of a cable station (or a lat pulldown) and grab an end with each hand.
- Back a few steps away from the weight stack until your arms are straight in front of you.

B

- Flare your elbows out, bend your arms, and pull the middle of the rope toward your eyes so your hands end up in line with your ears.
- Pause, then reverse back to the starting position.

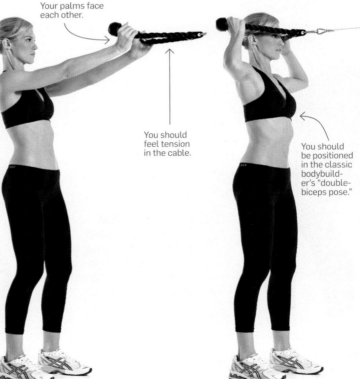

Your palms face each other.

You should feel tension in the cable.

You should be positioned in the classic bodybuilder's "double-biceps pose."

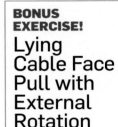

BONUS EXERCISE!

Lying Cable Face Pull with External Rotation

- If you can't maintain an upright posture while performing the cable face pull, try it while lying faceup on a flat bench.

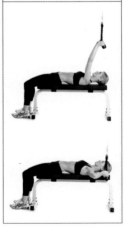

THE BEST STRETCH FOR YOUR BACK
Kneeling Swiss-Ball Lat Stretch

Why it's good: This stretch loosens your lats. When these muscles are tight, they rotate your upper arms inward, which contributes to poor posture.

Make the most of it: Hold this stretch for 30 seconds on each side, then repeat twice for a total of three sets. Perform this routine daily and up to three times a day if you're really tight.

- Kneel on the floor and place a Swiss ball about 2 feet in front of you. Place your hands on the ball, about 6 inches apart.
- Lean forward at your hips and press your shoulders toward the floor.

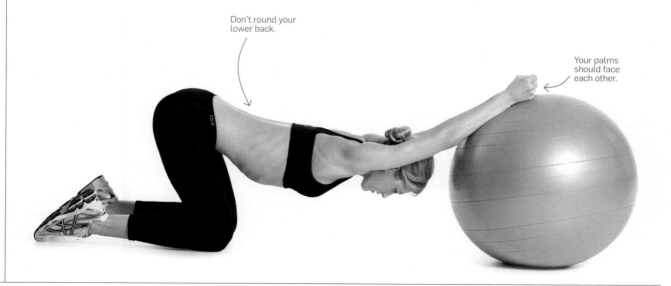

Don't round your lower back.

Your palms should face each other.

Back

THE ULTIMATE CHINUP WORKOUT

Whether you can't yet manage a single chinup or simply want to break out of your eight-rep rut, this training guide from Alwyn Cosgrove, CSCS, will provide the right plan for your body.

If you can't do more than one chinup . . .

EXERCISE 1: Band-Assisted Chinup
What to do: Do two sets of six repetitions, resting for 60 seconds between sets, before moving on to Exercise 2.

EXERCISE 2: Negative Chinup
What to do: Do two sets, resting for 60 seconds between them. Take as long as you can to lower your body—you should time yourself with a stopwatch—until your arms are straight. A key requirement: Try to lower yourself at the same rate from start to finish. When you're able to take 30 seconds to lower your body, or your combined lowering time for both sets is 45 seconds, add a third set. Complete all your sets, and then move on to Exercise 3.

EXERCISE 3: Kneeling Lat Pulldown
What to do:
- Choose the heaviest weight that allows you to complete four repetitions (but not five).
- Do 10 sets of two repetitions each, resting for 60 seconds between sets.
- Perform each repetition as quickly as possible.
- Each week, reduce each rest period by 15 seconds.
- In week 5, do one set of as many repetitions as you can.
- In week 6, start the process over again.

When you can do at least two chinups . . .

It's time to upgrade your routine. Your best option is a method called diminished-rest interval training. Instead of trying to do more repetitions, you'll focus on reducing your rest times between sets. Eventually, you'll eliminate the rest times altogether—and as a result, you'll be able to do more reps continuously.

What to do: Simply take the number of chinups you can complete with perfect form and divide that number in half. That's the number of repetitions you'll do in each set. So if you can do two chinups, you'll do one-rep sets. If you can do five chinups, you'll do three-rep sets. (Round up if the dividend isn't a whole number.) Once you've determined your repetition range, complete three sets with 60 seconds of rest after each. Do this workout twice a week, spacing the sessions at least 3 days apart. Each week, reduce each rest period by 15 seconds. Once each rest period is zero, do an additional set at each workout.

Once you can do 10 chinups . . .

You'll probably be tempted to stick with the status quo—three sets of 10 repetitions each workout, say. However, you won't improve very quickly that way. Instead, build pure strength by adding additional weight and doing fewer repetitions. You'll automatically increase the number of reps you can complete with just your body weight.

What to do: To perform this workout, you'll need a TKO dip belt (available at www.elitefts.com). This is a strap that goes around your waist and that allows you to attach a weight plate to it. Now do the workout below. For each set, use the heaviest weight that allows you to complete the prescribed number of repetitions. So as the number of reps you perform decreases, the amount of weight you use increases. Do each workout three times a week; rest for 60 seconds between sets.

	SET 1	SET 2	SET 3	SET 4	SET 5	SET 6
WEEK 1	8	6	4	8	6	4
WEEK 2	7	5	3	7	5	3
WEEK 3	6	4	2	6	4	2
WEEK 4	5	3	1	5	3	1

Once you reach week 5, start the process over, using the same number of sets and reps that you did in week 1 but adjusting the weight so that it corresponds to your current strength level. You should expect to use more weight for each set in weeks 5 through 8 than you did in the corresponding sets of weeks 1 through 4.

SCULPT THE PERFECT BACK

Tone and strengthen your back in almost no time with this 15-minute routine, courtesy of Craig Ballantyne, MS, CSCS, *Women's Health* fitness advisor and owner of TurbulenceTraining.com. It fully trains your lats but really zeroes in on the muscles of your middle and upper back. These are the common weak spots that lead to poor posture. Strengthening these muscles not only helps you stand tall but also improves the stability of your shoulders. The end result: Your entire upper half will both look better and work better.

What to do: Choose one movement from each exercise group (A, B, C, and D). Then do one set of each exercise in succession, resting for 60 seconds between sets. So you'll do one set of Exercise A, rest for 60 seconds, do one set of Exercise B, rest for another 60 seconds, and so on. Once you've completed one set of all four exercises, rest for 2 minutes and repeat the entire circuit two more times. Perform this workout once or twice a week.

EXERCISE GROUP A

For any of the exercises except the negative chinup, do as many reps as you can up until the point at which you really start to struggle. On each rep, take 3 seconds to lower your body back to the starting position. For the negative chinup, do five reps in which you take 5 seconds to lower your body each time.

Negative chinup
  (page 98)

Band-assisted chinup
  (page 98)

Chinup (page 96)

Neutral-grip chinup
  (page 99)

Mixed-grip chinup
  (page 100)

Pullup (page 99)

EXERCISE GROUP B

Do as many repetitions as you can up until the point at which you really start to struggle. (This is usually about two repetitions short of failure.) On each repetition, take 2 seconds to lower your body back to the starting position.

Inverted row
  (page 72)

Modified inverted row
  (page 74)

Underhand-grip
  inverted row
  (page 74)

Elevated-feet inverted
  row (page 74)

Inverted row with feet
  on Swiss ball
  (page 74)

Towel-grip inverted
  row (page 75)

EXERCISE GROUP C

Do 12 repetitions of this exercise. On each repetition, take 2 seconds to lower the weights back to the starting repetition.

Rear lateral raise
  (page 83)

Overhand-grip rear
  lateral raise
  (page 84)

Underhand-grip rear
  lateral raise
  (page 84)

Crossover rear lateral
  raise (page 85)

EXERCISE GROUP D

Do 10 repetitions of this exercise. On each repetition, take 2 seconds to lower your arms back to the starting repetition.

Swiss-ball Y raise
  (page 87)

Incline Y raise
  (page 86)

Swiss-ball T raise
  (page 88)

Incline T raise
  (page 88)

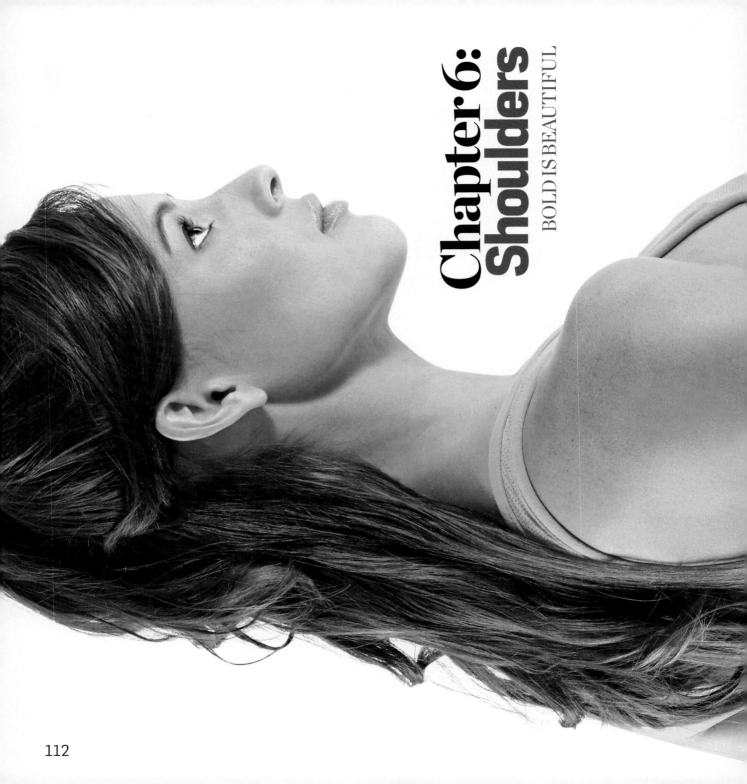

Chapter 6: Shoulders

BOLD IS BEAUTIFUL

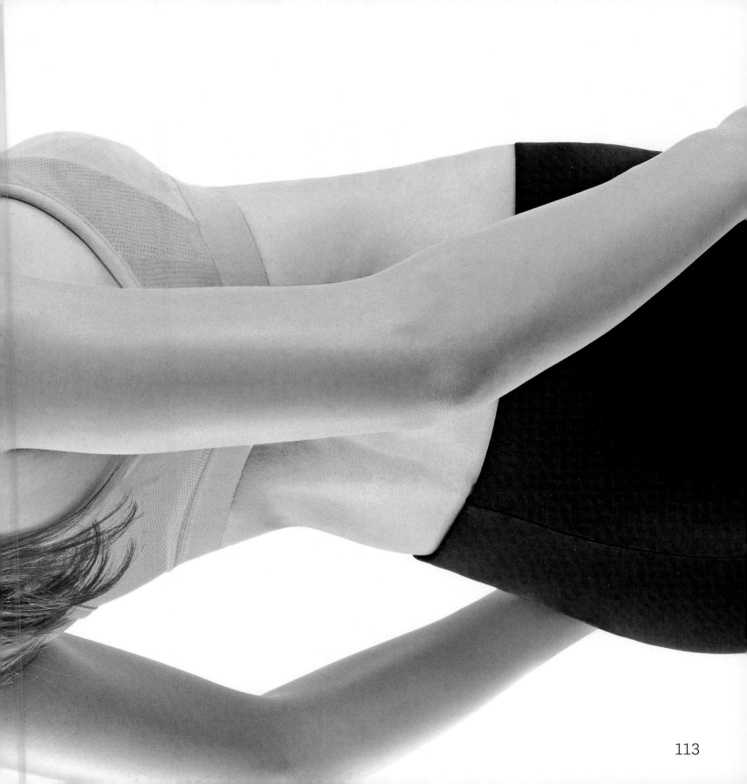

Shoulders

A great set of shoulders can work magic: They make your waist look slimmer, accentuate already-fit arms, and instantly transform any sleeveless top into an eye-catcher. They're also among the easiest muscles for you to define, since the shoulder region is one of the last places your body deposits fat. (How often do you hear people complain about "shoulder fat"?)

Plus, strong shoulders help you strengthen and firm the rest of your upper body. That's because your shoulders assist in most exercises for your chest, back, triceps, and biceps. So you might say they're your muscle-building MVP.

Bonus Benefits

A pain-free upper body! Shoring up weaknesses in the muscles that surround your shoulder joint reduces your risk for neck and shoulder pain.

You'll stand taller! Weakness in the rotator cuff, the network of muscles on the back side of the shoulder joint, allows muscles on the front side of the joint to pull your shoulders forward, causing a slumped posture. But you can shift this balance of power by building a strong rotator cuff—so that you once again stand tall and proud.

Extra power! Whenever you throw or swing, your arms rotate from the shoulder joints. Strong shoulder muscles make it easier to move your arms with more power.

Meet Your Muscles

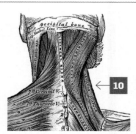

Levator Scapula
People would consider the levator scapula [10] to be a neck muscle. And indeed, this ropelike muscle runs down the back of your neck and attaches to the inside edge of your shoulder blade. However, it works with your upper trapezius to help shrug your shoulder, which is why you can strengthen it with the barbell and dumbbell shrugs.

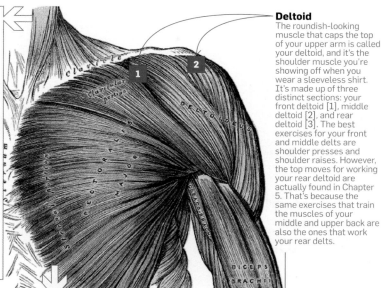

Deltoid
The roundish-looking muscle that caps the top of your upper arm is called your deltoid, and it's the shoulder muscle you're showing off when you wear a sleeveless shirt. It's made up of three distinct sections: your front deltoid [1], middle deltoid [2], and rear deltoid [3]. The best exercises for your front and middle delts are shoulder presses and shoulder raises. However, the top moves for working your rear deltoid are actually found in Chapter 5. That's because the same exercises that train the muscles of your middle and upper back are also the ones that work your rear delts.

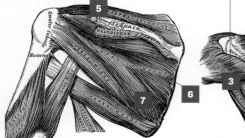

Serratus Anterior
Your serratus anterior [9] starts next to the outer edge of your pectorals, on the surface of your upper eight ribs. It wraps around your rib cage until it connects to the undersurface of your shoulder blade, along the inner edge. This muscle's job is to help stabilize and rotate your shoulder blade. You can make it stronger with the serratus shrug and the serratus chair shrug.

Rotator Cuff
Your rotator cuff muscles are a network of four muscles that attach your shoulder blade to your shoulder joint. They are the supraspinatus [5], the infraspinatus [6], the teres minor [7], and the subscapularis [8]. While these muscles are activated in just about every upper-body exercise—they contract to help stabilize your shoulder joint—they also need to be worked directly with shoulder rotation exercises.

Upper Trapezius
Although the trapezius as a whole is categorized as a back muscle, the upper portions of your traps [4] are best developed with exercises such as the lateral raise and the shoulder shrug, both of which are featured in this chapter.

MUSCLE MISTAKE
Your Shoulders Hurt, but You Lift Anyway
Think of it this way: When your car gets a flat tire, you don't risk driving on it, since that could permanently damage the rims. It's the same way with your shoulders. But just avoiding the offending exercise isn't good enough. After all, a flat tire doesn't fix itself if you simply park the car in your garage. You need to take action. If you notice recurring shoulder pain, see an orthopedist or a physical therapist.

Shoulders | PRESSES

In this chapter, you'll find 40 exercises that target the muscles of your shoulders. Throughout, you'll notice that certain exercises have been given the designation Main Move. Master this basic version of a movement, and you'll be able to do all of its variations with flawless form.

SHOULDER PRESSES
These exercises target your front deltoids, middle deltoids, and triceps. They also activate your upper traps, rotator cuff, and serratus anterior, which assist in the movement or act as stabilizers.

MAIN MOVE
Barbell Shoulder Press

A

- Grab a barbell with an overhand grip that's just beyond shoulder width, and hold it at shoulder level in front of your body.

- Stand with your feet shoulder-width apart.

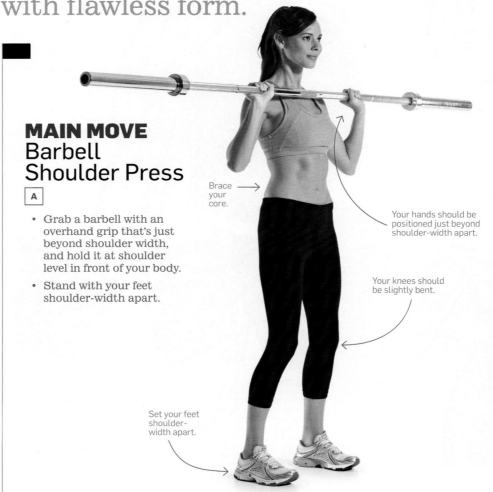

Brace your core.

Your hands should be positioned just beyond shoulder-width apart.

Your knees should be slightly bent.

Set your feet shoulder-width apart.

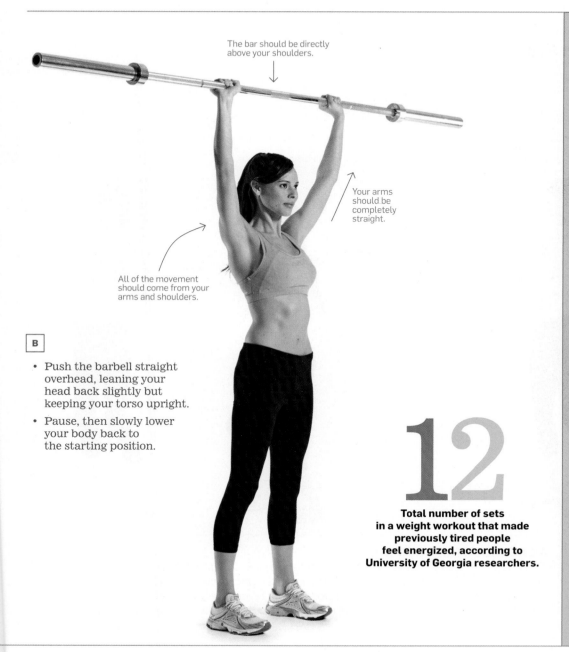

The bar should be directly above your shoulders.

Your arms should be completely straight.

All of the movement should come from your arms and shoulders.

B

- Push the barbell straight overhead, leaning your head back slightly but keeping your torso upright.

- Pause, then slowly lower your body back to the starting position.

12

Total number of sets in a weight workout that made previously tired people feel energized, according to University of Georgia researchers.

What about the Back Rest?

People often do the shoulder press seated, with their backs braced against a back rest. This provides a stable surface from which to lift, allowing the use of heavier weights. However, greater loads also mean increased stress on the shoulder joint in the "at-risk position"—the point at which your elbows are bent 90 degrees with your palms facing forward. This is the portion of the lift in which you're most likely to suffer a shoulder injury. Avoid that fate by skipping the back rest.

Shoulders | PRESSES

VARIATION #1
Barbell Push Press

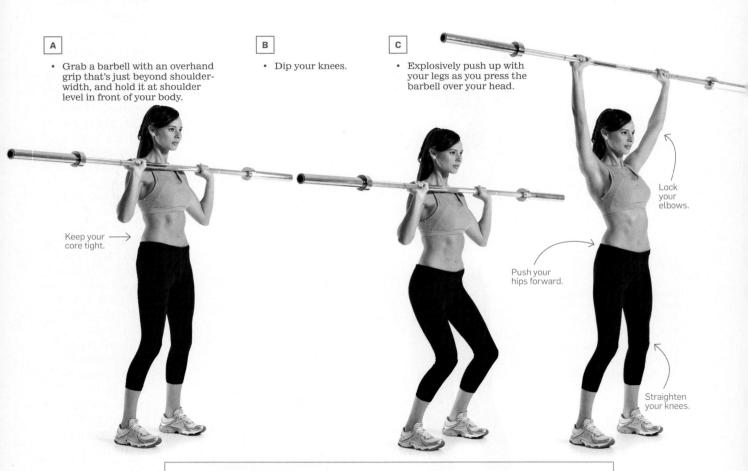

A

- Grab a barbell with an overhand grip that's just beyond shoulder-width, and hold it at shoulder level in front of your body.

Keep your core tight. →

B

- Dip your knees.

C

- Explosively push up with your legs as you press the barbell over your head.

Lock your elbows.

Push your hips forward.

Straighten your knees.

MORE WEIGHT, LESS RISK

If you want to press heavier weights, try the push press. It doesn't carry the same injury risk as doing a shoulder press against a back rest (see "What about the Back Rest?" on the previous page). That's because your legs help you push through the at-risk position, reducing the strain on your shoulders.

VARIATION #2
Barbell Split Jerk

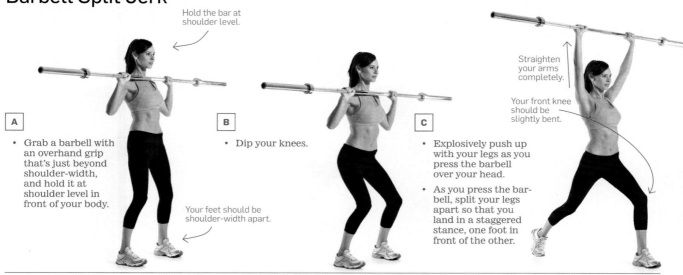

Hold the bar at shoulder level.

A

- Grab a barbell with an overhand grip that's just beyond shoulder-width, and hold it at shoulder level in front of your body.

Your feet should be shoulder-width apart.

B

- Dip your knees.

C

- Explosively push up with your legs as you press the barbell over your head.
- As you press the barbell, split your legs apart so that you land in a staggered stance, one foot in front of the other.

Straighten your arms completely.

Your front knee should be slightly bent.

VARIATION #3
Seated Barbell Shoulder Press

The barbell should be directly over your shoulders.

A

- Sit at the end of a bench with your torso upright.

Brace your abs.

Your feet should be flat on the floor.

B

- Press the barbell over your head.

Don't bend forward. Your torso should be completely upright.

Keep your lower back naturally arched as you perform the movement.

Shoulders |

MAIN MOVE
Dumbbell Shoulder Press

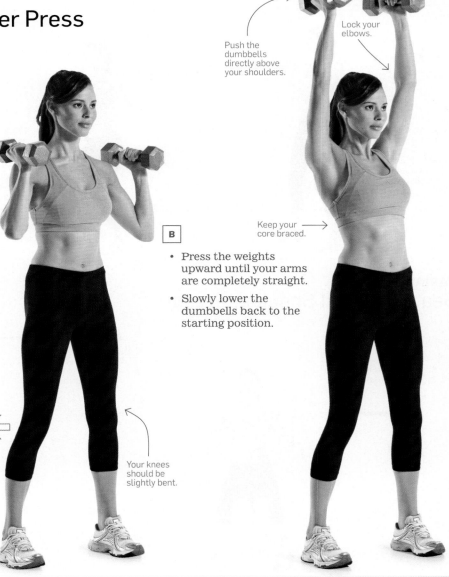

Push the dumbbells directly above your shoulders.

Lock your elbows.

Keep your core braced.

A

- Stand holding a pair of dumbbells just outside your shoulders, with your arms bent and palms facing each other.

- Set your feet shoulder-width apart, and slightly bend your knees.

B

- Press the weights upward until your arms are completely straight.

- Slowly lower the dumbbells back to the starting position.

Your knees should be slightly bent.

TRAINER'S TIP
Make sure to push the dumbbells in a straight line, rather than pushing them up and toward each other as many people do—a habit that increases the risk for shoulder injuries.

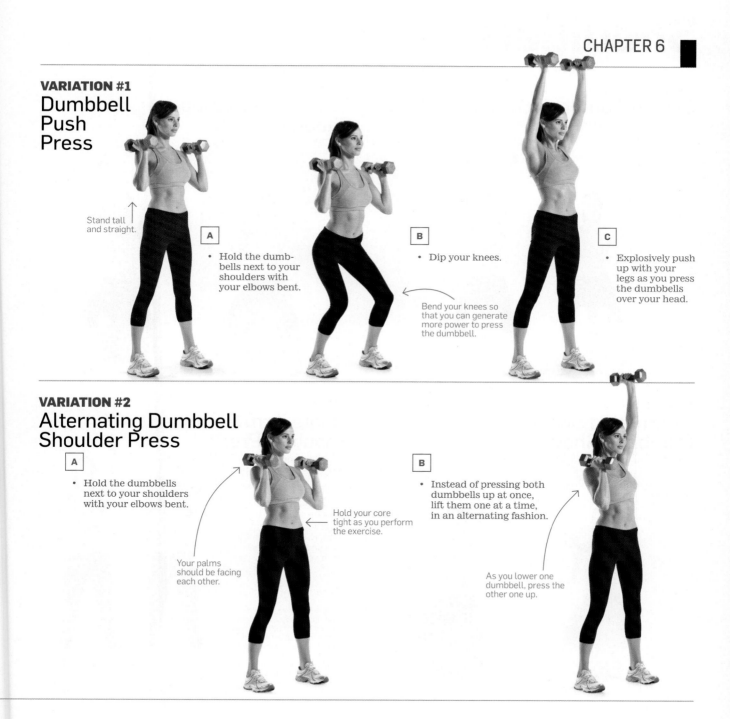

VARIATION #1
Dumbbell Push Press

Stand tall and straight.

A
- Hold the dumb-bells next to your shoulders with your elbows bent.

B
- Dip your knees.

Bend your knees so that you can generate more power to press the dumbbell.

C
- Explosively push up with your legs as you press the dumbbells over your head.

VARIATION #2
Alternating Dumbbell Shoulder Press

A
- Hold the dumbbells next to your shoulders with your elbows bent.

Hold your core tight as you perform the exercise.

Your palms should be facing each other.

B
- Instead of pressing both dumbbells up at once, lift them one at a time, in an alternating fashion.

As you lower one dumbbell, press the other one up.

121

Shoulders | PRESSES

VARIATION #3
Seated Dumbbell Shoulder Press
- Sit at the end of a bench with your torso upright.

Your lower back should be naturally arched.

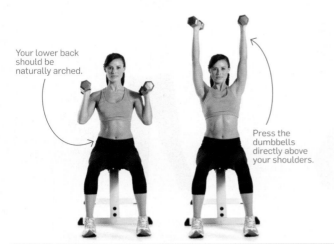

Press the dumbbells directly above your shoulders.

VARIATION #4
Swiss-Ball Dumbbell Shoulder Press
- Sit on a Swiss ball with your torso upright.

Your palms should be facing each other.

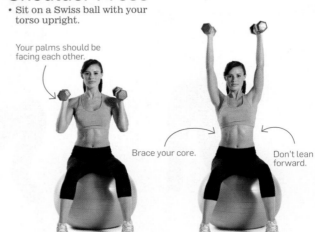

Brace your core.

Don't lean forward.

VARIATION #5
Alternating Swiss-Ball Dumbbell Shoulder Press
- Sit on a Swiss ball with your torso upright.
- Instead of pressing both dumbbells up at once, lift them one at a time, in an alternating fashion.

As you lower one dumbbell, press the other up.

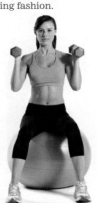
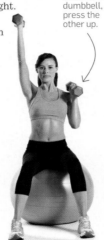

VARIATION #6
Single-Arm Dumbbell Shoulder Press
- Perform a dumbbell shoulder press using only one dumbbell at a time.
- Complete the prescribed number of reps with your right arm, then immediately do the same number with your left arm.

Let your free hand hang to your side or place it on your hip.

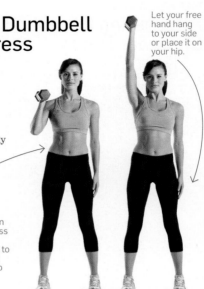

Because using just one dumbbell causes uneven weight distribution across your body, this exercise increases the challenge to your core, making those muscles work harder to keep you balanced.

VARIATION #7
Dumbbell Alternating Shoulder Press and Twist

- Hold the dumbbells next to your shoulders with your elbows bent.

- Rotate your torso to the right as you press the dumbbell in your left hand at a slight angle above your shoulder.
- Reverse the movement back to the start, rotate to your left, and press the dumbbell in your right hand upward. Alternate back and forth.

Rotating your torso activates your obliques, core muscles that are often weak.

Press the dumbbell up diagonally.

Your palms should be facing each other.

Straighten your left arm completely.

Keep your abs braced as you rotate your torso. This will limit the amount your lower spine can twist, protecting you from injury.

Pivot your feet.

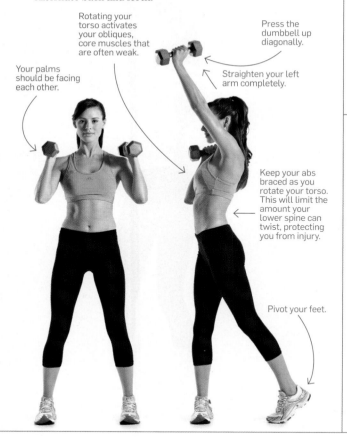

Floor Inverted Shoulder Press

- Assume a pushup position, but move your feet forward and raise your hips so that your torso is nearly perpendicular to the floor.
- Your hands should be slightly wider than your shoulders, and your arms should be straight.
- Without changing your body posture, lower your body until your head nearly touches the floor.
- Pause, then return to the starting position by pushing your body back up until your arms are straight.

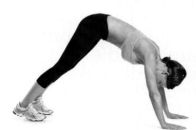

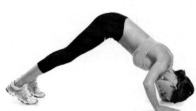

Inverted Shoulder Press

- Assume a pushup position, but place your feet on a bench and push your hips up so that your torso is nearly perpendicular to the floor.
- Without changing your body posture, lower your body until your head nearly touches the floor.

Your arms should be straight.

Your hands should be slightly wider than shoulder width apart.

While the inverted shoulder press is technically a pushup, the tweak to your form shifts more of the workload to your shoulders and triceps, reducing the demand on your chest.

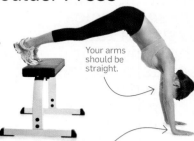

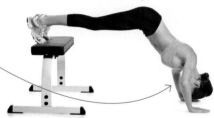

123

Shoulders | RAISES

SHOULDER RAISES

These exercises target your front and middle deltoids. However, the different variations shift the section of the muscle that works the hardest. What's more, shoulder raises work your rear deltoids, upper traps, rotator cuff, and serratus anterior, since these muscles assist in raising the weight or act as stabilizers on nearly every version of this exercise.

MAIN MOVE
Front Raise

A

- Grab a pair of dumbbells and let them hang at arm's length next to your sides, with your palms facing each other.

B

- Raise your arms straight in front of you until they're parallel to the floor and perpendicular to your torso.
- Pause, then slowly lower the dumbbells back to the starting position.

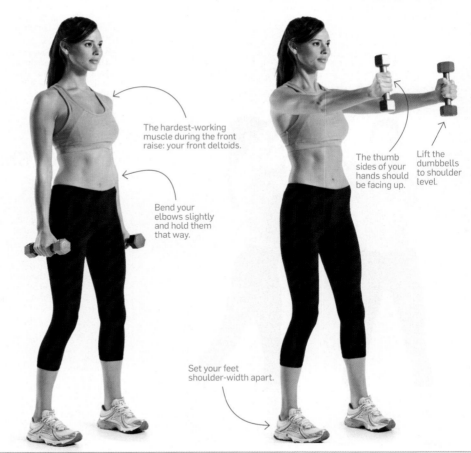

The hardest-working muscle during the front raise: your front deltoids.

Bend your elbows slightly and hold them that way.

The thumb sides of your hands should be facing up.

Lift the dumbbells to shoulder level.

Set your feet shoulder-width apart.

VARIATION #1
Weight-Plate Front Raise

A

- Instead of holding two dumbbells, grab the sides of a weight plate with both hands.

B

- Raise the weight to shoulder level.

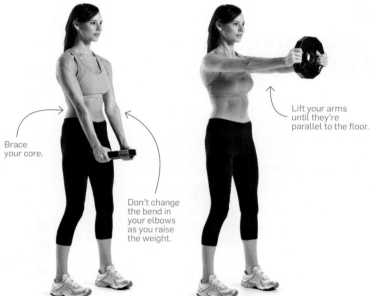

Brace your core.

Don't change the bend in your elbows as you raise the weight.

Lift your arms until they're parallel to the floor.

17

Percent more reps per three sets people could do when they were well-hydrated, according to University of Connecticut researchers. Remember, your muscles are about 80 percent water.

VARIATION #2
Cable Front Raise

A

- Attach a rope handle to the low pulley of a cable station, and stand facing away from the weight stack.
- Hold the handle with your right hand, your arm hanging next to your side and your palm facing your thigh.

B

- Without changing the bend in your elbow, raise your arm straight out in front of you until it's parallel to the floor.
- Pause, then slowly lower back to the starting position.
- Complete the prescribed number of repetitions with your right arm, then immediately switch hands and do the same number with your left arm.

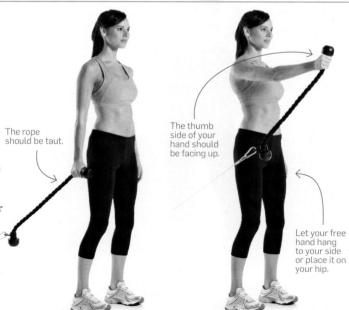

The rope should be taut.

The thumb side of your hand should be facing up.

Let your free hand hang to your side or place it on your hip.

MAIN MOVE
Lateral Raise

A

- Grab a pair of dumbbells and let them hang at arm's length next to your sides.
- Stand tall, with your feet shoulder-width apart.
- Turn your arms so that your palms are facing forward, and bend your elbows slightly.

B

- Without changing the bend in your elbows, raise your arms straight out to your sides until they're at shoulder level.
- Pause for 1 second at the top of the movement, then slowly lower the weights back to the starting position.

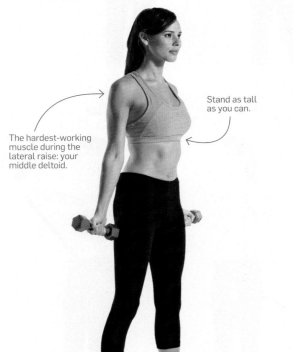

Stand as tall as you can.

The hardest-working muscle during the lateral raise: your middle deltoid.

Set your feet shoulder-width apart.

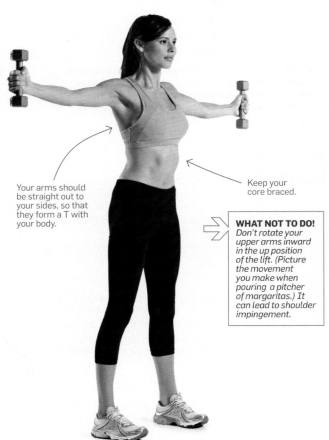

Your arms should be straight out to your sides, so that they form a T with your body.

Keep your core braced.

WHAT NOT TO DO!
Don't rotate your upper arms inward in the up position of the lift. (Picture the movement you make when pouring a pitcher of margaritas.) It can lead to shoulder impingement.

VARIATION #1
Alternating Lateral Raise with Static Hold

- Stand holding a pair of dumbbells straight out from your sides, as you would in the "up" position of a lateral raise.

- Lower and raise one arm, then lower and raise the other. That's one repetition.

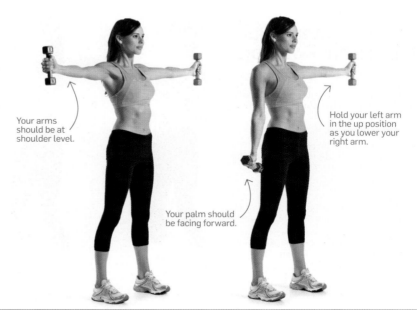

Your arms should be at shoulder level.

Hold your left arm in the up position as you lower your right arm.

Your palm should be facing forward.

VARIATION #2
Leaning Lateral Raise

- Hold a dumbbell in your left hand, at arm's length next to your side.
- Stand with your right leg next to a sturdy object such as a power rack.
- Place your left foot next to your right.
- Grab the power rack with your right hand, and allow your right arm to straighten so that you're leaning to your left.

- Without changing the bend in your elbow, raise your left arm straight out to your side until it's at shoulder level.
- Lower and repeat.
- Complete the prescribed number of repetitions with your left arm, then immediately do the same number with your right arm.

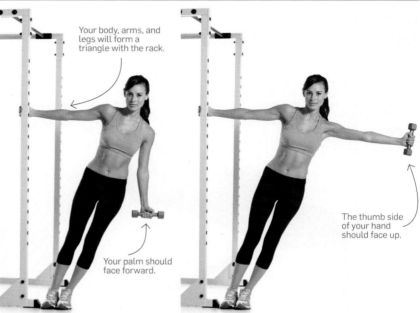

Your body, arms, and legs will form a triangle with the rack.

Your palm should face forward.

The thumb side of your hand should face up.

Shoulders | RAISES

Bent-Arm Lateral Raise and External Rotation

A

- Grab a pair of dumbbells and hold them at arm's length with your palms turned toward each other.
- Bend your elbows 90 degrees.
- Without changing the bend in your elbows, raise your upper arms out to the sides until they're parallel to the floor.

B

- Rotate your upper arms up and back so that your forearms are pointing toward the ceiling.
- Pause, then reverse the movement and return to the starting position.

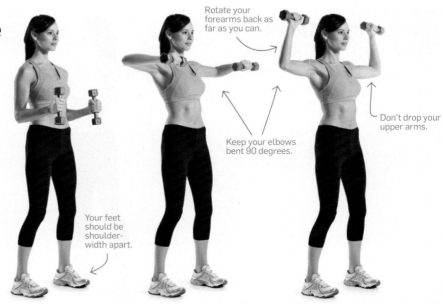

Rotate your forearms back as far as you can.

Don't drop your upper arms.

Keep your elbows bent 90 degrees.

Your feet should be shoulder-width apart.

Side-Lying Lateral Raise

A

- Grab a dumbbell in your right hand and lie on your left side on an incline bench that's set to 15 degrees.
- Hold the dumbbell next to your right side with your palm facing your thigh.

Your right elbow should be slightly bent.

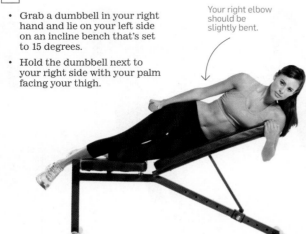

B

- Without changing the bend in your elbow, raise your arm until it's in line with your shoulder as you rotate your palm outward.
- Lower the weight and repeat.

Your arm should be perpendicular to your body.

Your palm should be facing forward.

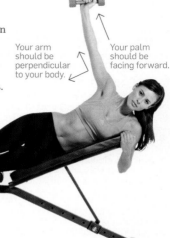

Combo Shoulder Raise

Since the combo shoulder raise is a combination of the front raise and the lateral raise, it targets both your front and middle deltoids.

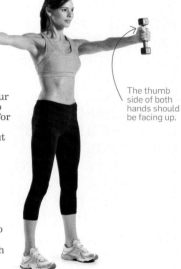

A

- Grab a pair of dumbbells and hold them at arm's length next to your thighs.
- Turn your left palm so that it's facing the side of your thigh, and your right palm so that it's facing forward.

Your right palm should be facing forward.

Your left palm should be facing your thigh.

B

- Simultaneously raise your right arm straight out to your side, as you would for a lateral raise, and lift your left arm straight out in front of you, as you would for a front raise.
- When both arms are at shoulder level, pause, and lower back to the starting position.
- On your next rep, rotate your arms so that you do a lateral raise with your left and a front raise with your right.

The thumb side of both hands should be facing up.

Scaption

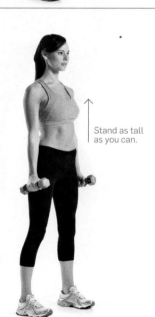

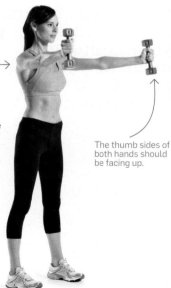

Your arms should form a horizontal Y shape.

A

- Standing with your feet shoulder-width apart, hold a pair of dumbbells at arm's length next to your sides.
- Your palms should be facing each other and your elbows slightly bent.

Stand as tall as you can.

B

- Without changing the bend in your elbows, raise your arms at a 30-degree angle to your body (so that they form a Y) until they're at shoulder level.
- Pause, then slowly lower the weights back to the starting position.

The thumb sides of both hands should be facing up.

Shoulders | SHRUGS

SHOULDER SHRUGS

Most of these exercises target your upper traps and levator scapulae. You work these muscles anytime you shrug your shoulders toward your ears. However, the last two exercises in this section target your serratus anterior. In these movements, you perform a "reverse shrug," pushing your shoulders down as you raise the rest of your body upward.

MAIN MOVE
Barbell Shrug

A

- Grab a barbell with an overhand grip that's just beyond shoulder-width apart, and let the bar hang at arm's length in front of your waist.

- Keeping your back naturally arched, lean forward at your hips.

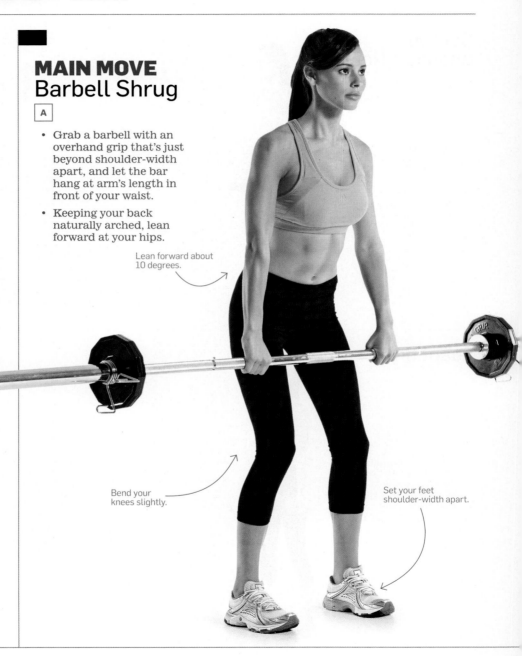

Lean forward about 10 degrees.

Bend your knees slightly.

Set your feet shoulder-width apart.

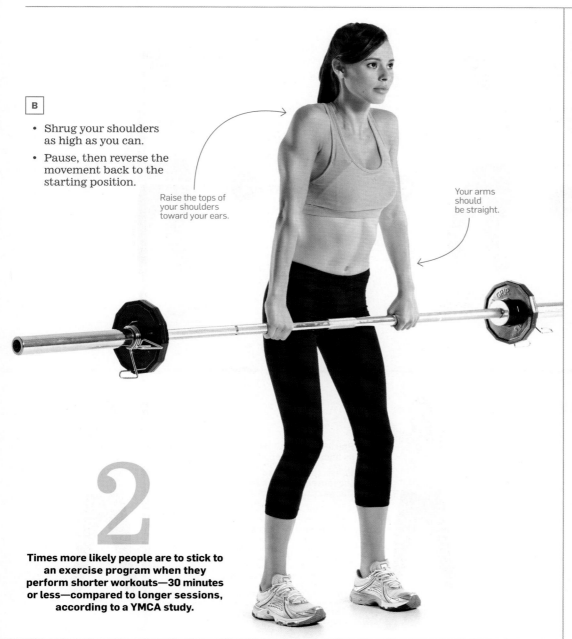

B

- Shrug your shoulders as high as you can.
- Pause, then reverse the movement back to the starting position.

Raise the tops of your shoulders toward your ears.

Your arms should be straight.

MUSCLE MISTAKE
You're Still Doing Upright Rows

Turns out, about two-thirds of people are at high risk for shoulder impingement when performing this popular upper-trap exercise. This is a painful condition in which the muscles or tendons of your rotator cuff become entrapped in your shoulder joint. Impingement most often occurs when your upper arms are simultaneously at shoulder level or higher and rotated inward—the exact position they're in at the top of the upright row.

2

Times more likely people are to stick to an exercise program when they perform shorter workouts—30 minutes or less—compared to longer sessions, according to a YMCA study.

Shoulders | SHRUGS

VARIATION #1
Wide-Grip Barbell Shrug

A

- Hold the barbell with an overhand grip that's about twice shoulder width.

Lean forward at your hips about 10 degrees.

B

- Shrug your shoulders as high as you can.

Using a wider grip increases the demand on your middle traps and rhomboids.

Keep your arms straight as you shrug.

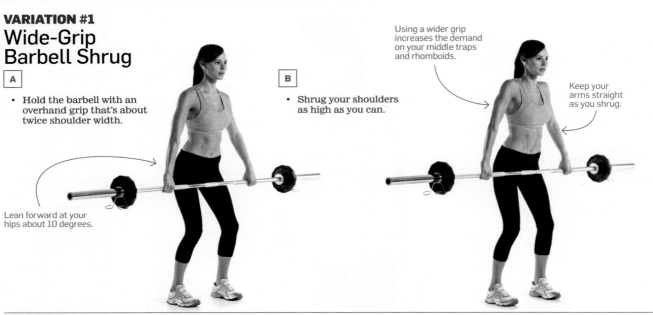

VARIATION #2
Overhead Barbell Shrug

A

- Hold a barbell above your head with an underhand grip that's about twice shoulder width.
- Your arms should be completely straight.

Lock your elbows and keep them that way.

Your feet should be shoulder-width apart.

B

- Shrug your shoulders as high as you can.
- Pause, then reverse the movement back to the starting position.

SHRUG FOR BALANCE
Holding the weight above your head as you shrug works your upper traps while reducing the emphasis on your levator scapulae. (The levator scapulae are frequently overused compared to the upper traps.) For many people, this can lead to better posture, since these muscles are often imbalanced.

Try to raise the tops of your shoulders as close to your ears as you can. The movement is slight; you'll feel it, but it's hard to see.

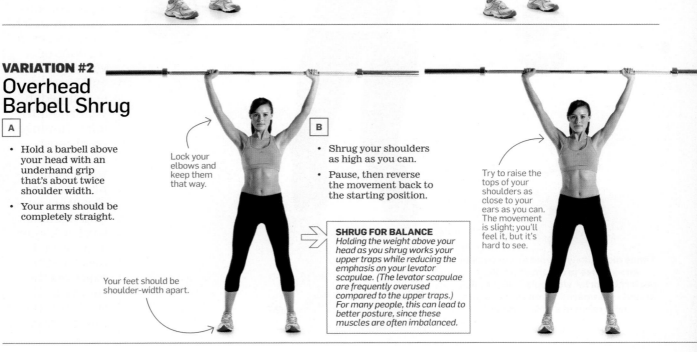

MAIN MOVE
Dumbbell Shrug

- Grab a pair of dumbbells and let them hang at arm's length next to your sides, your palms facing each other.

B

- Shrug your shoulders as high as you can.
- Pause in the up position, then slowly lower the dumbbells back to the start.

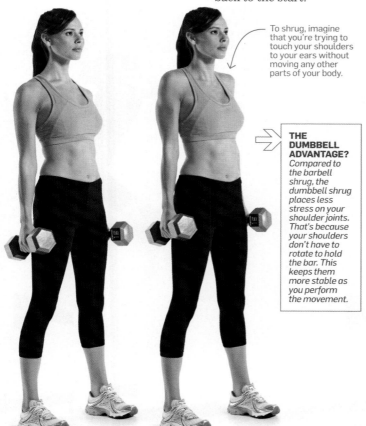

To shrug, imagine that you're trying to touch your shoulders to your ears without moving any other parts of your body.

THE DUMBBELL ADVANTAGE?
Compared to the barbell shrug, the dumbbell shrug places less stress on your shoulder joints. That's because your shoulders don't have to rotate to hold the bar. This keeps them more stable as you perform the movement.

VARIATION
Overhead Dumbbell Shrug

- Hold a pair of dumbbells straight above your shoulders, with your arms completely straight and your palms facing out.

- Shrug your shoulders as high as you can.
- Pause, then reverse the movement back to the starting position.

Keep your arms straight.

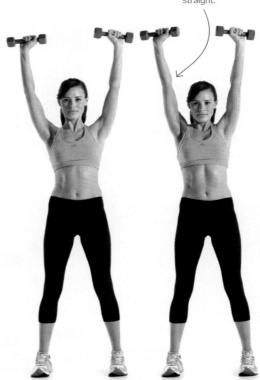

Shoulders | SHRUGS

MAIN MOVE
Serratus Shrug

Imagine that you're "shrugging" your shoulders down instead of up.

A

- Grab the bars of a dip station and lift yourself so your arms are fully extended.

- Bend your knees and cross your ankles behind you.

A MUSCLE YOU SHOULDN'T NEGLECT
As its name suggests, the serratus shrug targets your serratus anterior. Weakness in this muscle promotes poor posture and can also lead to shoulder impingement during shoulder presses. Use this "shrug" to make your serratus strong.

Keep your torso upright.

B

- Without changing your arm position, press your shoulders down as you lift your upper body.

- Pause for 5 seconds, then return to the starting position and repeat. That's one rep. As you progress, try to hold each repetition for a longer period of time.

Lock your elbows.

Let your torso sink between your shoulders.

Bend your knees.

Cross your ankles behind you.

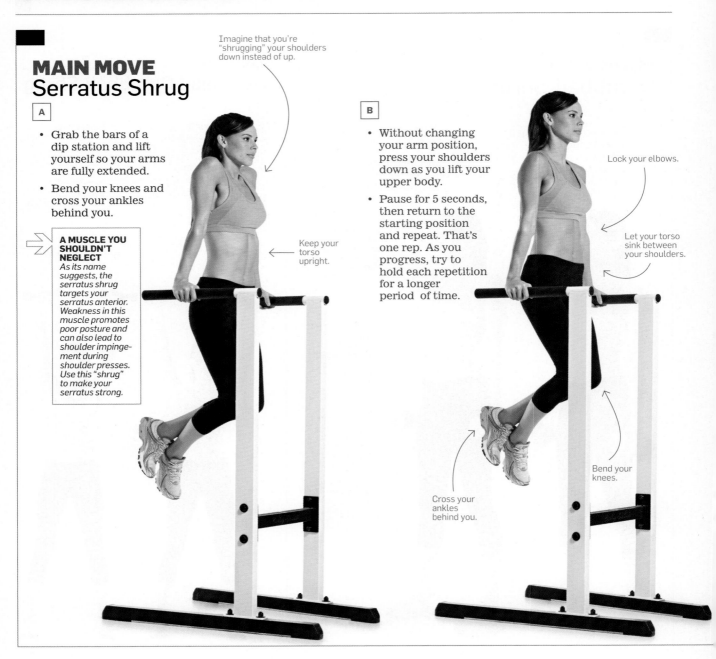

VARIATION

Serratus Chair Shrug

- Sit upright on a chair or bench and place your hands flat on the sitting surface next to your hips.
- Completely straighten your arms.

- Press your shoulders down as you lift your upper body.
- Pause for 5 seconds, then lower your body back to the starting position. That's one rep.

WORK YOUR SERRATUS ANYWHERE! *You can do this version of the exercise at your desk or even on your couch while watching TV.*

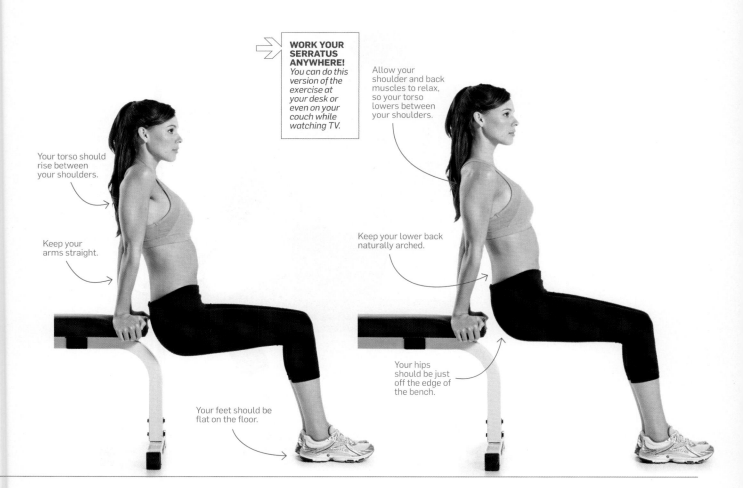

Your torso should rise between your shoulders.

Keep your arms straight.

Your feet should be flat on the floor.

Allow your shoulder and back muscles to relax, so your torso lowers between your shoulders.

Keep your lower back naturally arched.

Your hips should be just off the edge of the bench.

Shoulders | ROTATIONS

SHOULDER ROTATIONS
These exercises target your rotator cuff muscles, particularly your infraspinatus and teres minor.

MAIN MOVE
Seated Dumbbell External Rotation

A

- Grab a dumbbell in your left hand and sit on a bench.
- Place your left foot on the bench with your knee bent.
- Bend your left elbow 90 degrees and place the inside portion of it on your left knee.

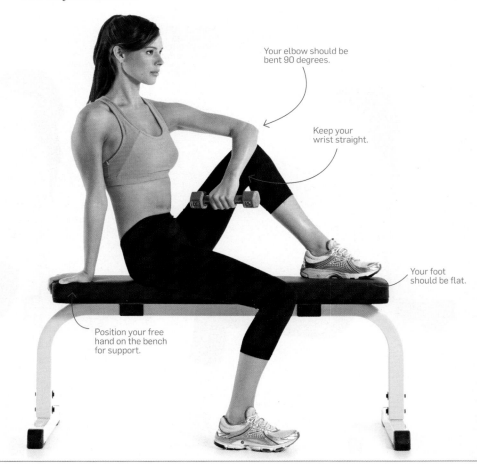

Your elbow should be bent 90 degrees.

Keep your wrist straight.

Your foot should be flat.

Position your free hand on the bench for support.

B

- Without changing the bend in your elbow, rotate your upper arm and forearm up and back as far as you can.
- Pause, then return to the starting position.
- Complete the prescribed number of repetitions with your left arm, then immediately do the same number with your right arm.

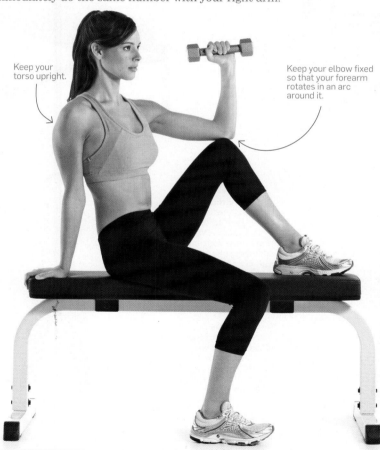

Keep your torso upright.

Keep your elbow fixed so that your forearm rotates in an arc around it.

Embrace External Rotation

External rotation is when you rotate your upper arms outward (or "externally"). For a visual, raise your arm as if you're about to give someone a high-five. Notice how your upper arm rotated outward? That's external rotation. And it's important because it targets the three rotator cuff muscles—your supraspinatus, infraspinatus, and teres minor—that attach to the outside of your upper arm. This helps create balance with your lats and pecs, which attach to the *inside* of your upper arm. If these muscles overpower your rotator cuff, they can permanently rotate your arms inward, causing caveman-like posture. External rotation is your exercise weapon against that.

Shoulders | ROTATIONS

VARIATION
Lying External Rotation

- Grab a dumbbell in your right hand and lie on your left side on an incline bench.
- Place a folded-up towel on the right side of your torso and then position your right elbow on the towel, with your arm bent 90 degrees.
- Let your forearm hang down in front of your abs.

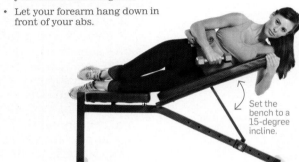

Set the bench to a 15-degree incline.

- Rotate your upper arm up and back as far as you can, without allowing your elbow to lose contact with the towel.
- Pause, then slowly lower the weight back to the starting position.
- Complete the prescribed number of repetitions with your right arm, then immediately lie on your right side and do the same number of reps with your left arm.

Your arm should be bent 90 degrees.

Keep your elbow fixed as you rotate your arm.

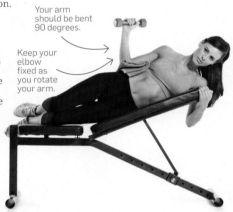

Dumbbell Diagonal Raise

- Grab a dumbbell in your right hand and hold it next to the outside of your left hip, your palm facing your hip.
- Your elbow should be slightly bent.

Your right palm should be in front of your pocket.

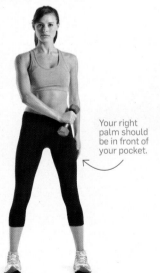

- Without changing the bend in your elbow, raise the dumbbell up and across your body until your hand is above your head and your palm is facing forward.
- Reverse the movement to return to the starting position.
- Complete the prescribed number of repetitions with your right arm, then immediately do the same number with your left arm.

Keep your elbow slightly bent.

Let your free arm hang at arm's length or place it on your hip.

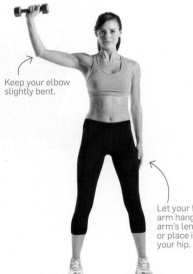

Cable Diagonal Raise

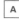

- Attach a stirrup handle to the low pulley of a cable station.
- Standing with your right side toward the weight stack, grab the handle with your left hand and position it in front of your right hip, with your elbow slightly bent.

- Without changing the bend in your elbow, pull the handle up and across your body until your hand is above your head.
- Lower the handle to the starting position.
- Complete the prescribed number of repetitions with your left arm, then immediately do the same number with your right arm.

Is a Shoulder Injury in Your Future?

Determine your risk with this test: Hold your arm so that your elbow is bent at a right angle and your upper arm is parallel to the floor, like you're giving a high-five. Without changing the position of your upper arm or moving your shoulder, rotate your forearm as far as you can forward and down and then reverse the movement in the other direction. You want to be able to rotate your forearm 180 degrees. If you fall short, use the sleeper stretch (page 143) to improve your flexibility.

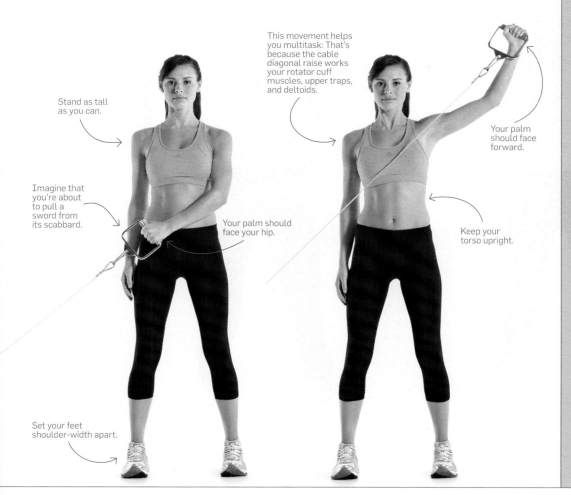

Stand as tall as you can.

Imagine that you're about to pull a sword from its scabbard.

Your palm should face your hip.

This movement helps you multitask: That's because the cable diagonal raise works your rotator cuff muscles, upper traps, and deltoids.

Your palm should face forward.

Keep your torso upright.

Set your feet shoulder-width apart.

Shoulders |

MAIN MOVE
Cable External Rotation

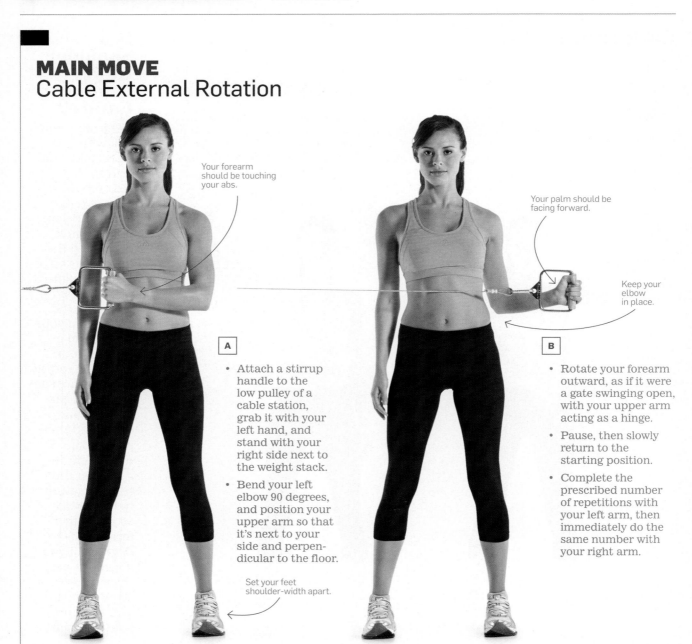

Your forearm should be touching your abs.

Your palm should be facing forward.

Keep your elbow in place.

Set your feet shoulder-width apart.

A
- Attach a stirrup handle to the low pulley of a cable station, grab it with your left hand, and stand with your right side next to the weight stack.
- Bend your left elbow 90 degrees, and position your upper arm so that it's next to your side and perpendicular to the floor.

B
- Rotate your forearm outward, as if it were a gate swinging open, with your upper arm acting as a hinge.
- Pause, then slowly return to the starting position.
- Complete the prescribed number of repetitions with your left arm, then immediately do the same number with your right arm.

VARIATION #1
45-Degree Cable External Rotation

A

- Stand at an angle to the weight stack.
- Hold your upper arm at a 45-degree angle to your body.

B

- Without changing the position of your upper arm, rotate your forearm up and back as far as you can.

Your upper arm should be at an angle between parallel to the floor and the side of your torso.

Don't raise or lower your elbow as you rotate your arm.

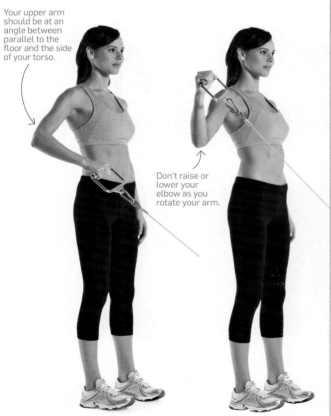

VARIATION #2
90-Degree Cable External Rotation

A

- Stand facing the weight stack.
- Hold your upper arm at a 90-degree angle to your body.

B

- Without changing the position of your upper arm, rotate your forearm up and back as far as you can.

Pull your shoulders down and hold them that way.

Keep your wrist straight.

Stand tall and straight.

Your palm should be facing behind you.

Your elbow should be bent 90 degrees.

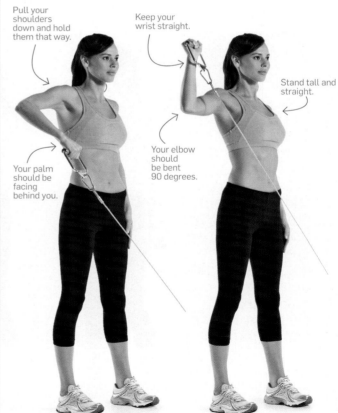

Shoulders

THE BEST SHOULDER EXERCISE YOU'VE NEVER DONE
Scaption and Shrug

This movement is the exercise that keeps on giving. That's because when you raise the dumbbells to perform scaption, you target your front deltoids, rotator cuff, and serratus anterior. Then comes the shrug. Like an overhead shrug, this version of the movement emphasizes your upper traps over your levator scapulae. This helps better balance the muscles that rotate your shoulder blades. The end result: Healthier shoulders and better posture.

A
- Stand holding a pair of dumbbells at arm's length next to your sides, your palms facing each other and your elbows slightly bent.

B
- Without changing the bend in your elbows, raise your arms at a 30-degree angle to your body (so that they form a "Y") until they're at shoulder level.

C
- At the top of the movement, shrug your shoulders upward.
- Pause, then slowly lower the weight back to the starting position.

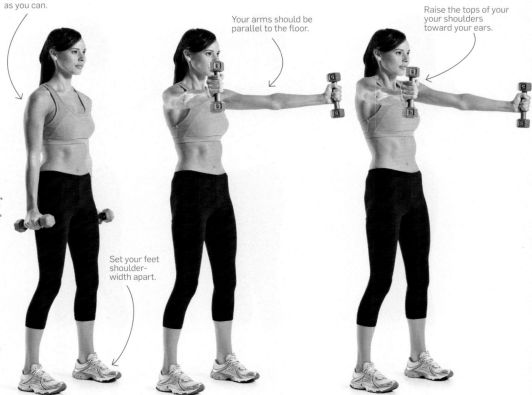

Stand as tall as you can.

Your arms should be parallel to the floor.

Raise the tops of your your shoulders toward your ears.

Set your feet shoulder-width apart.

THE BEST STRETCH FOR YOUR SHOULDERS
Sleeper Stretch

Why it's good:
It loosens your rotator cuff muscles. A stiff rotator cuff can lead to shoulder strain.

Make the most of it: Hold the stretch for 30 seconds, and repeat three times. Perform this routine two or three times a day to improve flexibility, or three times a week to maintain flexibility.

A

- Lie on the floor on your left side with your left upper arm on the floor and your elbow bent 90 degrees.
- Adjust your torso so that your right shoulder is slightly behind your left, not directly over it.
- Your left forearm should point toward the ceiling.

B

- Gently push your left hand toward the floor until you feel a comfortable stretch in the back of your left shoulder.
- Hold for the prescribed amount of time, then roll over and repeat the stretch for your right shoulder.

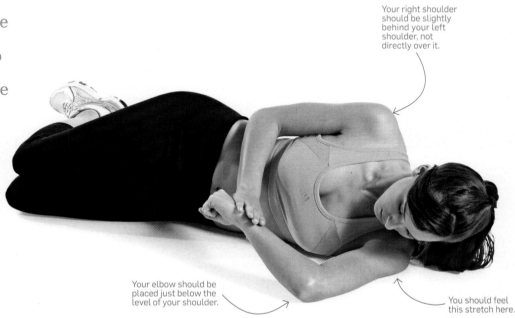

Your right shoulder should be slightly behind your left shoulder, not directly over it.

Your elbow should be placed just below the level of your shoulder.

You should feel this stretch here.

Shoulders

SCULPT PERFECT SHOULDERS

This 4-week total-body workout from Nick Tumminello, owner of Performance University in Baltimore, prioritizes your shoulders—to improve your posture and leave you looking great in a sleeveless top.

What to do: Do each Weight Workout (Workout A, Workout B, and Workout C) once a week, resting at least a day between each session. Perform each trio (1A, 1B, and 1C) or pair (2A, 2B) of exercises as a mini-circuit. That is, complete one set of each exercise in a succession, without resting. After you've done one set of each move, rest for the indicated amount of time, then repeat the circuit until you've finished all of the prescribed sets. Once you've done at least two or three sets (your choice) of exercises 1A, 1B, and 1C, move on to next group of exercises.

WORKOUT A

EXERCISE	SETS	REPS	REST
1A. Goblet squat (page 204)	2–3	15–20	0
1B. Dumbbell shoulder press (page 120)	2–3	10–15	0
1C. Thrusters (page 343)	2–3	10–15	1–2 min
2A. Single-leg hip raise (page 240)	1–2	15–20	0
2B. Swiss-ball Y-T-W-L raises (page 87–91)	1–2	10–12	1 min

WORKOUT B

EXERCISE	SETS	REPS	REST
1A. Incline pushup (page 38)	2–3	15–20	0
1B. (Incline) pushup plus (page 64)	2–3	15–20	0
1C. Plank (page 278)	2–3	20–40 sec hold	1–2 min
2A. Dumbbell side lunge (page 221)	1–2	10–15	0
2B. Seated dumbbell external rotation (page 136)	1–2	12–15	1 min

WORKOUT C

EXERCISE	SETS	REPS	REST
1A. Single-leg dumbbell straight-leg deadlift (page 257)	2–3	12–15	0
1B. Dumbbell row (page 78)	2–3	12–15	0
1C. Dumbbell alternating shoulder press and twist (page 123)	2–3	10–12	1–2 min
2A. Reverse dumbbell lunge (page 217)	1–2	10–15	0
2B. Side plank (page 284)	1–2	15–25 sec hold	1 min

Chapter 7: Arms
THE MUSCLES THAT GET YOU NOTICED

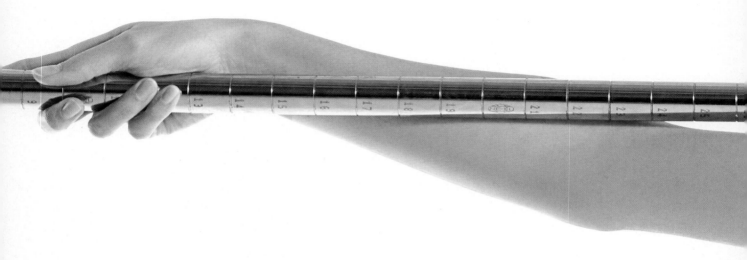

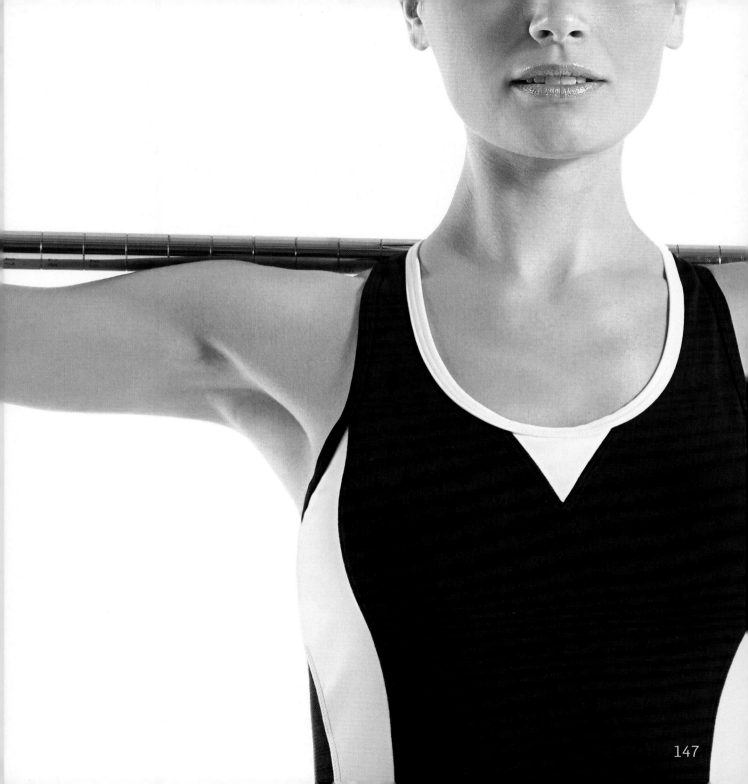

Arms

Your arms are like built-in publicists for all the hard work you do in the gym. That's because they're the only major muscles you can expose almost anywhere, anytime. If your biceps and triceps are well-defined, people will assume the rest of you is toned as well.

The best part is that a sculpted set of arms isn't as hard to achieve as you might think. The reason: Just about every upper-body exercise—whether it's for your chest, back, or shoulders—also involves your arms. After all, these exercises require that you use your arms to help move the weights. So work hard on your other upper-body muscles, and your arms will benefit by default. Then you can simply use the specific biceps, triceps, and forearm exercises in this chapter to give them a little extra love.

Bonus Benefits

Life is easier! Stronger biceps allow you to carry just about any object with less effort. So whether you're toting groceries or holding a baby, you'll notice the difference.

Damage control! Your triceps protect your elbow joints by acting as shock absorbers, lessening stress whenever your elbows are forced to flex suddenly, such as in breaking your fall if you trip or bracing yourself when biking a bumpy path.

Tighter muscle, everywhere! Your arms assist in exercises for all the muscles of your upper body. So if the smaller muscles of your arms give out too early, you'll be shortchanging the bigger muscles of your chest, back, and shoulders. Make sure your arms are strong, and you'll benefit all over.

Meet Your Muscles

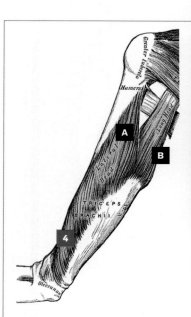

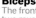

Biceps

The front of your upper arm owes its bulge to two muscle groups: your biceps brachii and your brachialis.

Your biceps brachii [1] originates at your shoulder and attaches to your forearm. Its duties are to bend your elbow and to rotate your forearm—a movement known as supination. Any type of arm curl works this muscle, as do chinups and rows.

Your brachialis [2] starts in the middle of your upper-arm bone and also attaches to your forearm. It assists your biceps brachii in bending your elbow.

The brachioradialis [3] originates on your upper-arm bone, near your elbow, and attaches close to your wrist. So it helps your biceps brachii bend your elbow and rotate your forearm, but it contributes little to the size of your biceps.

The biceps brachii is composed of two separate sections, or heads, that unite just before they attach to a forearm bone called the radius. The brachialis attaches to your ulna, the longer of the two forearm bones.

Triceps

The muscle on the back of your upper arm is called the triceps brachii [4]. When well-defined, it forms a horseshoe-like shape. Considering its name—triceps—it should be no surprise that the muscle is composed of three different sections, or heads. All three heads start on the back of either your upper arm or your shoulder blade, and then unite so that they attach together on your forearm. As a result, the primary job of your triceps is to straighten your arm. So this muscle is engaged in any exercise in which you straighten your arm against resistance: triceps extensions, triceps pressdowns and, of course, chest and shoulder presses.

The outer segment of your triceps is called the lateral head [A].

The middle segment of your triceps is called the medial head (not shown; hidden by the lateral head).

The inner segment of your triceps is called the long head [B].

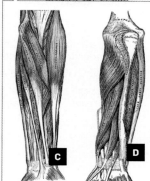

Forearms

Your wrist and finger flexors [C] are located on the inside of your forearm. They allow you to bend your wrist forward, and they can be trained with exercises such as wrist curls.

Your wrist extensors [D] are located on the outside, or "top," of your forearm. They allow you to bend your wrist backward, and they can be trained with exercises such as wrist extensions.

Biceps | ARM CURLS

In this chapter, you'll find 74 exercises that target the muscles of your arms. These exercises are divided among three major sections: Biceps, Triceps, and Forearms. Within each section, you'll notice that certain exercises have been given the designation Main Move. Master this basic version of a movement, and you'll be able to do all of its variations with flawless form.

ARM CURLS

These exercises target your biceps brachii, brachialis, and brachioradialis. Your upper-back and rear-shoulder muscles also come into play, since they keep your shoulders stable as you curl a weight in front of your body.

MAIN MOVE
EZ-Bar Curl

- Grab an EZ-curl bar with an underhand, shoulder-width grip.
- Your palms should angle inward.
- Let the bar hang at arm's length in front of your waist.

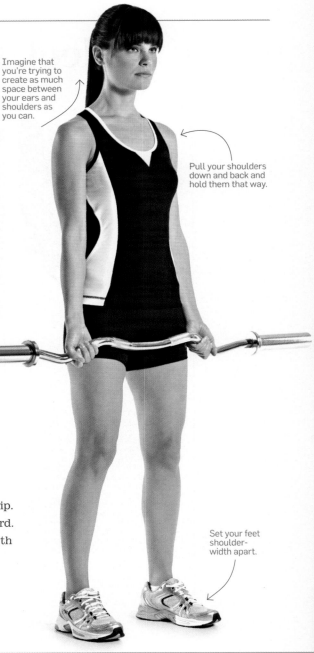

Imagine that you're trying to create as much space between your ears and shoulders as you can.

Pull your shoulders down and back and hold them that way.

Set your feet shoulder-width apart.

2.5

Times more strength lifters gained when lowering a weight slowly and lifting it fast compared to performing each rep at a slow speed from start to finish, according to a George Washington University study.

Keep your chest up.

Stand as tall as you can for the entire exercise.

B

- Without moving your upper arms, bend your elbows and curl the bar as close to your shoulders as you can.

- Pause, then slowly lower the weight back to the starting position.

- Each time you return to the starting position, completely straighten your arms.

HOW DO YOU MEASURE UP?

No, you probably don't want bigger arms. But if you're overweight, measuring their circumference can be a useful way to track your total-body fat loss efforts and stay motivated. That's because as you lose flab, your arms will shrink and start to look more toned. For the most accurate results, take your measurements before breakfast and exercising. Extend your arm straight in front of you and wrap a measuring tape around the largest portion of your upper arm. Record the circumference, then measure your other arm.

Biceps | ARM CURLS

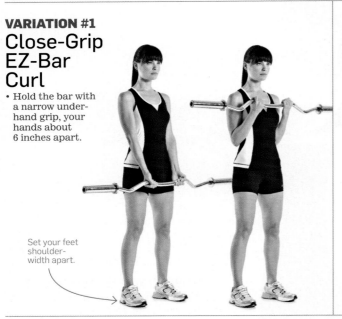

VARIATION #1
Close-Grip EZ-Bar Curl

- Hold the bar with a narrow underhand grip, your hands about 6 inches apart.

Set your feet shoulder-width apart.

VARIATION #2
Wide-Grip EZ-Bar Curl

- Hold the bar with an underhand grip that's about 1½ times shoulder width.

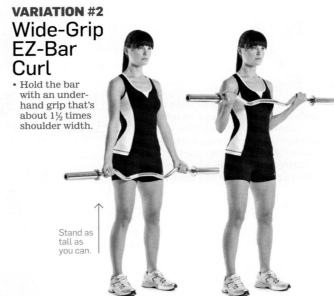

Stand as tall as you can.

VARIATION #3
Swiss-Ball Preacher Curl

A

- Kneel over a Swiss ball and rest your upper arms on it.
- Hold the bar with a narrow underhand grip, your elbows bent about 5 degrees.

Your elbows should be slightly bent.

B

- Without moving your upper arms off the ball, curl the weight toward your shoulders.

Your lower back should be naturally arched.

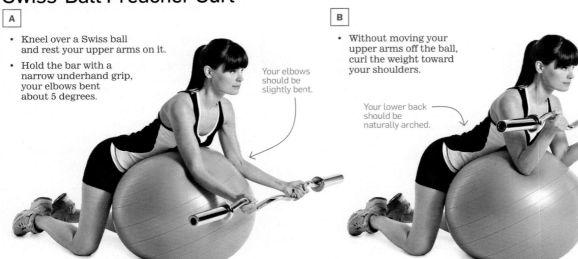

VARIATION #4
EZ-Bar Preacher Curl
- Rest your upper arms on the sloping pad of a preacher bench and hold the bar in front of you, your elbows bent about 5 degrees.
- Without moving your upper arms, bend your elbows and curl the bar toward your shoulders.

Your hands should be about 6 inches apart.

Keep your upper arms on the pad.

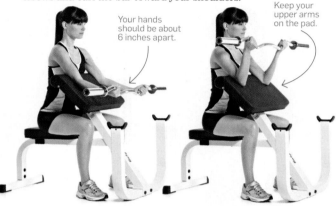

VARIATION #5
Reverse EZ-Bar Curl
- Hold the bar with an overhand, shoulder-width grip.

Your palms should be angled toward each other facing your thighs.

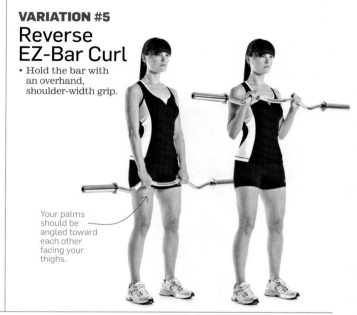

VARIATION #6
Telle Curl

Stand tall and straight.

Hold your upper and lower arms in place when you bend over.

Your elbows should be bent about 90 degrees.

Keep your lower back naturally arched.

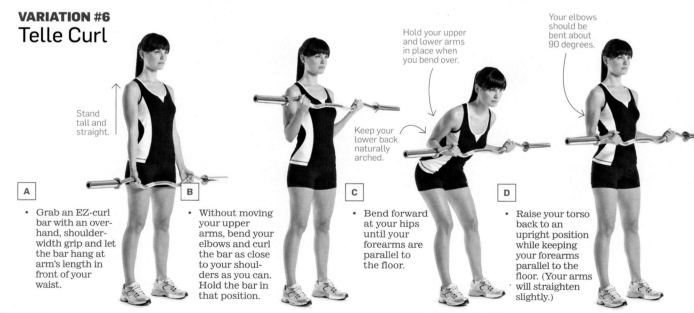

A
- Grab an EZ-curl bar with an overhand, shoulder-width grip and let the bar hang at arm's length in front of your waist.

B
- Without moving your upper arms, bend your elbows and curl the bar as close to your shoulders as you can. Hold the bar in that position.

C
- Bend forward at your hips until your forearms are parallel to the floor.

D
- Raise your torso back to an upright position while keeping your forearms parallel to the floor. (Your arms will straighten slightly.)

Biceps | ARM CURLS

MAIN MOVE
Standing Dumbbell Curl

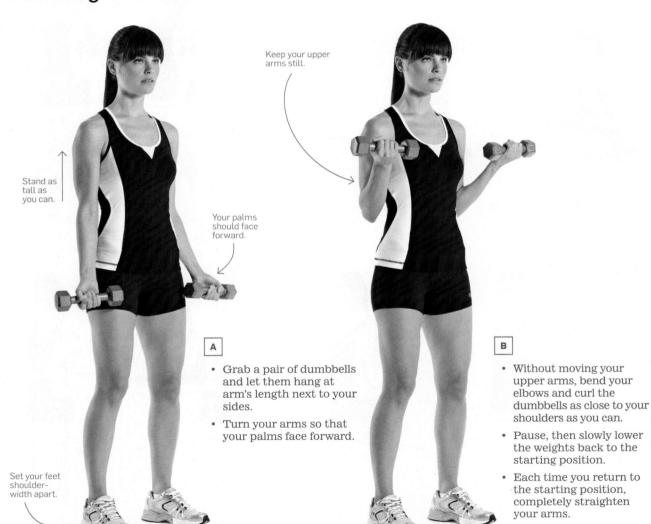

Keep your upper arms still.

Stand as tall as you can.

Your palms should face forward.

Set your feet shoulder-width apart.

A

- Grab a pair of dumbbells and let them hang at arm's length next to your sides.
- Turn your arms so that your palms face forward.

B

- Without moving your upper arms, bend your elbows and curl the dumbbells as close to your shoulders as you can.
- Pause, then slowly lower the weights back to the starting position.
- Each time you return to the starting position, completely straighten your arms.

VARIATION #1

Twisting Standing Dumbbell Curl

Besides using this method while standing, you can also use the twisting technique with any of the other body positions listed on the next page.

Your arms should be straight.

Don't move your upper arms.

Your palms should be facing each other.

Keep your chest up.

Your palms should be facing your shoulders.

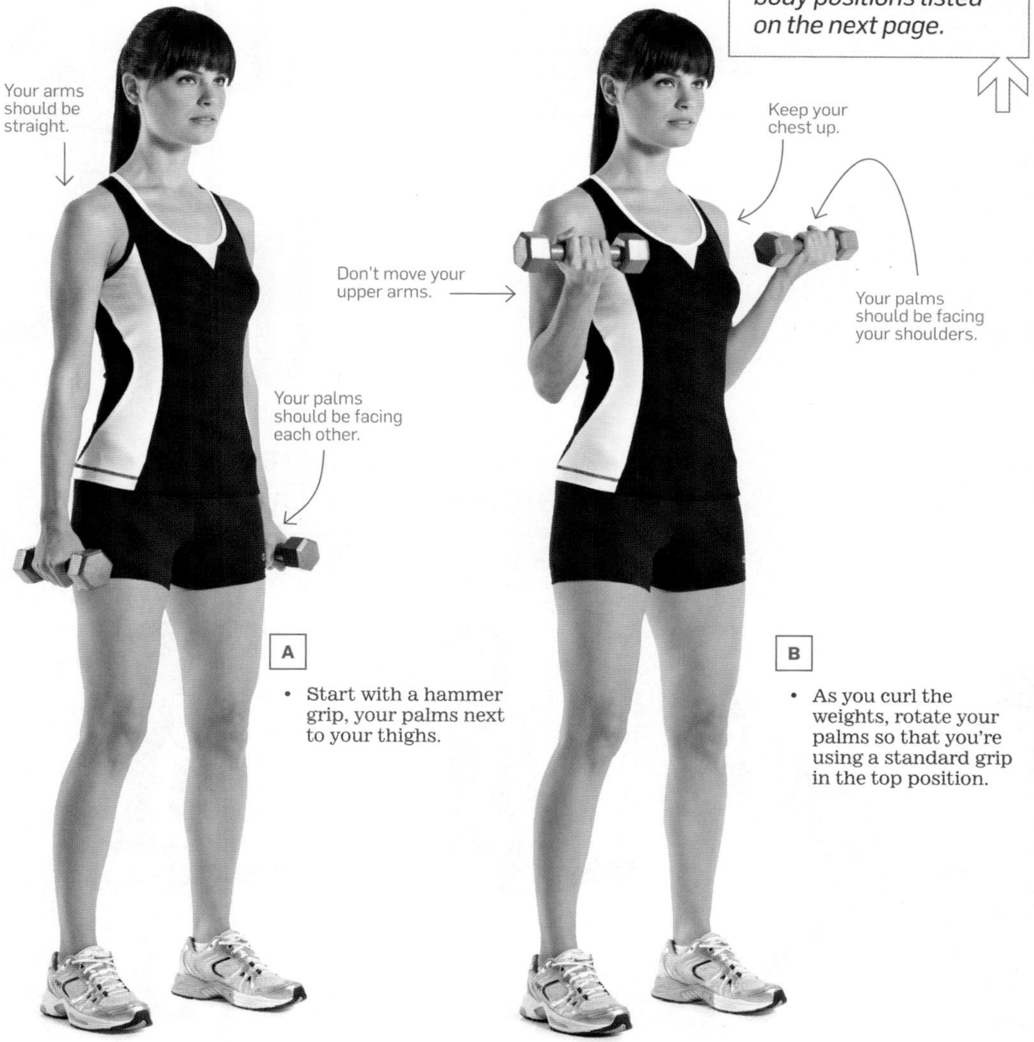

A

- Start with a hammer grip, your palms next to your thighs.

B

- As you curl the weights, rotate your palms so that you're using a standard grip in the top position.

More Ways to Curl!

Instead of curling both dumbbells at once, lift them one at a time, in an alternating fashion. Simply raise and lower one dumbbell, then repeat with the other. You may be able to do more reps this way since one arm rests each time the other curls the dumbbell. So your biceps won't fatigue as fast. Another approach for variety: Simultaneously raise one dumbbell as you lower the other. You can use these techniques with any of the body positions and grips listed on the next page, as well as just about any other curl.

Biceps | ARM CURLS

VARIATIONS #2-25

Mix and match any of five grips with any of five body positions for 25 different versions of this biceps exercise. Here, you'll see five examples of how the grips and body positions can be paired. But vary the combos frequently for best results.

BODY POSITION #1: INCLINE
Incline Offset-Thumb Dumbbell Curl

- Lie faceup on a bench that's set to a 45-degree incline.

- Lying on an incline causes your arms to hang behind your body, which emphasizes the long head of your biceps brachii to a greater degree.

Use an offset-thumb grip.

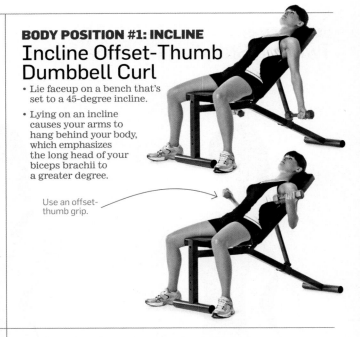

BODY POSITION #2: DECLINE
Decline Hammer Curl

- Lie with your chest against a bench that's set to a 45-degree incline.

- This position causes your arms to hang in front of your body, placing more emphasis on your brachialis.

Don't move your upper arms.

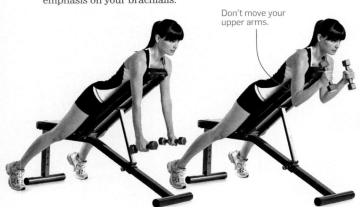

BODY POSITION #3: SEATED
Seated Reverse Dumbbell Curl

- Sit tall on a bench or Swiss ball.

- Performing the exercise in a seated position may make you less likely to rock your torso back and forth—or "cheat"—as you curl the weights.

Keep your chest up and your shoulders pulled down and back.

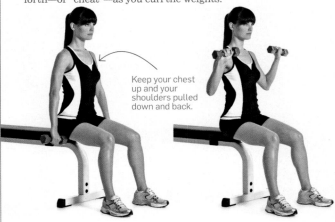

BODY POSITION #4: STANDING

Standing Dumbbell Curl

- Stand with your feet shoulder-width apart. (For complete instructions, see the standing dumbbell curl, also listed as the Main Move on page 154.)

- Anytime you're standing, you engage more core muscles than when you're sitting.

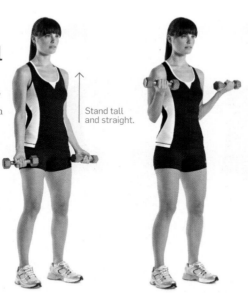

Stand tall and straight.

BODY POSITION #5: SPLIT STANCE

Split-Stance Offset-Pinky Dumbbell Curl

- Place one foot in front of you on a bench or step that's just higher than knee level.

- Putting one foot on a bench forces your hip and core muscles to work harder in order to keep your body stable.

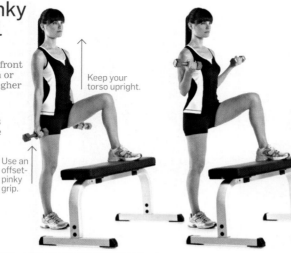

Keep your torso upright.

Use an offset-pinky grip.

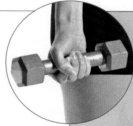

Standard Grip
Your palms face forward, and you grip the handle in the middle.

This is the default dumbbell curl grip.

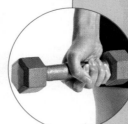

Offset-Pinky Grip
Your palms face forward, and each pinky finger touches the inside head of a dumbbell.

This shifts the way the weight is distributed, providing more variety.

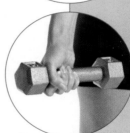

Offset-Thumb Grip
Your palms face forward, and each thumb touches the outside head of a dumbbell.

This forces your biceps brachii to work harder to keep your forearm rotated outward as you curl the weight.

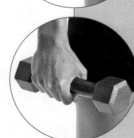

Hammer Grip
Your palms face each other.

This causes your brachialis muscle to work harder for the entire movement.

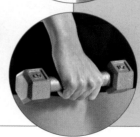

Reverse Grip
Your palms face behind you.

This exercise targets your brachioradialis but decreases the activity of your biceps brachii. You'll really feel it in your forearms.

Biceps | ARM CURLS

VARIATION #26
Standing Zottman Curl

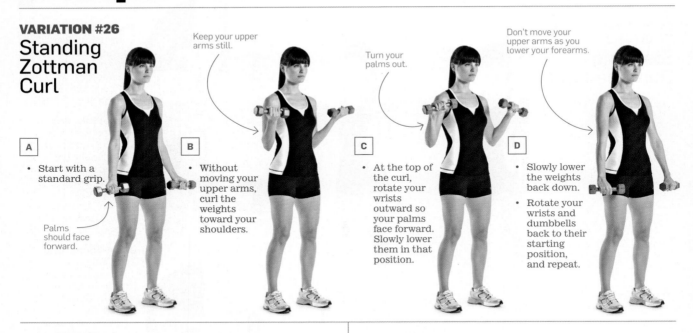

Keep your upper arms still.

Turn your palms out.

Don't move your upper arms as you lower your forearms.

A

- Start with a standard grip.

Palms should face forward.

B

- Without moving your upper arms, curl the weights toward your shoulders.

C

- At the top of the curl, rotate your wrists outward so your palms face forward. Slowly lower them in that position.

D

- Slowly lower the weights back down.
- Rotate your wrists and dumbbells back to their starting position, and repeat.

VARIATION #27
Static Curl

- Grab a dumbbell with your right hand and stand behind a raised incline bench.
- Place the back of your upper arm across the top of the bench.
- Lower the dumbbell until your arm is bent about 20 degrees.
- Hold that position for 40 seconds to build more muscle, or hold for 6 to 8 seconds for greater gains in strength. Then repeat with your left arm. That's one set.

The mid-part of your upper arm should be the only part touching the bench.

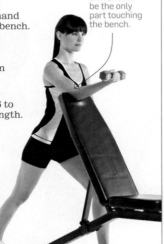

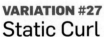
PICK THE RIGHT WEIGHT
Choose the heaviest dumbbell that allows you to hold for the length of time that matches your goal. So if you're building strength, you'll use a heavier weight than if you're focusing on faster muscle growth.

VARIATION #28
Dumbbell Curl with Static Hold

A

- Grab a pair of dumbbells and let them hang at arm's length next to your sides, your palms facing forward.
- Raise your left forearm so your elbow is bent 90 degrees and hold it there.

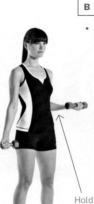

B

- Perform a set of dumbbell curls with your right arm. After you've finished all your reps, switch arms, performing the static hold with your right arm and curling with your left.

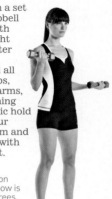

Hold the position where your elbow is bent at 90 degrees.

VARIATION #29
Hammer Curl to Press

A

- Let the dumbbells hang at arm's length at your sides, your palms facing each other.

Stand as tall as you can.

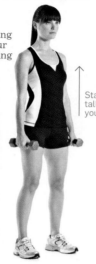

B

- Curl the dumbbells toward your shoulders.

Keep your upper arms still.

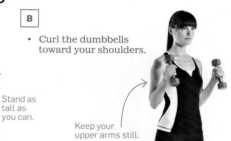

C

- Press the dumbbells above your head until your arms are straight.

The dumbbells should be directly over your shoulders.

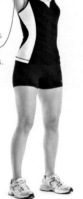

VARIATION #30
Split-Stance Hammer Curl to Press

A

- Stand tall, with one foot in front of you and placed on a bench or step that's just higher than knee level.
- Let the dumbbells hang at arm's length at your sides, your palms facing each other.

Brace your core.

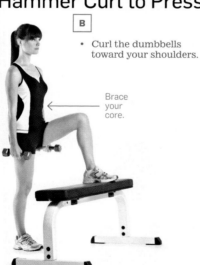

B

- Curl the dumbbells toward your shoulders.

C

- Press the dumbbells above your head until your arms are straight.

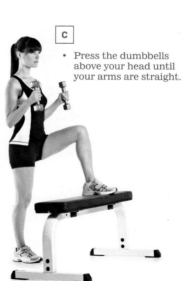

Your torso should be upright.

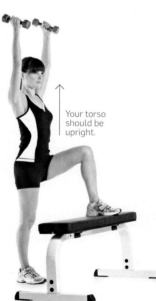

Biceps | ARM CURLS

Cable Alternating Flex Curl

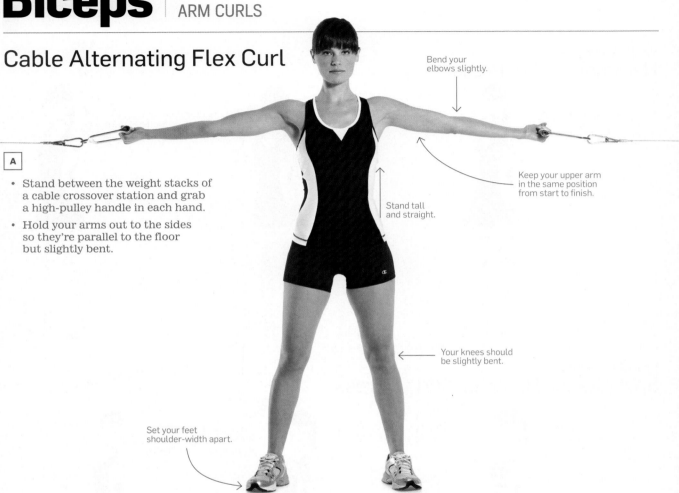

Bend your elbows slightly.

A

- Stand between the weight stacks of a cable crossover station and grab a high-pulley handle in each hand.
- Hold your arms out to the sides so they're parallel to the floor but slightly bent.

Keep your upper arm in the same position from start to finish.

Stand tall and straight.

Your knees should be slightly bent.

Set your feet shoulder-width apart.

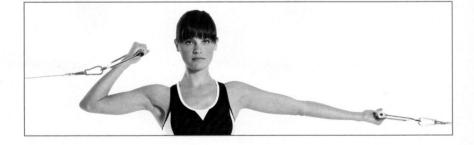

B

- Without moving your left arm, curl your right hand toward your head.
- Slowly allow your right arm to straighten, then repeat the move with your left arm.

Cable Curl

 A

- Attach a straight bar to the low pulley of a cable station.
- Grab the bar with a shoulder-width, underhand grip and hold it at arm's length.

 B

- Without allowing your upper arms to move, curl the bar as close to your chest as you can.
- Pause, then lower back to the starting position.

Cable Hammer Curl

 A

- Attach a rope to a low-pulley cable and stand 1 to 2 feet in front of the weight stack.
- Grab an end of the rope in each hand, your palms facing each other.

 B

- With your elbows tucked at your sides, slowly curl your fists up toward your shoulders.
- Pause, then lower back to the starting position.

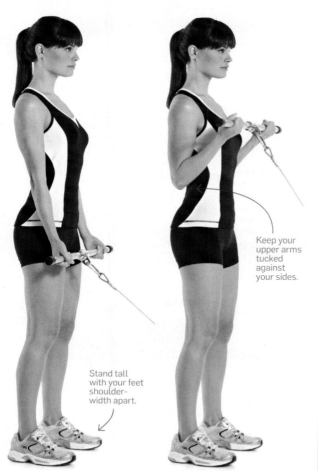

Keep your upper arms tucked against your sides.

Stand tall with your feet shoulder-width apart.

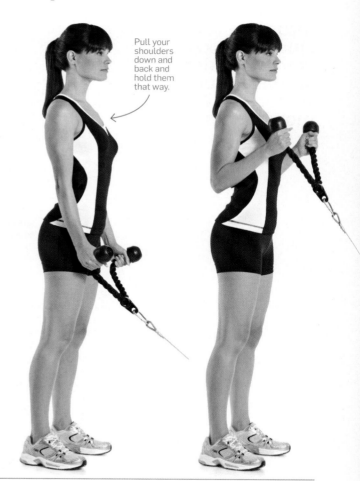

Pull your shoulders down and back and hold them that way.

Triceps |

ARM EXTENSIONS

These exercises target your triceps brachii. Your upper-back and rear-shoulder muscles come into play, too, since they keep your shoulders stable as you perform the movements.

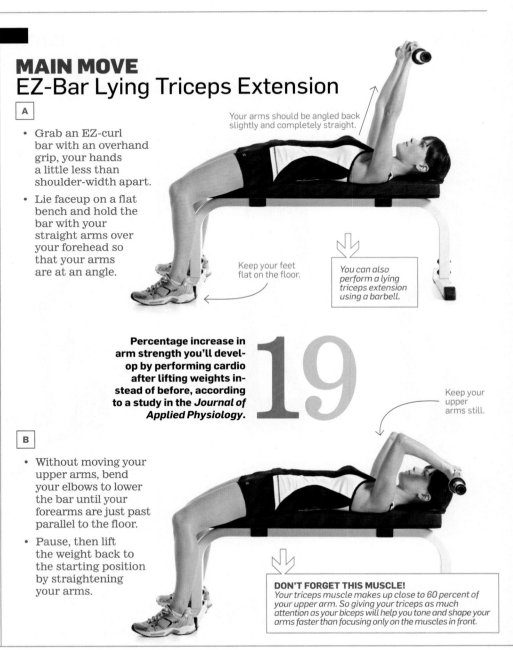

MAIN MOVE
EZ-Bar Lying Triceps Extension

A

- Grab an EZ-curl bar with an overhand grip, your hands a little less than shoulder-width apart.

- Lie faceup on a flat bench and hold the bar with your straight arms over your forehead so that your arms are at an angle.

Your arms should be angled back slightly and completely straight.

Keep your feet flat on the floor.

You can also perform a lying triceps extension using a barbell.

Percentage increase in arm strength you'll develop by performing cardio after lifting weights instead of before, according to a study in the *Journal of Applied Physiology*.

19

B

- Without moving your upper arms, bend your elbows to lower the bar until your forearms are just past parallel to the floor.

- Pause, then lift the weight back to the starting position by straightening your arms.

Keep your upper arms still.

DON'T FORGET THIS MUSCLE!
Your triceps muscle makes up close to 60 percent of your upper arm. So giving your triceps as much attention as your biceps will help you tone and shape your arms faster than focusing only on the muscles in front.

VARIATION #1
Incline EZ-Bar Lying Triceps Extension

- Instead of lying on a flat bench, perform the movement on an incline bench. Set the backrest to a 30-degree angle.

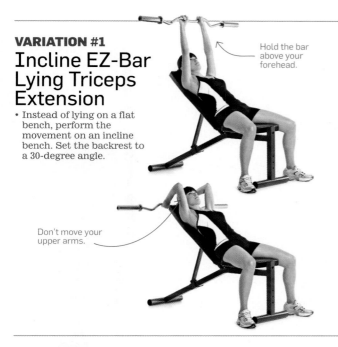

Hold the bar above your forehead.

Don't move your upper arms.

VARIATION #2
Swiss-Ball EZ-Bar Lying Triceps Extension

- Instead of lying on a flat bench, perform the movement while lying with your middle and upper back placed firmly on a Swiss ball. Raise your hips so that your body forms a straight line from your knees to your shoulders.

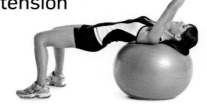

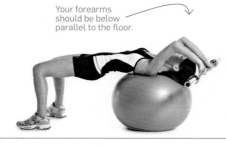

Your forearms should be below parallel to the floor.

VARIATION #3
Static Lying Triceps Extension

- Lower the bar until your elbows are bent 90 degrees.

- Hold that position for 40 seconds to build more muscle, or hold for 6 to 8 seconds for greater gains in strength. That's one set.

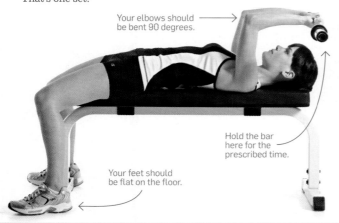

Your elbows should be bent 90 degrees.

Hold the bar here for the prescribed time.

Your feet should be flat on the floor.

VARIATION #4
Lying Triceps Extension to Close-Grip Bench Press

- Start by doing an EZ-bar lying triceps extension, performing as many reps as you can until you start to struggle. Then, without changing the position of your hands, immediately switch to a bench press. Complete as many reps as you can with perfect form.

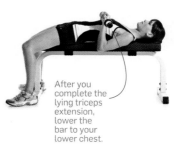

After you complete the lying triceps extension, lower the bar to your lower chest.

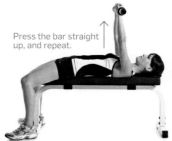

Press the bar straight up, and repeat.

MAIN MOVE
EZ-Bar Overhead Triceps Extension

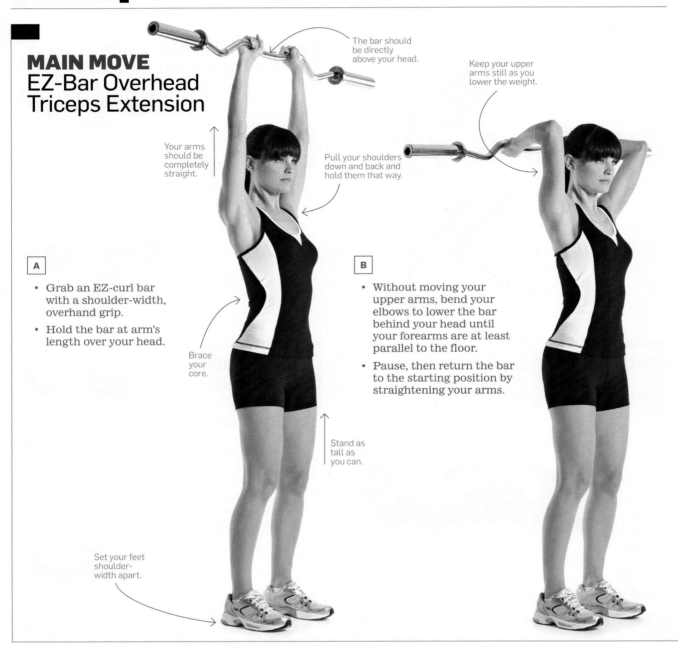

The bar should be directly above your head.

Keep your upper arms still as you lower the weight.

Your arms should be completely straight.

Pull your shoulders down and back and hold them that way.

A

- Grab an EZ-curl bar with a shoulder-width, overhand grip.
- Hold the bar at arm's length over your head.

Brace your core.

Stand as tall as you can.

Set your feet shoulder-width apart.

B

- Without moving your upper arms, bend your elbows to lower the bar behind your head until your forearms are at least parallel to the floor.
- Pause, then return the bar to the starting position by straightening your arms.

VARIATION #1
Seated EZ-Bar Overhead Triceps Extension

A

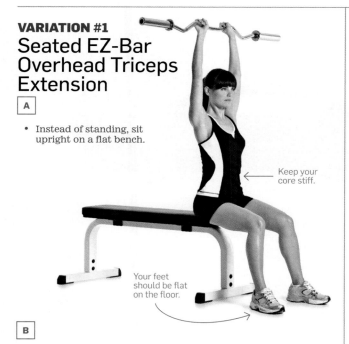

- Instead of standing, sit upright on a flat bench.

Keep your core stiff.

Your feet should be flat on the floor.

B

- Without moving your upper arms, bend your elbows and lower the bar.

Your forearms should be at least parallel to the floor.

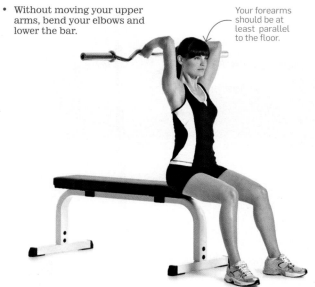

VARIATION #2
Swiss-Ball EZ-Bar Overhead Triceps Extension

A

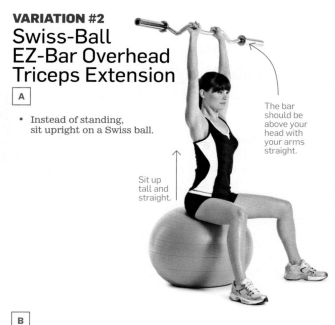

- Instead of standing, sit upright on a Swiss ball.

The bar should be above your head with your arms straight.

Sit up tall and straight.

B

- Keep your upper arms still, bend your elbows, and lower the bar until your forearms are at least parallel to the floor.

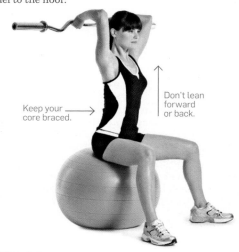

Keep your core braced.

Don't lean forward or back.

Triceps | ARM EXTENSIONS

MAIN MOVE
Dumbbell Lying Triceps Extension

A

- Grab a pair of dumbbells and lie faceup on a flat bench.
- Hold the dumbbells over your head with straight arms, your palms facing each other.

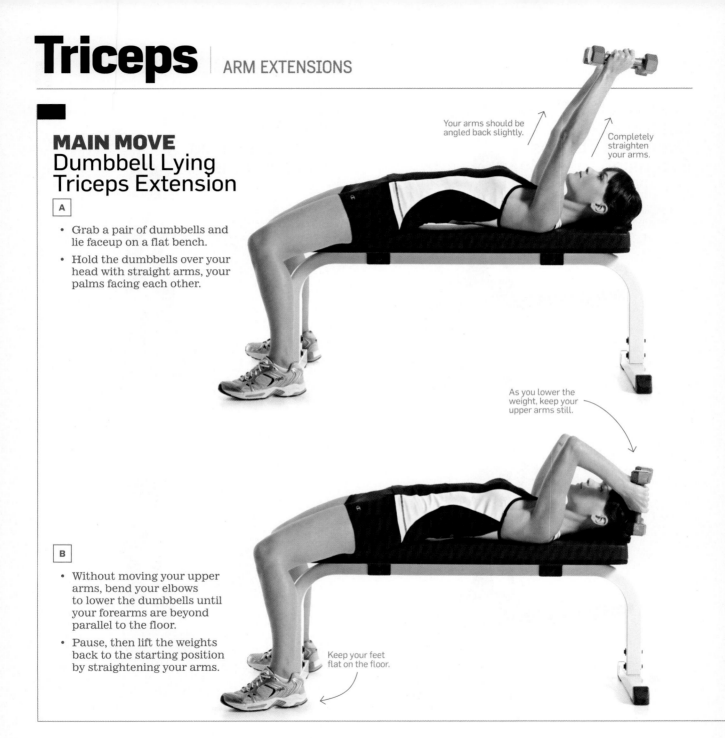

Your arms should be angled back slightly.

Completely straighten your arms.

As you lower the weight, keep your upper arms still.

B

- Without moving your upper arms, bend your elbows to lower the dumbbells until your forearms are beyond parallel to the floor.
- Pause, then lift the weights back to the starting position by straightening your arms.

Keep your feet flat on the floor.

VARIATION #1
Alternating Dumbbell Lying Triceps Extension

- Grab a pair of dumbbells and lie on your back on a flat bench, with your palms facing each other and your arms straight.

- Instead of lowering both dumbbells at once, lower them one at a time, in an alternating fashion.

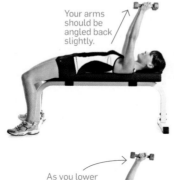
Your arms should be angled back slightly.

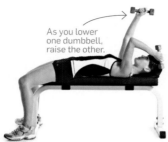
As you lower one dumbbell, raise the other.

VARIATION #2
Swiss-Ball Dumbbell Lying Triceps Extension

- Instead of lying on a flat bench, perform the movement with your middle and upper back placed firmly on a Swiss ball, and raise your hips so they're in line with your torso.

- Without moving your upper arms, bend your elbows to lower the dumbbells until your forearms are beyond parallel to the floor.

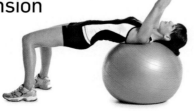

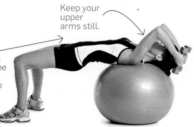

Keep your upper arms still.

Your body should form a straight line from your shoulders to your knees.

VARIATION #3
Lying Dumbbell Pullover to Extension

A

- Grab a pair of dumbbells and lie faceup on a flat bench.

- Hold the dumbbells directly over your shoulders.

- Your palms should be facing each other.

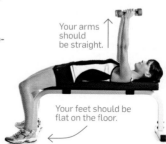
Your arms should be straight.

Your feet should be flat on the floor.

B

- Without moving your upper arms, bend your elbows to lower the dumbbells until your forearms are parallel to the floor.

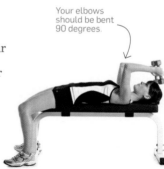
Your elbows should be bent 90 degrees.

C

- Without changing the bend in your elbows, lower the dumbbells back beyond your head as far as you comfortably can.

- Pause, then reverse through each phase of the movement, back to the starting position.

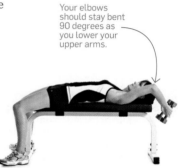
Your elbows should stay bent 90 degrees as you lower your upper arms.

Triceps | ARM EXTENSIONS

MAIN MOVE
Dumbbell Overhead Triceps Extension

Your arms should be completely straight.

Your forearms should be at least parallel to the floor.

Don't move your upper arms.

Brace your core.

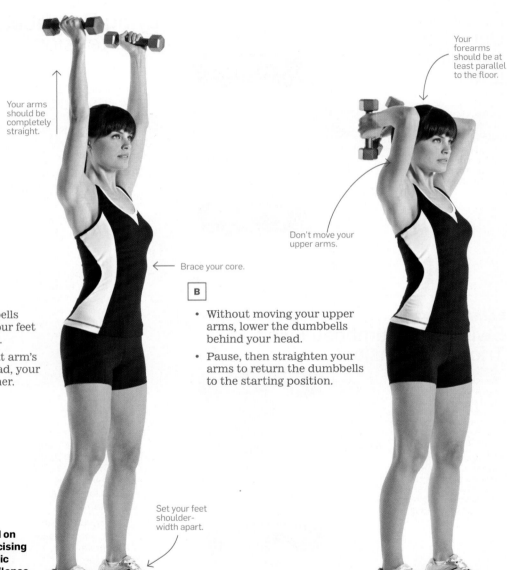

A

- Grab a pair of dumbbells and stand tall with your feet shoulder-width apart.
- Hold the dumbbells at arm's length above your head, your palms facing each other.

B

- Without moving your upper arms, lower the dumbbells behind your head.
- Pause, then straighten your arms to return the dumbbells to the starting position.

Set your feet shoulder-width apart.

2

Times better people did on cognitive tests after exercising while listening to music compared to sweating in silence, according to an Ohio State University study.

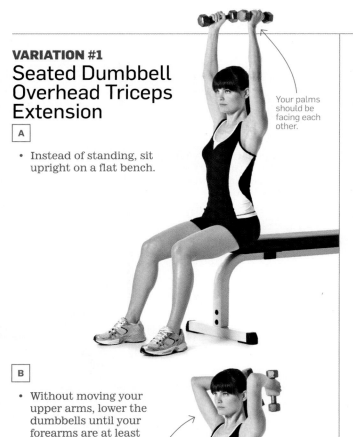

VARIATION #1
Seated Dumbbell Overhead Triceps Extension

A

- Instead of standing, sit upright on a flat bench.

Your palms should be facing each other.

B

- Without moving your upper arms, lower the dumbbells until your forearms are at least parallel to the floor.

Your upper arms shouldn't move as you lower the weight.

VARIATION #2
Swiss-Ball Dumbbell Overhead Triceps Extension

- Instead of standing, sit upright on a Swiss ball.
- Without moving your upper arms, lower the dumbbells until your forearms are at least parallel to the floor.
- Pause, then straighten your arms to return the dumbbells to the starting position.

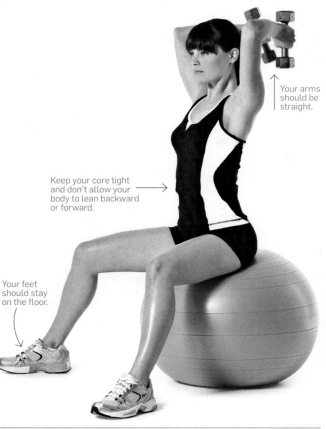

Your arms should be straight.

Keep your core tight and don't allow your body to lean backward or forward.

Your feet should stay on the floor.

Triceps | ARM EXTENSIONS

Cable Overhead Triceps Extension

A

- Attach a rope handle to the high pulley of a cable station.
- Grab the rope and stand with your back to the weight stack.
- Stand in a staggered stance, one foot in front of the other.
- Bend at your hips until your torso is nearly parallel to the floor.
- Hold an end of the rope in each hand behind your head, with your elbows bent 90 degrees.

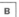

B

- Without moving your upper arms, push your forearms forward until your elbows are locked.
- Pause, then return to the starting position.

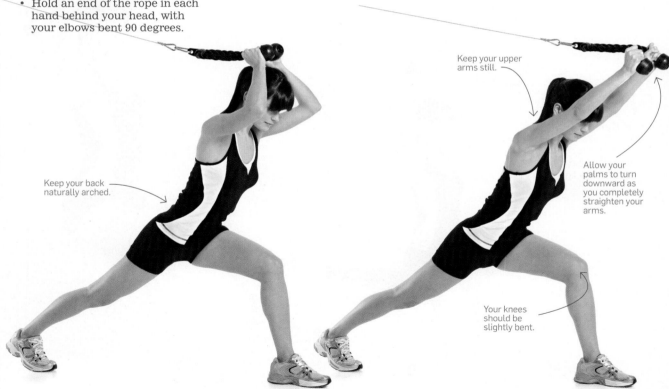

Keep your back naturally arched.

Keep your upper arms still.

Allow your palms to turn downward as you completely straighten your arms.

Your knees should be slightly bent.

MAIN MOVE
Triceps Pressdown

TRAINER'S TIP
If you use too much weight in the triceps pressdown, you'll involve your back and shoulder muscles, defeating the purpose. One strategy to avoid that mistake: Imagine you're wearing tight suspenders that hold your shoulders down as you do the exercise. Can't keep them down? You need to use a lighter weight.

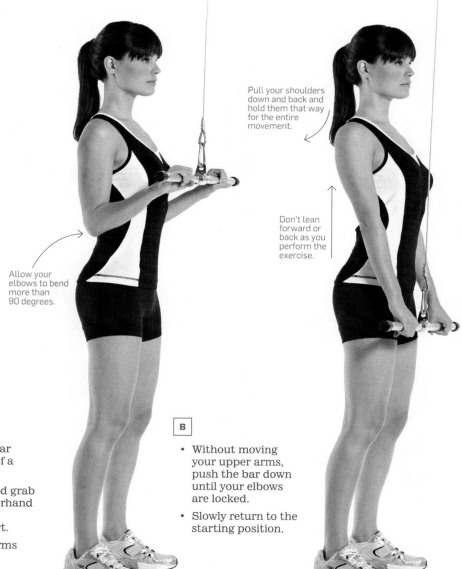

Pull your shoulders down and back and hold them that way for the entire movement.

Allow your elbows to bend more than 90 degrees.

Don't lean forward or back as you perform the exercise.

A

- Attach a straight bar to the high pulley of a cable station.
- Bend your arms and grab the bar with an overhand grip, your hands shoulder-width part.
- Tuck your upper arms next to your sides.

B

- Without moving your upper arms, push the bar down until your elbows are locked.
- Slowly return to the starting position.

Triceps | ARM EXTENSIONS

VARIATION #1
Underhand-Grip Triceps Pressdown
• Hold the bar with an underhand grip.

Your palms should be facing up.

Straighten your arms completely.

Stand as tall as you can.

VARIATION #2
Rope Triceps Pressdown
• Hold an end of the rope with each hand.

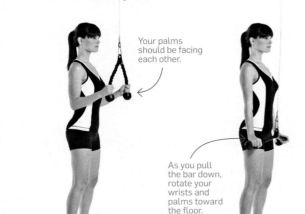

Your palms should be facing each other.

As you pull the bar down, rotate your wrists and palms toward the floor.

VARIATION #3
Single-Arm Rope Triceps Pressdown

A
• Hold an end of the rope with your right hand, your palm facing in.

B
• Complete the prescribed number of reps with your right arm, then immediately do the same number with your left arm.

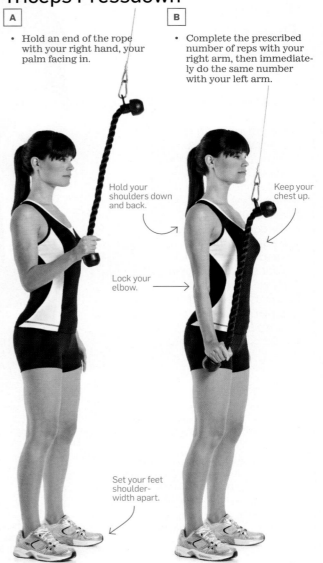

Hold your shoulders down and back.

Keep your chest up.

Lock your elbow.

Set your feet shoulder-width apart.

Dumbbell Kickback

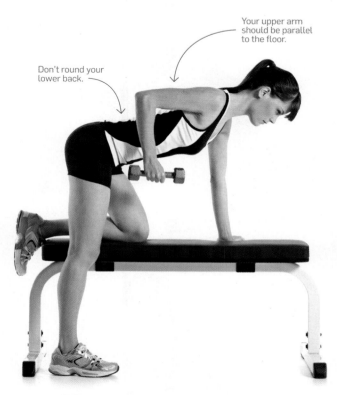

Don't round your lower back.

Your upper arm should be parallel to the floor.

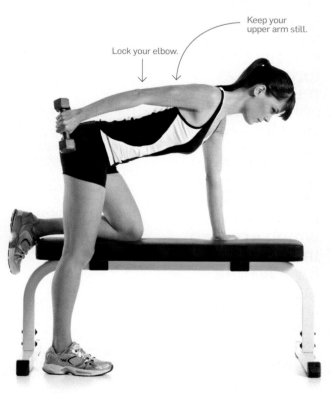

Lock your elbow.

Keep your upper arm still.

A

- Place your left hand and left knee on a flat bench.
- Your lower back should be naturally arched and your torso parallel to the floor.
- Hold your right upper arm so that it's parallel to the floor, with your elbow bent.

B

- Without moving your right upper arm, raise your forearm until your arm is completely straight.
- Reverse the movement back to the starting position.

Forearms | WRIST AND HAND EXERCISES

These exercises target either your wrist flexors or wrist extensors, forearm muscles that contribute to grip strength. The muscles of your hands, fingers, and thumbs, which are also important for a strong grip, are trained with many of the exercises as well.

Wrist Curl

A

- Grab a pair of dumbbells with an underhand, shoulder-width grip.
- Kneel in front of a bench.
- Place your forearms on the bench so that your palms are facing up and your hands are hanging off the bench.
- Allow your wrists to bend backward from the weight of the dumbbells.

B

- Curl your wrists upward by raising your palms toward your body.
- Reverse the movement to return to the starting position.

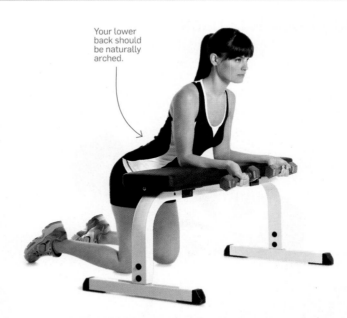

Your lower back should be naturally arched.

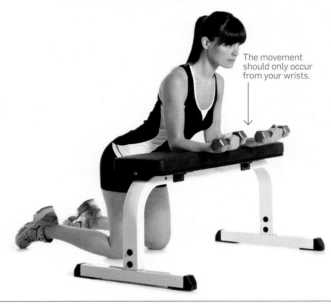

The movement should only occur from your wrists.

Wrist Extension

 A

- Grab a pair of dumbbells with an overhand, shoulder-width grip.
- Kneel in front of a bench.
- Place your forearms on the bench so that your palms are facing down and your hands are hanging off the bench.
- Allow your wrists to bend forward from the weight of the dumbbells.

B

- Extend your wrists upward by raising the backs of your hands toward your body.
- Reverse the movement to return to the starting position.

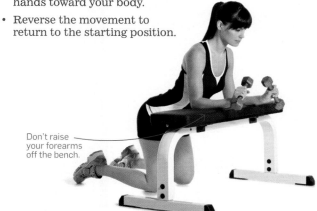

Don't raise your forearms off the bench.

Bar Hold

- Set a barbell on a rack at the level of your hips, and load it with a heavy weight.
- Grab the bar with an overhand grip that's beyond shoulder-width. (The wider your grip, the harder the bar is to hold—in a good way.)
- Dip your knees to lift the bar off the rack, then hold it for the appropriate amount of time for your goal. For maximum strength, choose the heaviest weight you can hold for about 20 seconds. To build more muscle, choose the heaviest that you can hold for about 60 seconds.

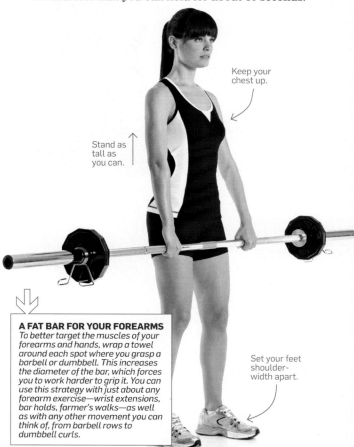

Keep your chest up.

Stand as tall as you can.

Set your feet shoulder-width apart.

A FAT BAR FOR YOUR FOREARMS
To better target the muscles of your forearms and hands, wrap a towel around each spot where you grasp a barbell or dumbbell. This increases the diameter of the bar, which forces you to work harder to grip it. You can use this strategy with just about any forearm exercise—wrist extensions, bar holds, farmer's walks—as well as with any other movement you can think of, from barbell rows to dumbbell curls.

Forearms | WRIST AND HAND EXERCISES

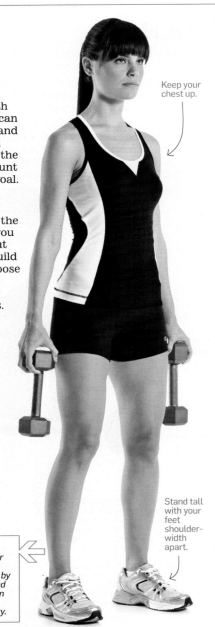

Hex Dumbbell Hold

- Grab the top of a hex dumbbell with each hand. (You can also work each hand separately.) Hold the dumbbell for the appropriate amount of time for your goal.

- For maximum strength, choose the heaviest weight you can hold for about 20 seconds. To build more muscle, choose the heaviest that you can hold for about 60 seconds.

To make the hex dumbbell hold harder, try to perform an arm curl while grasping the weight in this manner.

HOLD FOR MUSCLE
Simply holding barbells or dumbbells strengthens your wrists and forearms by as much as 25 percent and 16 percent, respectively, in 12 weeks, according to a study at Auburn University.

Keep your chest up.

Stand tall with your feet shoulder-width apart.

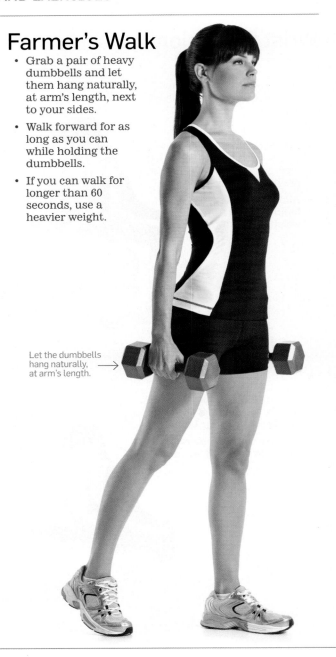

Farmer's Walk

- Grab a pair of heavy dumbbells and let them hang naturally, at arm's length, next to your sides.

- Walk forward for as long as you can while holding the dumbbells.

- If you can walk for longer than 60 seconds, use a heavier weight.

Let the dumbbells hang naturally, at arm's length.

Plate Pinch Curl

A

- Grab a pair of light weight plates in your right hand.
- Hold the two plates together with your fingers and thumb by pinching the plates. (If you have the option, you should pinch the smooth side of the plates.)
- Let the plates hang at arm's length next to your sides.

Pinch the plates together.

B

- Without moving your upper arms, bend your elbows and curl the weights as close to your shoulders as you can.
- Slowly lower the weights back to the starting position.

Keep your upper arm still.

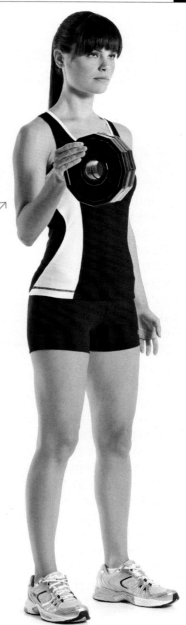

19

Average number of points people were able to lower their systolic blood pressure after 8 weeks of doing exercises to improve grip strength, according to a study in the *European Journal of Applied Physiology*. Diastolic blood pressure decreased by 5 points.

Arms

THE BEST ARM EXERCISES YOU'VE NEVER DONE
Triple-Stop EZ-Bar Curl

What makes these moves so special? They require you to stop for 10 seconds at three different positions as you perform the movement. Pausing at each point increases strength at that joint angle and 10 degrees in either direction. So this helps eliminate any weak points you might have. It also keeps your muscles under tension for more than 30 seconds each set, a key for building muscle. You can apply the technique to nearly any variation of the arm curl or arm extension.

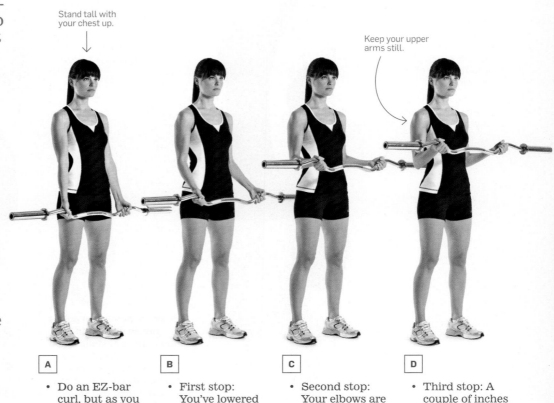

Stand tall with your chest up.

Keep your upper arms still.

A
- Do an EZ-bar curl, but as you lower the bar, pause for 10 seconds each at the three positions shown. One complete repetition is one set.

B
- First stop: You've lowered the bar about 2 inches.

C
- Second stop: Your elbows are bent 90 degrees.

D
- Third stop: A couple of inches before your arms are straight.

Triple-Stop Lying Dumbbell Triceps Extension

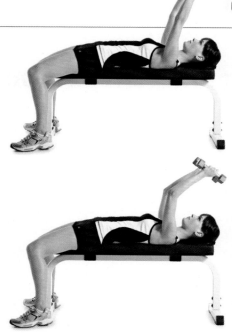

 A

- Do a lying dumbbell triceps extension, but pause for 10 seconds each at the three positions shown. One complete repetition is one set.

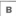 **B**

- First stop: You've lowered the weights about 4 inches.

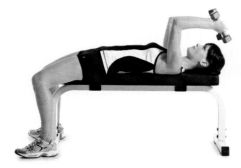

 C

- Second stop: Your elbows are bent about 90 degrees.

 D

- Third stop: Lower the weights to the bottom position of the exercise.

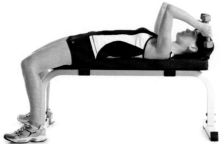

Arms

THE BEST STRETCH FOR YOUR BICEPS
Biceps Stretch

Why it's good:
This stretch loosens your biceps. When these muscles are stiff, your arms look permanently bent. Biceps stiffness also negatively affects the range of motion of your shoulders.

Make the most of it: Hold this stretch for 30 seconds for each arm, then repeat twice for a total of three sets. Perform this routine daily.

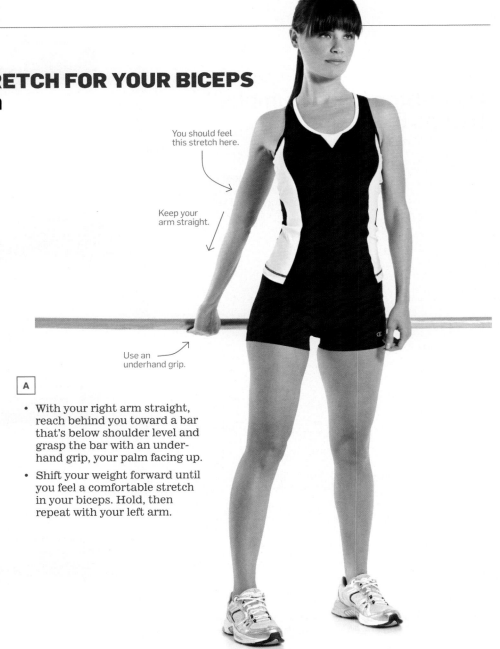

You should feel this stretch here.

Keep your arm straight.

Use an underhand grip.

A

- With your right arm straight, reach behind you toward a bar that's below shoulder level and grasp the bar with an underhand grip, your palm facing up.
- Shift your weight forward until you feel a comfortable stretch in your biceps. Hold, then repeat with your left arm.

THE BEST STRETCH FOR YOUR TRICEPS
Overhead Triceps Stretch

Why it's good:
This stretch loosens your triceps. When this muscle is tight, you may have trouble reaching over your head. That's because triceps tightness compromises your shoulder's range of motion.

Make the most of it: Hold this stretch for 30 seconds for each arm, then repeat twice for a total of three sets. Perform this routine daily.

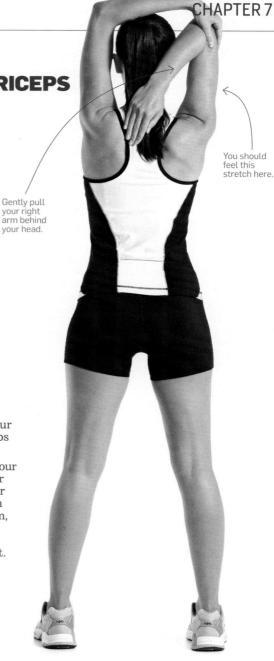

Gently pull your right arm behind your head.

You should feel this stretch here.

- Reach over your head with your right arm, then bend your elbow so that your hand drops behind your head.

- Grasp your right elbow with your left hand and gently pull your right arm farther behind your head. When you feel a stretch in the back of your upper arm, hold the position for the prescribed amount of time. Then switch arms and repeat.

Arms

SCULPT PERFECT ARMS

The key to a great arm workout: Keep it simple. And in fact, the best approach is to save exercises that target your arms for the end of your workout. After all, your arms are involved in every upper-body exercise. So if they tire out early, you won't be able to work the muscles of your chest, back, and shoulders as hard. Try this total-arm workout from Charles Staley, author of *Escalating Density Training*. It's designed to give your arms the work they need to firm up fast, without requiring that you ever increase the duration of your workout. Instead, you'll simply do more work in less time—a little-known secret for shaping your muscles.

What to do: Choose one exercise from the Biceps section of this chapter, and one exercise from the Triceps section. For each, select the heaviest weight that allows you to complete 10 repetitions. (Just ballpark it.) Then start your stopwatch, and do five reps of the decline hammer curl, followed by five reps of the triceps exercise. Rest for as little or as long as you want, and repeat. Continue to alternate back and forth in this manner for 10 minutes. At any time, you can drop your reps as desired. So as you fatigue, you might just do a set of three reps or two reps—go by feel. However, make sure to keep track of the total reps you perform in the 10 minutes. Then, in your next workout, try to beat that number. Repeat this routine every 4 days.

BONUS WORKOUT: THE BICEPS SHAPER

Your biceps muscles are composed of both fast-twitch and slow-twitch muscle fibers. So to completely train your arms, you need to make sure you work all of these fibers. Try this three-move routine twice a week for 4 weeks. It hits your fast-twitch fibers with heavy weights and low repetitions, a combination of your fast- and slow-twitch fibers with medium weights and repetitions, and your slow-twitch fibers with light weights and high repetitions. You'll perform the first exercise with your arms behind your body, the second with your arms in line with your body, and the third with your arms in front of your body, to help hit the entire complex of fibers that make up your biceps.

What to do: Do this workout as a circuit, performing one set of each exercise after the next, with no rest in between. After you've completed one circuit, rest for 2 minutes, then repeat the routine one or two more times. Choose any exercise from the menu, but make sure that you don't use the same grip (standard, hammer, offset-pinky, offset-thumb) on any of the movements. And to keep your muscles growing, choose new exercises every 4 weeks. For even more variety, you can also switch the order of exercises. So you might place the Exercise 3 movement first in your workout, the Exercise 1 movement second, and the Exercise 2 movement last, and so forth.

EXERCISE 1
Choose any one of these movements, and do six repetitions.

Incline dumbbell curl (page 156)

Incline hammer curl (page 156)

Incline offset-pinky curl (page 156)

Incline offset-thumb curl (page 156)

EXERCISE 2
Choose any one of these movements, and do 12 repetitions.

Standing dumbbell curl (page 154)

Standing hammer curl (page 157)

Standing offset-pinky curl (page 157)

Standing offset-thumb curl (page 157)

EXERCISE 3
Choose any one of these movements, and do 25 repetitions.

Decline dumbbell curl (page 156)

Decline hammer curl (page 156)

Decline offset-pinky curl (page 156)

Decline offset-thumb curl (page 156)

BONUS WORKOUT: THE TOTAL-BODY ARMS WORKOUT

Shape your arms as you burn fat all over, with this total-body workout plan from Craig Ballantyne, MS, CSCS, owner of TurbulenceTraining.com. It's designed to work all your muscles, but one routine zeroes in on your triceps—using the single-arm shoulder press, close-hands pushup, and lying dumbbell triceps extension—and the other prioritizes your biceps, with both the kneeling underhand-grip lat pulldown and the dumbbell curl. The end-result: Toned arms—and a toned body.

What to do: Alternate between Workout A and Workout B three days a week, resting at least a day between each session. So if you plan to life on Monday, Wednesday, and Friday, you'd do Workout A on Monday and Friday, and Workout B on Wednesday. The next week, you'd do Workout B on Monday and Friday, and Workout A on Do this workout three days a week, resting at least a day between each session. For each routine, do the exercises as a circuit, performing one movement after the other without resting. Once you've completed the entire circuit, rest for 2 minutes, and repeat one to two times.

One special note on the close-hands pushup: Perform the exercise as directed, but if you can't complete at least six repetitions, do the same movement with your hands on an inclined surface (as you would for the incline pushup on page 36). Simply find a height that allows you to complete at least 6 repetitions before you start to struggle. Then each time you do the workout, perform as many reps of the close-hands pushup as you can using this same guideline. (For more explanation, see "How Much Weight Should I Use" on page 13.)

WORKOUT A

EXERCISE	REPS
1. Dumbbell deadlift (page 250) or barbell deadlift (page 248)	8
2. Single-arm dumbbell shoulder press (page 122)	8
3. Dumbbell split squat (page 209)	8
4. Close-hands pushup (page 38)	AMAP*
5. Lying dumbbell triceps extension (page 179)	12

*As many as possible

WORKOUT B

EXERCISE	REPS
1. Kneeling underhand-grip lat pulldown (page 105)	12
2. Swiss-ball leg curl (page 243)	15
3. Dumbbell stepup (page 262)	10
4. Swiss-ball rollout (page 292)	10
5. Dumbbell curl (page 154)	8

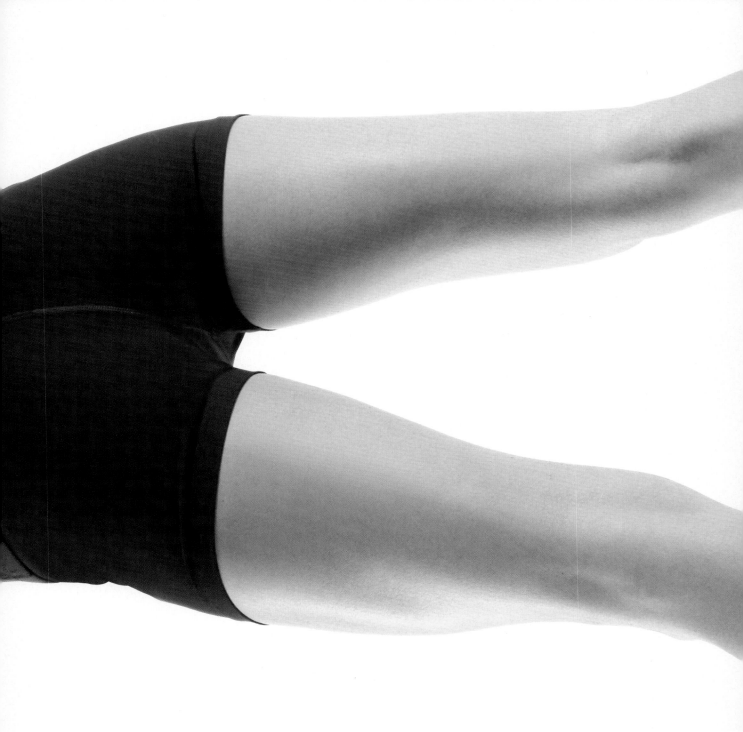

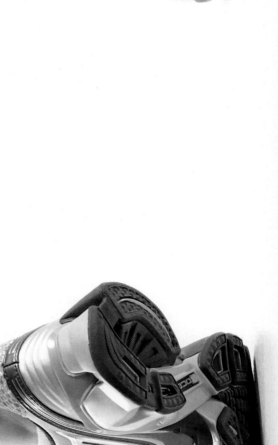

Chapter 8: Quadriceps & Calves

FIT LEGS, FIT BODY

Quads
& Calves

It can be tempting to skip exercises that work your quadriceps. No doubt this is because the movements that best train these muscles—squats and lunges—require a lot of effort. But, of course, that's exactly what makes them so worthwhile.

Take the squat, for example. It burns more calories per rep than almost any other exercise. And along with targeting your quadriceps, it hits all the other muscles in your lower body, too, including your hamstrings, glutes, and calves.

So sure, squats and lunges are hard, but embracing the quadriceps exercises in this chapter will reward you with strong, muscular legs and a leaner midsection. And for those who want to give their lower legs extra attention, this section also includes moves that focus *directly* on your calves.

Bonus Benefits

Great abs! Besides helping you burn belly flab, squats work the muscles of your core harder than many ab exercises do.

Better balance! Conditioning your quads also strengthens the ligaments and tendons within your legs—helping make your knees more stable and less susceptible to injury.

Stronger back! In a study of lifters who did both upper- and lower-body exercises, Norwegian scientists found that those who emphasized lower-body movements such as the squat and lunge gained the most upper-body strength.

Meet Your Muscles

Quadriceps
The main muscles on the front of your thigh are your quadriceps [1]. This muscle group has four distinct sections: the rectus femoris [A], vastus lateralis [B], vastus medialis [C], and vastus intermedius [not shown; hidden beneath the rectus femoris]. All of these segments come together at the quadriceps tendon [D] and attach just below your knee joint. As a whole, their main function is to straighten your knee. That's why squats and lunges are the best exercises for working your quadriceps: They require that you straighten your legs against a resistance, even if it's just your body weight.

Gastrocnemius
Your calf consists of two separate muscles, both located on the back of your lower leg. The muscle closest to the surface of the skin is called the gastrocnemius [3]. It's composed of two sections—one on the inside of your leg, the other on the outside. These sections start just above your knee and come together at your Achilles tendon [4], which attaches to the back of your heel.

Soleus
Your other calf muscle, the soleus [5], lies underneath your gastrocnemius. It starts just below your knee and joins up with the gastrocnemius at your Achilles tendon. The primary duty of both calf muscles is to extend your ankle. Think of this as the action of raising your heel when your foot is flat on the floor. So besides calf raises, any exercise that features some level of ankle extension—such as the squats or jumping movements—also work your calf muscles.

Hip Adductors
Your hip adductors [2] are the muscles on the inside of your thigh, or what's typically referred to as your groin. When your leg is straight out to the side, your hip adductors allow you to pull it back toward your body, a movement known as "hip adduction." (Creative name, huh?) These muscles are heavily involved in squats and lunges.

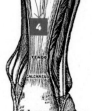

Quads & Calves | SQUATS

In this chapter, you'll find 99 exercises that target the muscles of your front thighs and lower legs. Throughout, you'll notice that certain exercises have been given the designation Main Move. Master this basic version of a movement, and you'll be able to do all of its variations with flawless form.

SQUATS

These exercises target your quadriceps. They also activate your core and just about every other muscle of your lower body, including your glutes, hamstrings, and calves. This makes the squat one of the best all-around exercises you can do.

MAIN MOVE
Body-Weight Squat

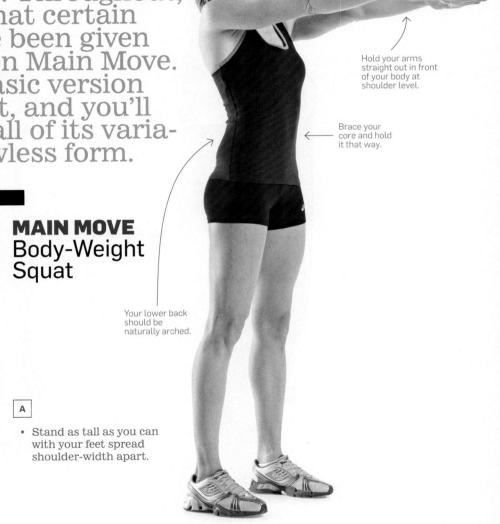

Hold your arms straight out in front of your body at shoulder level.

Brace your core and hold it that way.

Your lower back should be naturally arched.

A

- Stand as tall as you can with your feet spread shoulder-width apart.

529

**Most weight, in pounds,
ever squatted by a woman weighing
123 pounds or less.**

SET YOUR STANCE
Jump as high as you can three times in a row. Then look down at your foot placement. This is roughly where you want to place your feet when you squat.

Your torso should stay as upright as possible.

Don't let your lower back round.

Your arms should stay in the same position from start to finish.

Keep your core tight.

The tops of your thighs should be parallel to the floor or lower.

Keep your weight on your heels, not on your toes, for the entire movement. One gauge: If your weight is distributed correctly, you should be able to wiggle your toes at any moment during the lift.

B

- Lower your body as far as you can by pushing your hips back and bending your knees.
- Pause, then slowly push yourself back to the starting position.

The Secret to a Perfect Squat

Hone your squat technique with this muscle-memory trick from Mel Siff, PhD, author of *Supertraining* and one of the all-time great minds in the field of exercise science. It's an easy way to help your body and brain learn the proper movement of the lift.

What to do: Prior to your first set of squats, sit tall on a bench with your back upright and naturally arched, your shoulders pulled back, and your lower legs perpendicular to the floor and at least shoulder-width apart. Hold your arms straight out in front of your body at shoulder level so that they're parallel to the floor. Bend forward at your hips—without changing the arch in your back—and move your feet back toward you just enough that you're able to stand up slowly, without having to rock backward or forward or change your body posture. Pay attention: That's the position you should be in when you squat. Once standing, reverse the movement and slowly lower your body to the seated position. Repeat several times.

Quads & Calves | SQUATS

VARIATION #1
Prisoner Squat

- Place your fingers on the back of your head (as if you had just been arrested).

Pull your elbows and shoulders back.

Stick your chest out.

Push your hips back.

VARIATION #2
Body-Weight Squat with Knee Press-Out

- Place both legs between a 20-inch mini-band and position the band just below your knees.

- As you squat, focus on pushing your knees outward.

Your knees should stay over the centers of your feet as you squat.

If your knees fall inward when you squat, your hips have a glaring weakness. The good news: Pushing your knees outward against a resistance band can help better activate and strengthen these important muscles.

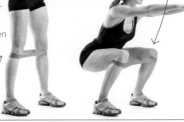

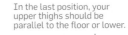

VARIATION #3
Body-Weight Wall Squat

PAUSE FOR POWER
The pause technique helps eliminate weaknesses throughout the entire range of motion of the squat.

Hold each position for 5 to 10 seconds.

In the last position, your upper thighs should be parallel to the floor or lower.

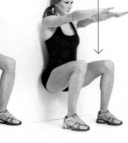

| A | B | C D | E |

- Lean back against a wall, with your feet about 2 feet away from it and shoulder-width apart.

- Keeping your back against the wall, bend your knees slightly so that your body descends a few inches. Now hold that position for 5 to 10 seconds.

- Continue to lower yourself a few inches at time, four more times.

- Once you've paused at all five positions, stand up and rest. That's one set.

192

VARIATION #4
Swiss-Ball Body-Weight Wall Squat

A

- Hold a Swiss ball behind you and stand so that the ball is pinned between your back and the wall.
- Place your feet about 2 feet in front of your body.

B

- Keeping your back in contact with the ball, lower your body until your upper thighs are at least parallel to the floor.

THE BEGINNER'S SQUAT
If you have trouble doing a standard body-weight squat, try the Swiss-ball version. It requires less core strength, which makes the exercise easier while helping you learn perfect form.

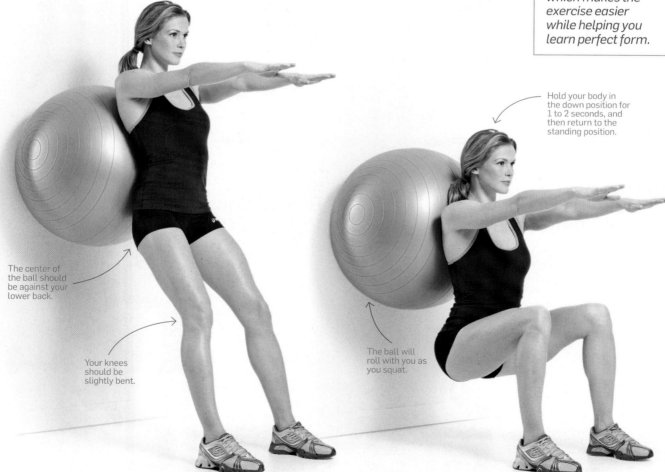

The center of the ball should be against your lower back.

Your knees should be slightly bent.

Hold your body in the down position for 1 to 2 seconds, and then return to the standing position.

The ball will roll with you as you squat.

Quads & Calves | SQUATS

VARIATION #5
Body-Weight Jump Squat

A

- Place your fingers on the back of your head and pull your elbows back so that they're in line with your body.

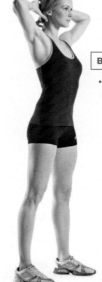

SQUAT FOR FAT LOSS
While the jump squat variation shown here is great for athletic performance, use a deeper squat when doing the exercise for fat loss. In fact, lower your body until your upper thighs are parallel to the floor (as shown in the iso-explosive body-weight jump squat below).

B

- Dip your knees in preparation to leap.

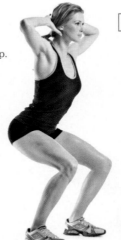

C

- Explosively jump as high as you can.
- When you land, immediately squat down and jump again.

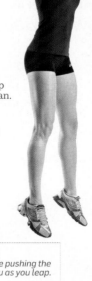

JUMP HIGHER
Imagine that you're pushing the floor away from you as you leap.

VARIATION #6
Iso-Explosive Body-Weight Jump Squat

- Place your fingers on the back of your head and pull your elbows back so that they're in line with your body.
- Push your hips back, bend your knees, and lower until your upper thighs are parallel to the floor.
- Pause for 5 seconds in the down position.
- After your pause, jump as high as you can.
- Land and reset.

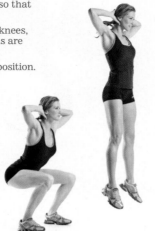

WORK YOUR LEGS ANYWHERE
The 5-second pause during this exercise eliminates all the elasticity in your muscles, which allows you to activate a maximum number of muscle fibers as you push yourself off the floor. This makes it a great exercise to use when you don't have access to weights.

VARIATION #7
Braced Squat

- Hold a weight plate in front of your chest with both hands, your arms completely straight.

TARGET YOUR BICEPS, TOO!
As you perform the braced squat, you can work your arms by doing a curl at the top of each repetition. With your arms outstretched, simply curl the plate toward your shoulders without moving your upper arms. Straighten your arms as you lower your body.

The braced squat overloads your core, helping to improve stability, strength, and performance. It's categorized as a body-weight exercise because the amount of weight you can use is limited due to shoulder fatigue from holding the plate in front of your body.

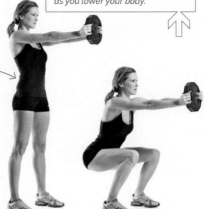

High Box Jump

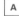

- Stand in front of a sturdy, secure box that's high enough so that you have to jump with great effort in order to land on top of it.
- Your feet should be shoulder-width apart.
- Dip your knees.

- Jump up onto the box with a soft landing.
- Step down and reset your feet.

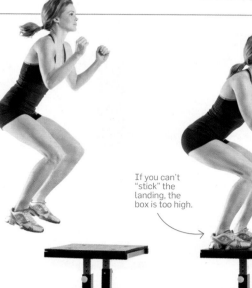

If you can't "stick" the landing, the box is too high.

Set your feet shoulder-width apart.

Depth Jump

- Stand at the edge of a 12-inch box.

ADD INCHES TO YOUR VERTICAL
The depth jump is one of the best drills for improving your vertical leap. Try it twice a week, doing four or five sets of three repetitions at the beginning of your workout. Rest for 60 to 90 seconds between sets.

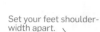

- Simply step off the box so that you land on both feet simultaneously (balls of feet first, followed by heels).

- When you make contact with the floor, jump as high as you can. That's one repetition.

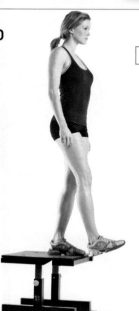

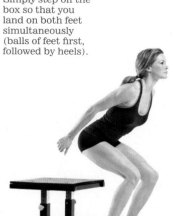

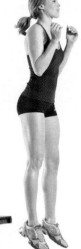

Quads & Calves | SQUATS

MAIN MOVE
Single-Leg Squat

A

- Stand on your left leg on a bench or box that's about knee height.
- Hold your arms straight out in front of you.

Keep your torso as upright as possible.

Flex your right ankle so that your toes are higher than your heel.

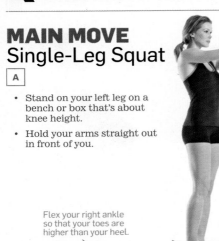

B

- Balancing on your left foot, bend your left knee and slowly lower your body until your right heel lightly touches the floor.
- Pause, then push yourself up.
- Complete the prescribed number of reps with your left leg, then immediately do the same number with your right.
- If this exercise is too hard, try the partial single-leg squat or the single-leg bench getup.

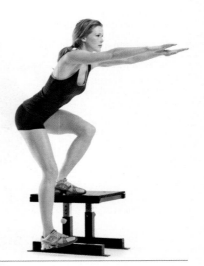

VARIATION #1
Single-Leg Bench Getup

A

- Sit tall on a bench with your back upright and naturally arched.
- Hold your arms straight out in front of your body at shoulder level, parallel to the floor.
- Raise your right foot off the floor.

Your lower back should be naturally arched.

B

- Without leaning foward, press your body to a standing position. (If you can't do this, try sliding your foot slightly back toward your body in the starting position.)
- Sit back down.

Push your hips forward.

Straighten your left knee.

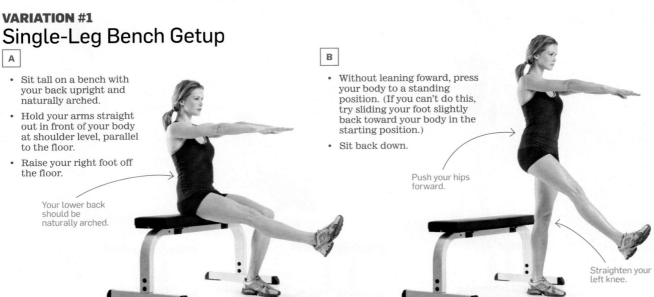

VARIATION #2
Partial Single-Leg Squat

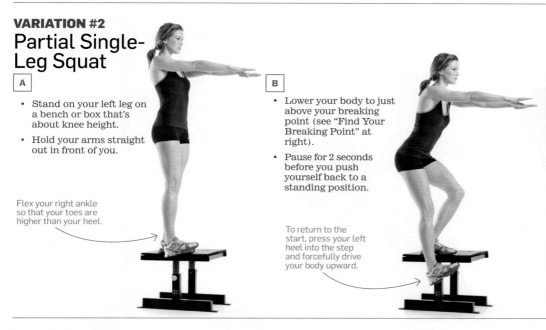

A

- Stand on your left leg on a bench or box that's about knee height.
- Hold your arms straight out in front of you.

Flex your right ankle so that your toes are higher than your heel.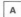

B

- Lower your body to just above your breaking point (see "Find Your Breaking Point" at right).
- Pause for 2 seconds before you push yourself back to a standing position.

To return to the start, press your left heel into the step and forcefully drive your body upward.

VARIATION #3
Pistol Squat

A

- Stand holding your arms straight out in front of your body at shoulder level, parallel to the floor.
- Raise your right leg off the floor, and hold it there.

Brace your core.

Your right leg should be straight.

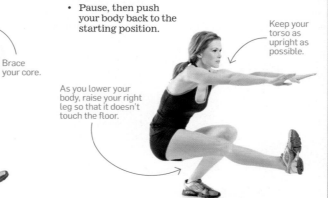

B

- Push your hips back and lower your body as far as you can.
- Pause, then push your body back to the starting position.

Keep your torso as upright as possible.

As you lower your body, raise your right leg so that it doesn't touch the floor.

Find Your Breaking Point

If you can't do at least three reps of the single-leg squat, try the partial single-leg squat. You'll first need to identify your breaking point. Your breaking point is the position you're in when you can no longer control the speed at which you lower your body. This could be after you've lowered yourself just an inch, or it could be after several inches. Determine its location, then follow the directions for the partial single-leg squat. As your strength improves, your breaking point will move lower. So retest it regularly.

Quads & Calves | SQUATS

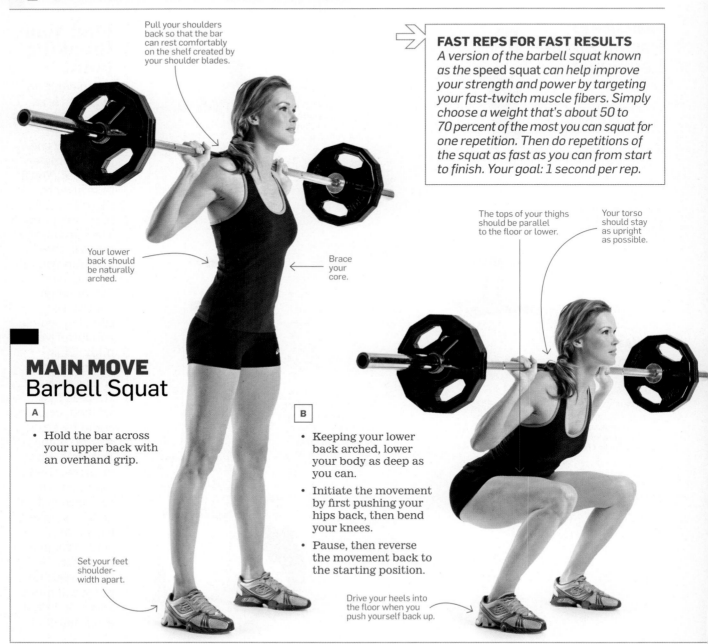

Pull your shoulders back so that the bar can rest comfortably on the shelf created by your shoulder blades.

FAST REPS FOR FAST RESULTS
A version of the barbell squat known as the speed squat *can help improve your strength and power by targeting your fast-twitch muscle fibers. Simply choose a weight that's about 50 to 70 percent of the most you can squat for one repetition. Then do repetitions of the squat as fast as you can from start to finish. Your goal: 1 second per rep.*

Your lower back should be naturally arched.

Brace your core.

The tops of your thighs should be parallel to the floor or lower.

Your torso should stay as upright as possible.

MAIN MOVE
Barbell Squat

A

- Hold the bar across your upper back with an overhand grip.

Set your feet shoulder-width apart.

B

- Keeping your lower back arched, lower your body as deep as you can.
- Initiate the movement by first pushing your hips back, then bend your knees.
- Pause, then reverse the movement back to the starting position.

Drive your heels into the floor when you push yourself back up.

VARIATION #1
Wide-Stance Barbell Squat

A

- Perform a squat with your feet set at twice shoulder width.

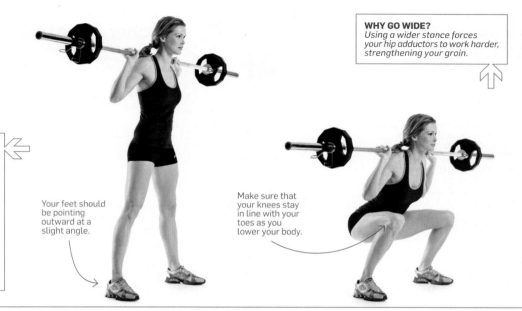

If your heels rise off the floor when you do a standard barbell squat, your hips are tight. But the wide-stance version of the exercise can help. Simply lower your body into the deepest position of the wide-stance squat that you can without allowing your heels to rise. Hold for 2 seconds. Try to lower your body a little farther with each workout. As your flexibility improves, narrow your stance and decrease the angle at which your toes point out.

Your feet should be pointing outward at a slight angle.

WHY GO WIDE?
Using a wider stance forces your hip adductors to work harder, strengthening your groin.

Make sure that your knees stay in line with your toes as you lower your body.

VARIATION #2
Barbell Front Squat

A

- Hold the bar with an overhand grip that's just beyond shoulder width.
- Raise your upper arms until they're parallel to the floor.
- Allow the bar to roll back so that it's resting on the fronts of your shoulders.

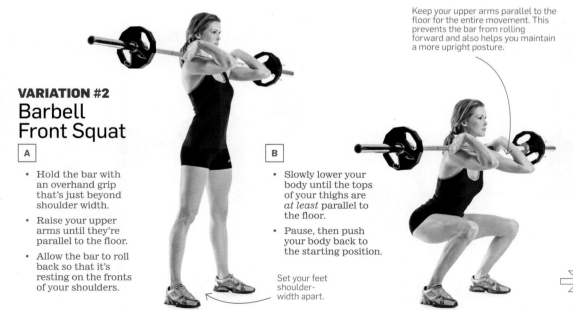

B

- Slowly lower your body until the tops of your thighs are *at least* parallel to the floor.
- Pause, then push your body back to the starting position.

Set your feet shoulder-width apart.

Keep your upper arms parallel to the floor for the entire movement. This prevents the bar from rolling forward and also helps you maintain a more upright posture.

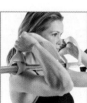

STRAPS
If your wrists aren't flexible enough to perform the traditional version of the barbell front squat, use this trick: Loop a pair of wrist straps around the bar—spaced shoulder-width apart—and cinch them tight. Then grasp the straps instead of bending your wrists back and resting the bar on your fingers.

Quads & Calves | SQUATS

VARIATION #3
Crossed-Arm Barbell Front Squat

- Set a bar on a squat rack and cross your arms in front of you so that each hand is on top of the bar.
- Step under the bar so that it's resting on the tops of your shoulders, and raise your arms so that the bar can't roll off them.
- Step back and perform a squat, keeping your arms in the same position for the entire movement.
- Push yourself back to a standing position.

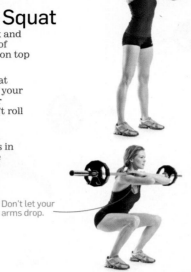

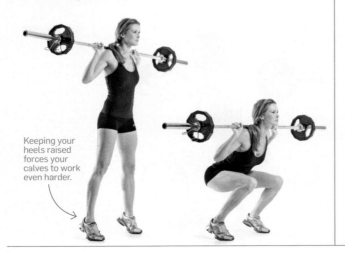

Don't let your arms drop.

VARIATION #4
Zercher Squat

- Hold the bar in the crooks of your arms—tightly against your chest—instead of across your back.
- Push yourself back to a standing position.

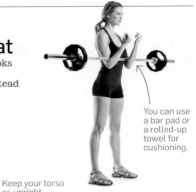

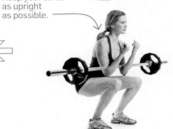

You can use a bar pad or a rolled-up towel for cushioning.

Keep your torso as upright as possible.

The Zercher squat not only strengthens your lower body but also works your biceps and front deltoids, muscles that have to stay contracted in order to hold the bar.

VARIATION #5
Barbell Siff Squat

- Before you squat, raise your heels as high as you can and hold them that way for the entire lift.

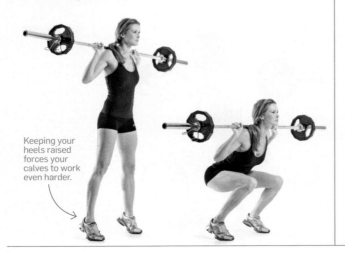

Keeping your heels raised forces your calves to work even harder.

VARIATION #6
Barbell Quarter Squat

- Lower your body only until your knees are bent about 60 degrees.

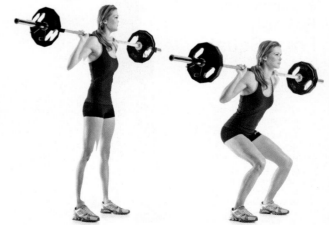

VARIATION #7
Barbell Squat with Heels Raised

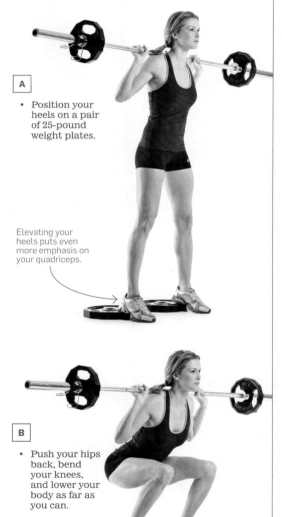

A

- Position your heels on a pair of 25-pound weight plates.

Elevating your heels puts even more emphasis on your quadriceps.

B

- Push your hips back, bend your knees, and lower your body as far as you can.

VARIATION #8
Barbell Hack Squat

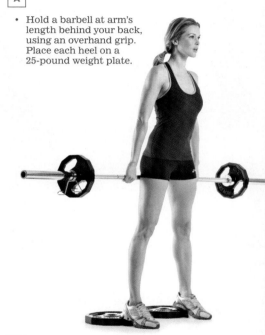

A

- Hold a barbell at arm's length behind your back, using an overhand grip. Place each heel on a 25-pound weight plate.

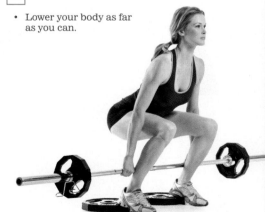

B

- Lower your body as far as you can.

Squat More– Instantly!

While it's best to use a full range of motion most of the time—as you do in other versions of the squat—the quarter squat allows you to lift about 20 percent more weight than you can when you squat lower. This reduces the involvement of your glutes and hamstrings and helps you overload lagging quads. Use the technique in stints of just 4 weeks at a time, though, in order to prevent muscle imbalances that occur when your quads become so strong that they overpower your hamstrings.

Quads & Calves | SQUATS

VARIATION #9
Barbell Jump Squat

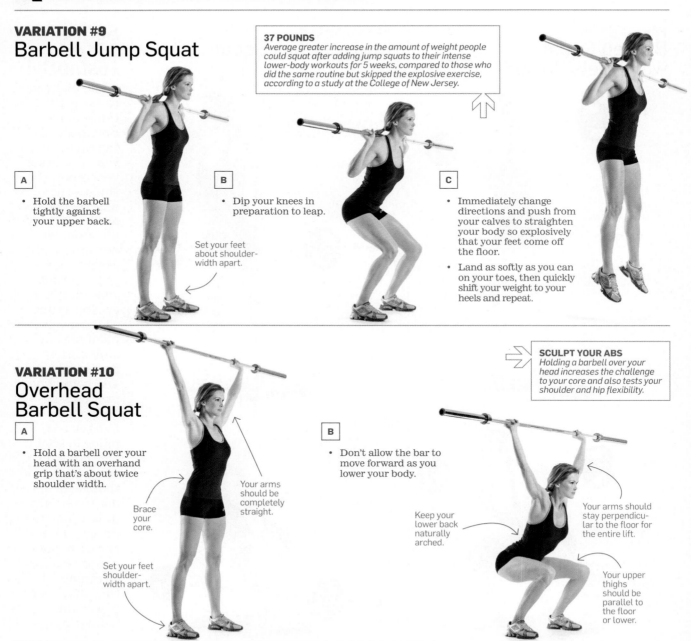

37 POUNDS
Average greater increase in the amount of weight people could squat after adding jump squats to their intense lower-body workouts for 5 weeks, compared to those who did the same routine but skipped the explosive exercise, according to a study at the College of New Jersey.

A

- Hold the barbell tightly against your upper back.

Set your feet about shoulder-width apart.

B

- Dip your knees in preparation to leap.

C

- Immediately change directions and push from your calves to straighten your body so explosively that your feet come off the floor.

- Land as softly as you can on your toes, then quickly shift your weight to your heels and repeat.

VARIATION #10
Overhead Barbell Squat

A

- Hold a barbell over your head with an overhand grip that's about twice shoulder width.

Brace your core.

Your arms should be completely straight.

Set your feet shoulder-width apart.

SCULPT YOUR ABS
Holding a barbell over your head increases the challenge to your core and also tests your shoulder and hip flexibility.

B

- Don't allow the bar to move forward as you lower your body.

Keep your lower back naturally arched.

Your arms should stay perpendicular to the floor for the entire lift.

Your upper thighs should be parallel to the floor or lower.

MAIN MOVE
Dumbbell Squat

A

- Hold a pair of dumbbells at arm's length next to your sides, your palms facing each other.

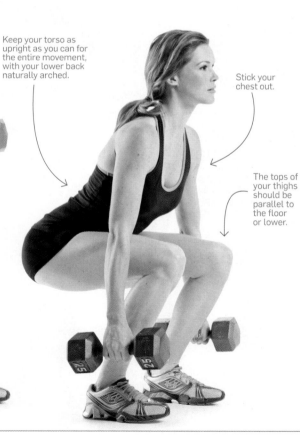

B

- Brace your abs, and lower your body as far as you can by pushing your hips back and bending your knees.
- Pause, then slowly push yourself back to the starting position.

KEEP YOUR HEAD UP
Looking down when you squat puts you at greater risk of injury, say scientists at Miami University of Ohio. The researchers found that gazing down during the movement causes your body to lean forward 4 to 5 degrees. This increases the strain on your lower back. Looking at yourself in the mirror can also cause a forward lean. Your best approach: Before you descend, find a mark that's stable and just above eye level, and stay focused on it throughout the movement.

Keep your torso as upright as you can for the entire movement, with your lower back naturally arched.

Stick your chest out.

The tops of your thighs should be parallel to the floor or lower.

Keep your weight on your heels, not on your toes, for the entire movement.

Quads & Calves | SQUATS

VARIATION #1
Goblet Squat

- Hold a dumbbell vertically next to your chest, with both hands cupping the dumbbell head. (Imagine that it's a heavy goblet.)

- Pause, then push yourself back to the starting position.

Don't be afraid to lower your body as deep as possible. Research shows that the most unstable knee angle during the squat is when your knees are bent 90 degrees—a few inches above the point where your upper thighs are parallel to the floor.

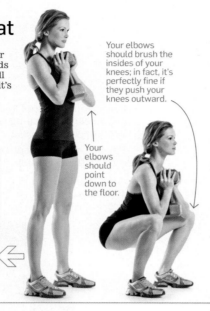

Your elbows should brush the insides of your knees; in fact, it's perfectly fine if they push your knees outward.

Your elbows should point down to the floor.

VARIATION #2
Wide-Stance Goblet Squat

- With both hands, hold a dumbbell vertically next to your chest.

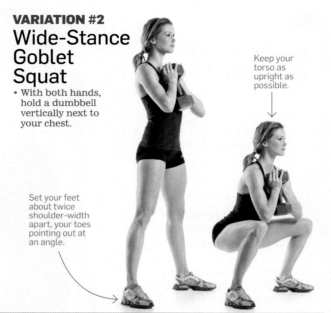

Keep your torso as upright as possible.

Set your feet about twice shoulder-width apart, your toes pointing out at an angle.

VARIATION #3
Sumo Squat

- Grasp a head of a heavy dumbbell in each hand, and hold the weight at arm's length in front of your waist.

Keep your lower back naturally arched for the entire movement.

Set your feet at about twice shoulder width, your toes turned out slightly.

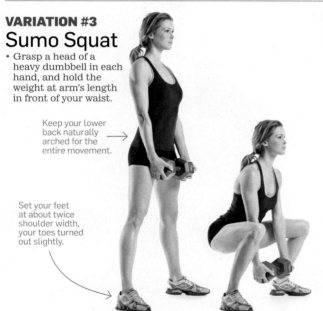

VARIATION #4
Dumbbell Front Squat

- Hold a pair of dumbbells so that your palms are facing each other, and rest one of the dumbbell heads on the meatiest part of each shoulder.

- Keep your body as upright as you can at all times.

- Don't allow your elbows to drop down as you squat.

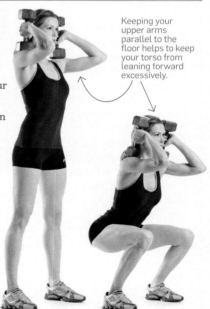

Keeping your upper arms parallel to the floor helps to keep your torso from leaning forward excessively.

VARIATION #5
Dumbbell Jump Squat

A

- Hold a pair of dumbbells at arm's length next to your sides, your palms facing each other.
- Dip your knees in preparation to leap.

JUMP HIGHER, RUN FASTER
You can boost your vertical leap and improve your speed with a simple jump squat routine, according to an 8-week study in the Journal of Strength and Conditioning. In the study, subjects used a weight that was 30 percent of the amount they could squat one time. Try it yourself: Twice a week, do five sets of six reps, resting 3 minutes after each set.

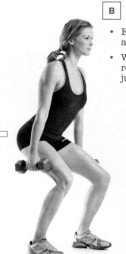

B

- Explosively jump as high as you can.
- When you land, reset quickly before jumping again.

Land as softly as you can on the balls of your feet, then lower your heels back to the floor.

VARIATION #6
Overhead Dumbbell Squat

A

- Hold a pair of dumbbells straight over your shoulders, your arms completely straight.

43

Percent reduction in knee pain after sufferers performed lower body exercises such as the squat for 4 months, according to a Tufts University study.

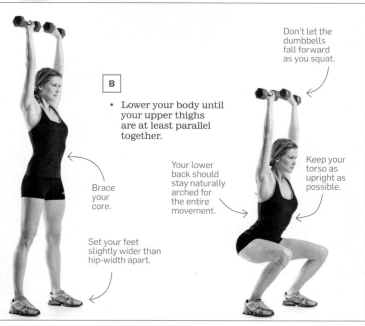

B

- Lower your body until your upper thighs are at least parallel together.

Don't let the dumbbells fall forward as you squat.

Brace your core.

Your lower back should stay naturally arched for the entire movement.

Keep your torso as upright as possible.

Set your feet slightly wider than hip-width apart.

MUSCLE MISTAKE
You Think Smith Machine Squats Are Superior

While the Smith machine—a squat rack with a bar that runs on guides—may look like a foolproof way to squat, it has a major flaw. The bar must travel straight up and down instead of in an arc as it does in a barbell squat. This places more stress on your lower back. What's more, Canadian scientists found that free-weight squats activate the quads almost 50 percent more than Smith machine squats.

Quads & Calves | SQUATS

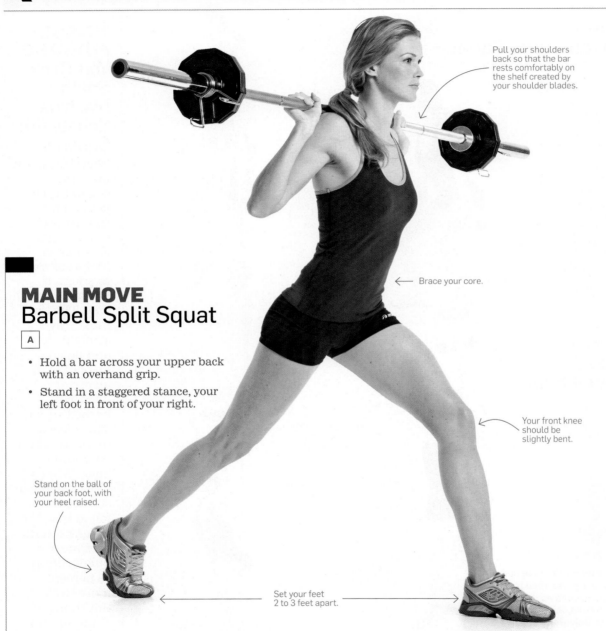

Pull your shoulders back so that the bar rests comfortably on the shelf created by your shoulder blades.

← Brace your core.

Your front knee should be slightly bent.

Stand on the ball of your back foot, with your heel raised.

Set your feet 2 to 3 feet apart.

MAIN MOVE
Barbell Split Squat

A

- Hold a bar across your upper back with an overhand grip.
- Stand in a staggered stance, your left foot in front of your right.

167

Percentage increase in core activity during the squat when people were reminded to keep their abs braced—as if they were about to be punched in the gut—according to a Utah State University study. The scientists say that hearing instructions reminds you that you may not be stiffening your core as much as you think. What's more, applying this to your workout subconsciously may work even better. The study subjects needed only one reminder. Consider this yours.

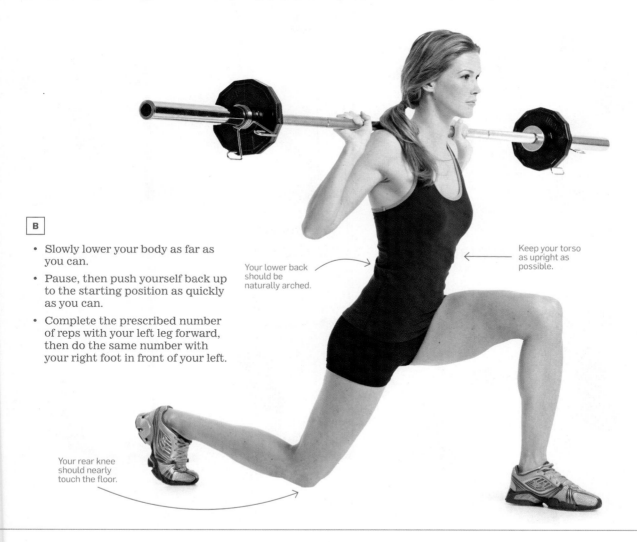

B

- Slowly lower your body as far as you can.

- Pause, then push yourself back up to the starting position as quickly as you can.

- Complete the prescribed number of reps with your left leg forward, then do the same number with your right foot in front of your left.

Your lower back should be naturally arched.

Keep your torso as upright as possible.

Your rear knee should nearly touch the floor.

Quads & Calves | SQUATS

VARIATION #1
Elevated-Front-Foot Barbell Split Squat
- Place your front foot on a 6-inch step or box.

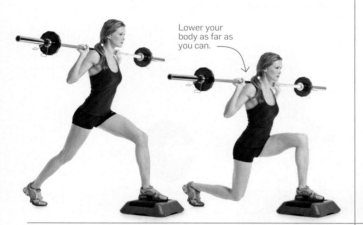

Lower your body as far as you can.

VARIATION #2
Elevated-Back-Foot Barbell Split Squat
- Place your back foot on a 6-inch step or box.

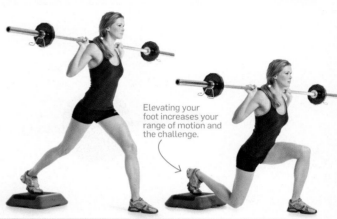

Elevating your foot increases your range of motion and the challenge.

VARIATION #3
Barbell Front Split Squat
- Hold the bar with an overhand grip that's just beyond shoulder width.
- Raise your upper arms until they're parallel to the floor.

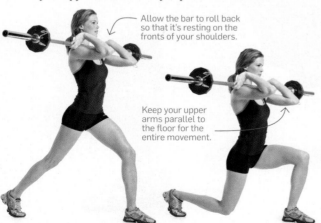

Allow the bar to roll back so that it's resting on the fronts of your shoulders.

Keep your upper arms parallel to the floor for the entire movement.

VARIATION #4
Barbell Bulgarian Split Squat
- Place just the instep of your back foot on a bench.

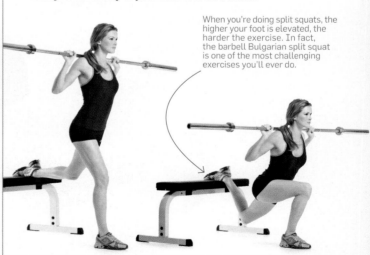

When you're doing split squats, the higher your foot is elevated, the harder the exercise. In fact, the barbell Bulgarian split squat is one of the most challenging exercises you'll ever do.

BODY-WEIGHT SPLIT SQUAT

You can do just about any version of the split squat without holding weights of any kind. Simply cross your arms in front of your chest or place your hands behind your ears or on your hips. The body-weight versions are ideal warmup exercises and are also valuable if weighted variations are too hard or if you don't have weights available.

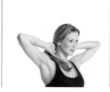

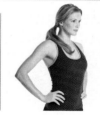

MAIN MOVE
Dumbbell Split Squat

TRAINER'S TIP
Just like in the two-legged version of the squat, be sure to brace your core as you perform this exercise.

A

- Hold a pair of dumbbells at arm's length next to your sides, your palms facing each other.

- Stand in a staggered stance, your left foot in front of your right.

B

- Slowly lower your body as far as you can.

- Pause, then push yourself back up to the starting position as quickly as you can.

- Complete the prescribed number of reps with your left foot forward, then do the same number with your right foot in front of your left.

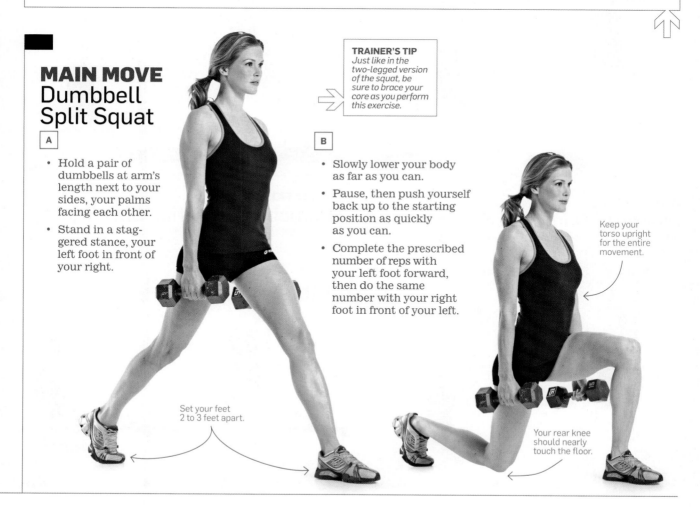

Keep your torso upright for the entire movement.

Set your feet 2 to 3 feet apart.

Your rear knee should nearly touch the floor.

Quads & Calves | SQUATS

VARIATION #1
Elevated-Front-Foot Dumbbell Split Squat
• Place your front foot on a 6-inch step or box.

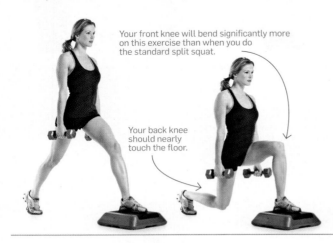

Your front knee will bend significantly more on this exercise than when you do the standard split squat.

Your back knee should nearly touch the floor.

VARIATION #2
Elevated-Back-Foot Dumbbell Split Squat
• Place your back foot on a 6-inch step or box.

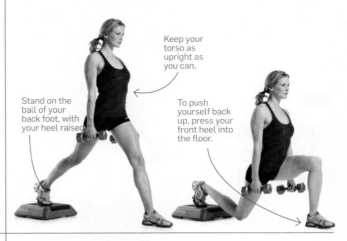

Keep your torso as upright as you can.

Stand on the ball of your back foot, with your heel raised.

To push yourself back up, press your front heel into the floor.

VARIATION #3
Overhead Dumbbell Split Squat
• Hold a pair of dumbbells directly over your shoulders, with your arms completely straight.

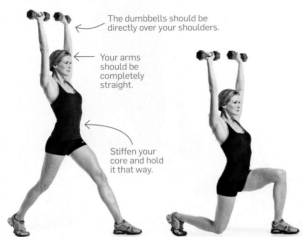

The dumbbells should be directly over your shoulders.

Your arms should be completely straight.

Stiffen your core and hold it that way.

VARIATION #4
Dumbbell Bulgarian Split Squat
• Place just the instep of your back foot on a bench.

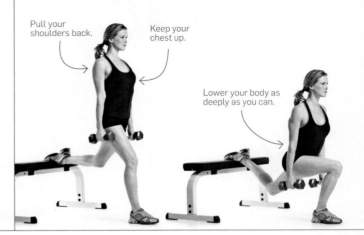

Pull your shoulders back.

Keep your chest up.

Lower your body as deeply as you can.

VARIATION #5

Dumbbell Split Jump

University of North Carolina scientists found that doing exercises like the split jump for 3 weeks can spike your vertical leap by up to 9 percent.

Keep your torso as upright as you can.

While in the air, scissor-kick your legs so you land with the opposite leg forward.

A
- From a standing position, lower your body into a split squat.

B
- Quickly switch directions and jump with enough force to propel both feet off the floor.

C
- Repeat, alternating back and forth with each repetition.

MUSCLE MISTAKE
You're Still Doing Leg Extensions

While the leg extension machine may seem like a safer alternative to squats and even lunges, it's actually quite the opposite. Case in point: Physiologists at the Mayo Clinic determined that leg extensions place significantly more stress on your knees than free-weight squats do. Why? Because the resistance is placed near your ankles, which leads to high amounts of torque being applied to your knee joint every time you lower the weight.

211

Quads & Calves

These exercises target your quadriceps. However, they also work just about all of the other muscles of your lower body, including your glutes, hamstrings, and calves.

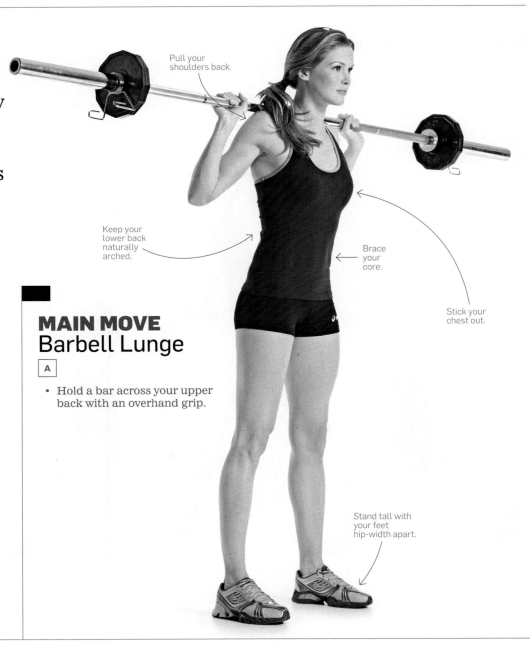

Pull your shoulders back.

Keep your lower back naturally arched.

Brace your core.

Stick your chest out.

Stand tall with your feet hip-width apart.

MAIN MOVE
Barbell Lunge

A

- Hold a bar across your upper back with an overhand grip.

1

Number of sets of an exercise needed to boost your levels of fat-burning hormones, according to a study at Ball State University.

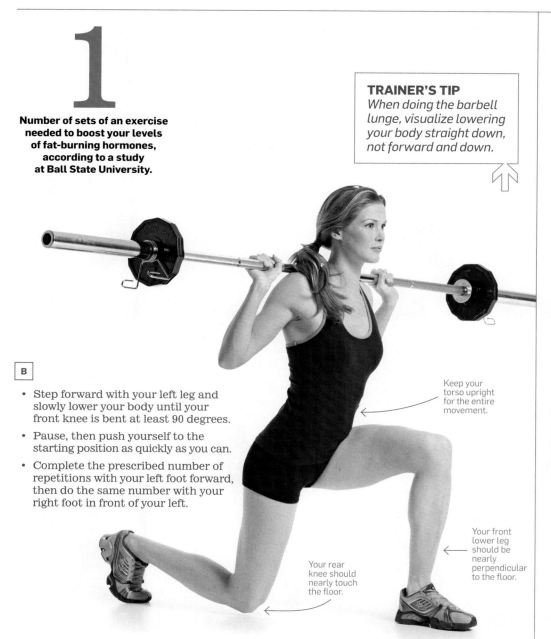

Keep your torso upright for the entire movement.

B

- Step forward with your left leg and slowly lower your body until your front knee is bent at least 90 degrees.

- Pause, then push yourself to the starting position as quickly as you can.

- Complete the prescribed number of repetitions with your left foot forward, then do the same number with your right foot in front of your left.

Your rear knee should nearly touch the floor.

Your front lower leg should be nearly perpendicular to the floor.

VARIATION #1
Alternating Barbell Lunge

- Instead of performing all of your reps with one leg before repeating with the other, alternate back and forth—doing one rep with your left, then one rep with your right.

VARIATION #2
Walking Barbell Lunge

- Instead of pushing your body backward to the starting position, raise up and bring your back foot forward so that you move forward (like you're walking) a step with every rep. Alternate the leg you step forward with each time.

VARIATION #3
Reverse Barbell Lunge

- Step backward with your right leg (instead of forward with your left). Then lower your body into a lunge. This looks the same in a photo as the barbell lunge. Do all your reps and repeat with your other leg. You can also use the alterating technique, stepping backward with a different leg each rep.

Quads & Calves | LUNGES

VARIATION #4
Barbell Box Lunge

- Place a 6-inch step or box about 2 feet in front of you.
- Step forward onto the box with your left leg, and then lower your body into a lunge.

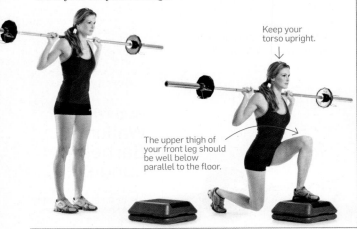

Keep your torso upright.

The upper thigh of your front leg should be well below parallel to the floor.

VARIATION #5
Reverse Barbell Box Lunge

- Stand on a 6-inch step or box.
- Step backward with your left leg into a lunge.

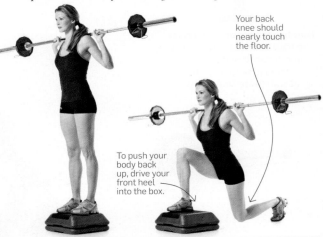

Your back knee should nearly touch the floor.

To push your body back up, drive your front heel into the box.

VARIATION #6
Barbell Stepover

A
- Place a 6-inch step or box about 2 feet in front of you, and stand with your feet hip-width apart.

B
- Step forward onto the step with your left foot as you lower your body into a lunge.

C
- Push yourself up so that you lift your right foot over the step and onto the floor in front of you.

D
- Lower yourself into a lunge.
- Reverse the movement to return to the starting position.

Don't allow your momentum to cause you to bend your torso forward; you should remain upright.

Drive your front heel into the box to push your body up.

VARIATION #7
Barbell Crossover Lunge

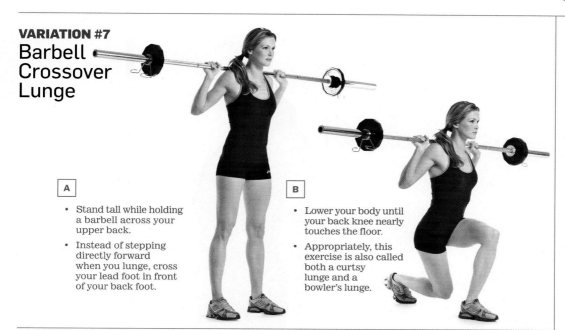

A

- Stand tall while holding a barbell across your upper back.
- Instead of stepping directly forward when you lunge, cross your lead foot in front of your back foot.

B

- Lower your body until your back knee nearly touches the floor.
- Appropriately, this exercise is also called both a curtsy lunge and a bowler's lunge.

VARIATION #8
Reverse Barbell Crossover Lunge

- Instead of stepping forward, step backward and cross your rear foot behind your front foot. These start and finish positions look identical to those in the photo of the barbell crossover lunge. This is also known as a drop lunge.

VARIATION #9
Barbell Side Lunge

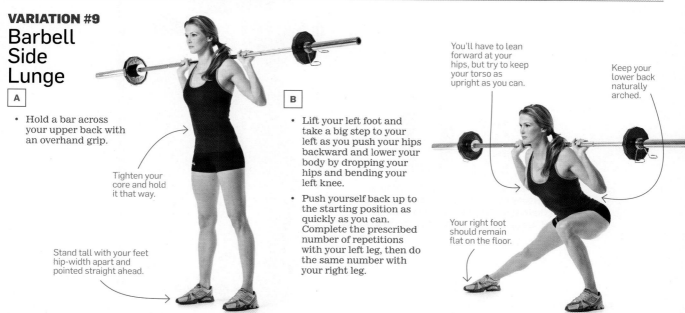

A

- Hold a bar across your upper back with an overhand grip.

Tighten your core and hold it that way.

Stand tall with your feet hip-width apart and pointed straight ahead.

B

- Lift your left foot and take a big step to your left as you push your hips backward and lower your body by dropping your hips and bending your left knee.
- Push yourself back up to the starting position as quickly as you can. Complete the prescribed number of repetitions with your left leg, then do the same number with your right leg.

You'll have to lean forward at your hips, but try to keep your torso as upright as you can.

Keep your lower back naturally arched.

Your right foot should remain flat on the floor.

215

Pull your
shoulders back.

Lift your
chest up.

Stand as
tall as
you can.

Brace your core
and hold it that
way for the
entire exercise.

MAIN MOVE
Dumbbell Lunge

- Grab a pair of dumbbells and hold
  them at arm's length next to your
  sides, your palms facing each other.

50

**Percent less likely people were to die
of heart disease when they first started working out
in their 40s compared to those who never
got off the couch, according to a German study.**

Stand tall with
your feet
hip-width apart.

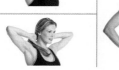

BODY-WEIGHT LUNGE

You can do just about any version of the lunge without holding weights of any kind. Simply cross your arms in front of your chest, or place your hands on your hips or behind your ears. These are ideal warmup exercises and are also valuable as great alternatives to the weighted variations.

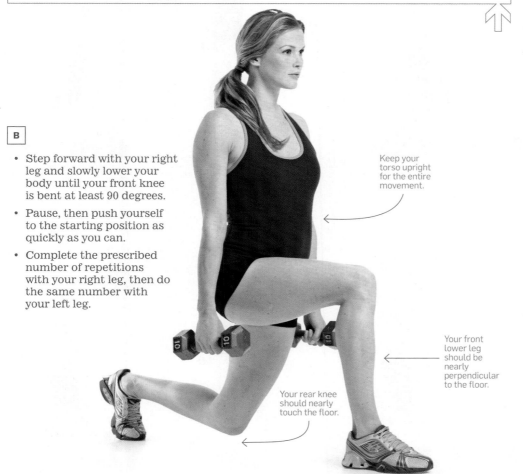

B

- Step forward with your right leg and slowly lower your body until your front knee is bent at least 90 degrees.

- Pause, then push yourself to the starting position as quickly as you can.

- Complete the prescribed number of repetitions with your right leg, then do the same number with your left leg.

Keep your torso upright for the entire movement.

Your front lower leg should be nearly perpendicular to the floor.

Your rear knee should nearly touch the floor.

VARIATION #1
Alternating Dumbbell Lunge

- Instead of performing all of your reps with one leg before repeating with the other, alternate back and forth— doing one rep with your left, then one rep with your right.

VARIATION #2
Walking Dumbbell Lunge

- Instead of pushing your body backward to the starting position, raise up and bring your back foot forward so that you move forward (like you're walking) a step with every rep. Alternate the leg you step forward with each time.

VARIATION #3
Reverse Dumbbell Lunge

- Step backward with your left leg. Then lower your body into a lunge. This looks the same in a photo as the dumbbell lunge. Do all your reps and repeat with your other leg. You can also use the alterating technique.

Quads & Calves | LUNGES

VARIATION #4
Dumbbell Box Lunge

- Place a 6-inch step or box about 2 feet in front of you.
- Step forward onto the box with your left leg, and then lower your body into a lunge.

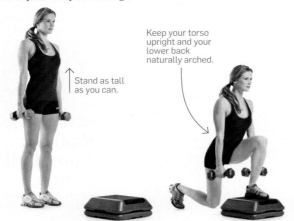

Stand as tall as you can.

Keep your torso upright and your lower back naturally arched.

VARIATION #5
Reverse Dumbbell Box Lunge

- Stand on a 6-inch step or box, and step backward with your left leg into a lunge.

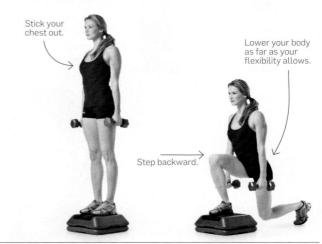

Stick your chest out.

Lower your body as far as your flexibility allows.

Step backward.

VARIATION #6
Dumbbell Stepover

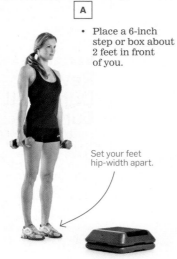

A
- Place a 6-inch step or box about 2 feet in front of you.

Set your feet hip-width apart.

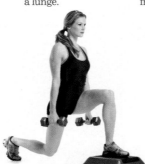

B
- Step forward onto the step with your left foot as you lower your body into a lunge.

C
- Push yourself up so that you lift your right foot over the step and onto the floor in front of you.

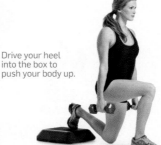

Drive your heel into the box to push your body up.

D
- Lower yourself into a lunge.
- Reverse the movement to return to the starting position.

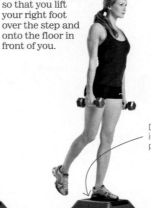

VARIATION #7
Reverse Dumbbell Box Lunge with Forward Reach

Hold the dumbbells so that your palms are facing each other.

Keep your lower back naturally arched.

- Stand on a 6-inch box or step, holding a pair of light dumbbells at your sides.
- Step backward into a lunge with your left leg as you lean forward at your hips and reach toward your feet. Reverse the movement to return to the starting position.

Step backward.

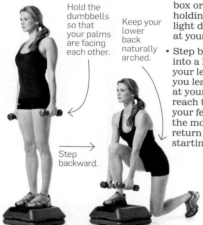

VARIATION #8
Dumbbell Crossover Lunge

- Instead of stepping directly forward when you lunge, cross your lead foot in front of your back foot, as if you were doing a curtsy.

Keep your torso as upright as possible.

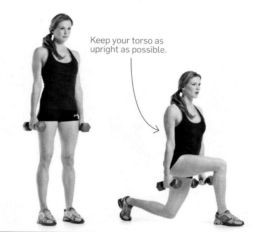

VARIATION #9
Reverse Dumbbell Crossover Lunge

- Instead of stepping forward, step backward and cross your rear foot behind your front foot.

VARIATION #10
Dumbbell Lunge and Rotation

- Grab a dumbbell and hold it by the ends, just below your chin.
- Step forward into a lunge. As you lunge, rotate your upper body toward the same side as the leg you're using to step forward.

If you're stepping forward with your left leg, rotate your torso to your left side. If you're stepping with your right, rotate to your right.

Brace your core and hold it that way for the entire movement.

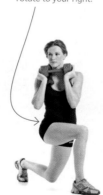

VARIATION #11
Overhead Dumbbell Lunge

- Hold a pair of dumbbells directly over your shoulders, with your arms completely straight.
- Step forward with your right leg into a lunge.

Don't allow the weight to carry you forward. Instead, think about dropping your hips straight down as you step forward. Keep your abs tight and your chest up.

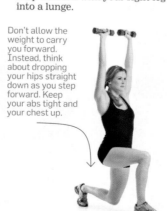

VARIATION #12
Overhead Dumbbell Reverse Lunge

- This time, step backward with your left leg into a lunge.

Quads & Calves | LUNGES

VARIATION #13
Offset Dumbbell Lunge

- Hold a dumbbell in your right hand next to your shoulder, with your arm bent.
- Step forward into a lunge with your right foot.
- Complete the prescribed number of reps on that side, then switch arms and lunge with your left leg for the same number of reps.

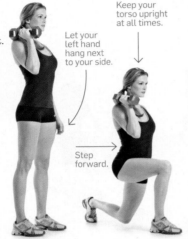

Let your left hand hang next to your side.

Keep your torso upright at all times.

Step forward.

STRENGTHEN YOUR CORE
Holding a weight on just one side of your body increases the demand placed on your core to keep your body stable.

VARIATION #14
Offset Dumbbell Reverse Lunge

- Hold a dumbbell in your left hand next to your shoulder, with your arm bent.
- Step backward into a lunge with your right foot.
- Complete the prescribed number of reps on that side, then switch arms and lunge backward with your left leg for the same number of reps.

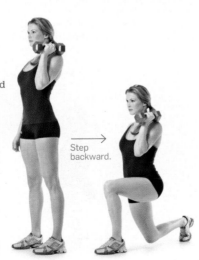

Step backward.

VARIATION #15
Dumbbell Rotational Lunge

A
- Hold a pair of dumbbells at arm's length next to your sides, your palms facing each other.
- Lift your left foot and step to the left and back, placing that foot so it's diagonal to your body and pointed toward 8 o'clock.

B
- Shift your weight onto your left leg, pivot on your right foot, and lower your body into a lunge as you simultaneously rotate your torso and the dumbbells to the left, over your front leg.
- Reverse the movement and push yourself back up to the start.
- Complete the prescribed number of reps with your left leg, then do the same number with your right leg. (Your right foot will point to 4 o'clock.)

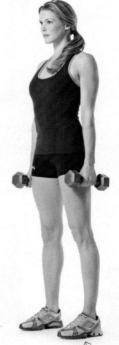

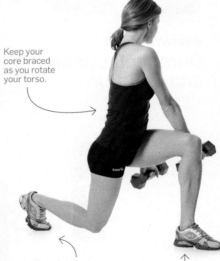

Keep your core braced as you rotate your torso.

Stand tall with your feet hip-width apart, pointing ahead to 12 o'clock.

Your right foot should rotate to point in the same direction as your left foot.

Your left foot should point to 8 o'clock in relation to your starting position.

VARIATION #16
Dumbbell Side Lunge

- Hold a pair of dumbbells at arm's length next to your sides, your palms facing each other.
- Lift your left foot and take a big step to your left as you push your hips backward and lower your body by dropping your hips and bending your left knee.
- Pause, then quickly push yourself back to the starting position.

Your right foot should remain flat on the floor.

Your feet should be pointed straight ahead in both the up and the down positions.

VARIATION #17
Dumbbell Diagonal Lunge

- Instead of stepping straight forward, lunge diagonally at a 45-degree angle.
- Complete all your reps, then switch legs and repeat.

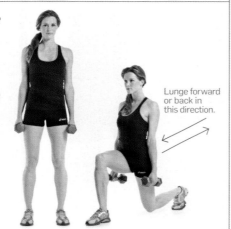

Lunge forward or back in this direction.

VARIATION #18
Reverse Dumbbell Diagonal Lunge

- You can also perform this exercise by lunging backward at a 45-degree angle.

VARIATION #19
Dumbbell Side Lunge and Touch

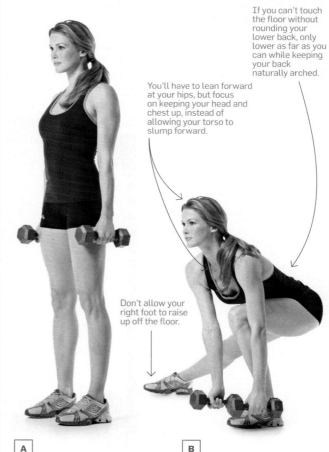

If you can't touch the floor without rounding your lower back, only lower as far as you can while keeping your back naturally arched.

You'll have to lean forward at your hips, but focus on keeping your head and chest up, instead of allowing your torso to slump forward.

Don't allow your right foot to raise up off the floor.

A
- Hold a pair of dumbbells at arm's length next to your sides.

B
- As you lower your body into a side lunge, bend forward at your hips and touch the dumbbells to the floor.

These exercises target your hip adductors, the muscles on the inside of your upper thigh.

MAIN MOVE
Standing Cable Hip Adduction

A

- Attach an ankle strap to the low pulley of a cable station, and then place the strap around your right ankle.
- Stand with your right side facing the weight stack.
- Take a big step away from the weight stack so that when you move your right leg toward the weight stack, the cable remains taut.
- Raise your right leg straight out to the side, toward the weight stack.

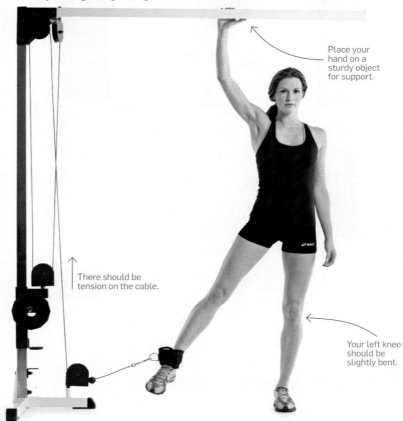

Place your hand on a sturdy object for support.

There should be tension on the cable.

Your left knee should be slightly bent.

- Without bending your knee, pull your right leg sideways so that it crosses in front of your left leg.
- Pause, then slowly return to the starting position. Complete the prescribed number of repetitions with your right leg, then do the same number with your left leg.

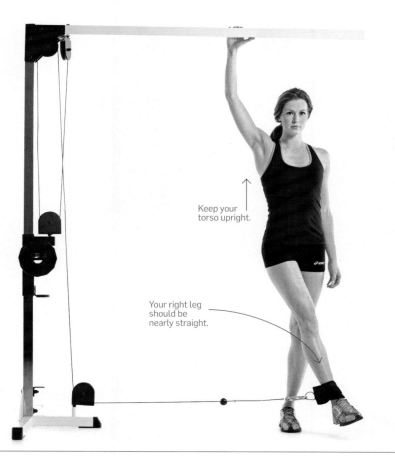

Keep your torso upright.

Your right leg should be nearly straight.

VARIATION #1
Valslide Hip Adduction

- Kneel on the floor and place each knee on a Valslide.

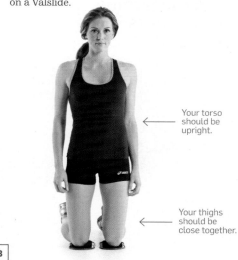

Your torso should be upright.

Your thighs should be close together.

B

- Push your knees out as far as you can.
- Pause, then pull your knees back together again.

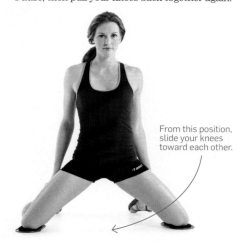

From this position, slide your knees toward each other.

223

Quads & Calves | CALF RAISES

The targets for these exercises are your gastrocnemius and soleus muscles.

MAIN MOVE
Standing Barbell Calf Raise

A

- Grab a barbell with an overhand grip and place it so that it rests comfortably across your upper back.
- Place the ball of each foot on a 25-pound weight plate.

B

- Rise up on your toes as high as you can.
- Pause, then slowly lower back to the starting position.

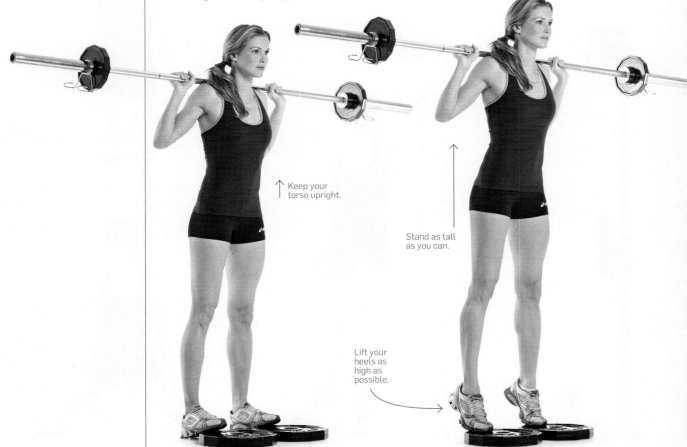

↑ Keep your torso upright.

Stand as tall as you can.

Lift your heels as high as possible.

VARIATION #1
Single-Leg Standing Dumbbell Calf Raise

A

- Grab a dumbbell in your right hand and stand on a step, block, or 25-pound weight plate.

- Cross your left foot behind your right ankle, and balance yourself on the ball of your right foot, with your right heel on the floor or hanging off a step.

Put your left hand on something stable—a wall or weight stack, for instance.

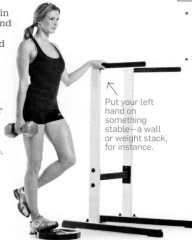

B

- Lift your right heel as high as you can. Pause, then lower and repeat.

- Complete the prescribed number of reps with your right leg, then do the same number with your left (while holding the dumbbell in your left hand).

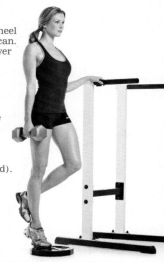

VARIATION #2
Single-Leg Bent-Knee Calf Raise

- Bend your knee, and hold it that way as you perform the exercise.

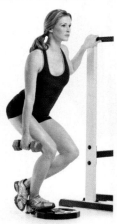
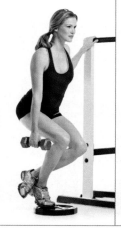

VARIATION #3
Single-Leg Donkey Calf Raise

- Keeping your back naturally arched, bend at your hips and lower your torso until your upper body is almost parallel to the floor.

- Complete the prescribed number of reps with your right leg, then do the same number with your left.

Don't round your lower back.

Place your hands on a sturdy object for support.

Raise your heel as high as you can.

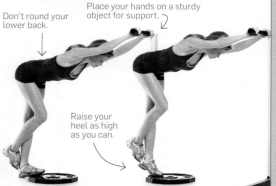

Bend for Great Calves

Of the two muscles that make up your calf, your soleus is more involved in extending your ankle when your knee is bent. Your gastrocnemius takes on a greater workload when your knee is straight. As a result, bent-leg calf raises target your soleus best, while standing calf raises—performed with your knee straight—zero in on your gastrocnemius. That's why if your calves don't seem to be growing, many experts recommend doing both versions of the exercise.

Quads & Calves

THE BEST QUADRICEPS EXERCISE YOU'VE NEVER DONE
Wide-Grip Overhead Barbell Split Squat

This movement is known as a "big bang" exercise since it works so many muscles at once. While your legs are the obvious emphasis during the split-squat portion of the move, holding the weight over your head challenges your shoulders, arms, upper back, and core, too. So it's a great strength and muscle builder, but it also burns tons of calories. If you're intimidated by holding a barbell overhead, start by performing it with just a broomstick or a pole instead.

A
- Hold a barbell straight over your head with an overhand grip that's about twice shoulder width.
- Stand in a staggered stance with your feet 2 to 3 feet apart.

B
- Slowly lower your body as far as you can.
- Pause, then push yourself back up to the starting position as quickly as you can.
- Complete the prescribed number of repetitions with your left leg forward, then do the same number with your right leg in front.

Lock your elbows.

Hold your shoulders down and back. You should try to create as much space between your shoulders and your ears as you can.

Brace your core.

Your left foot should be in front of your right one.

Don't allow the bar to move forward as you squat.

Your arms should be straight.

Keep your torso upright for the entire movement.

Bend the knee of your front leg.

Your rear knee should nearly touch the floor.

226

THE BEST CALF EXERCISE YOU'VE NEVER DONE
Farmer's Walk on Toes

This exercise not only works your calves but also improves your cardiovascular fitness. Choose the heaviest pair of dumbbells that allows you to perform the exercise for 60 seconds. If you feel like you could have gone longer, grab heavier weights on your next set.

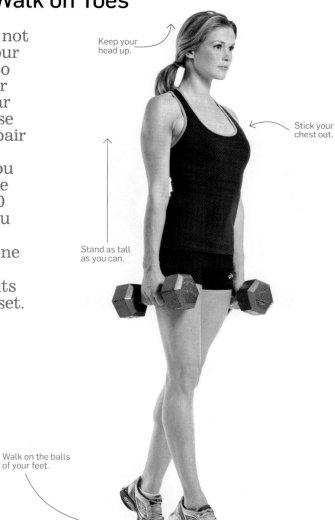

Keep your head up.

Stick your chest out.

Stand as tall as you can.

Walk on the balls of your feet.

A

- Grab a pair of heavy dumbbells and hold them at your sides at arm's length.

B

- Raise your heels and walk forward (or in a circle) for 60 seconds.

Quads & Calves

THE BEST STRETCH FOR YOUR QUADRICEPS
Kneeling Hip Flexor Stretch

Why it's good: This stretch loosens the muscles at the top of your thigh. When these muscles are tight, they pull your pelvis forward, which increases stress on your lower back and decreases the range of motion of your hips.

Make the most of it: Hold this stretch for 30 seconds on each side, then repeat twice for a total of three sets. Perform this routine daily, and up to three times a day if you're really tight.

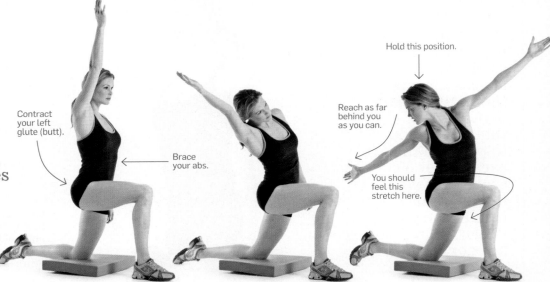

Contract your left glute (butt).

Brace your abs.

Hold this position.

Reach as far behind you as you can.

You should feel this stretch here.

A
- Kneel down on your left knee, with your right foot on the floor and your right knee bent 90 degrees.
- Reach up with your right hand as high as you can.

B
- Bend your torso to your right.

C
- Rotate your torso to the right as you reach with your right hand as far behind you as you can. Hold this position for the prescribed length of time.
- Kneel on your right knee, switch arms, and repeat.

10

Percentage reduction in the risk of groin injury for every degree that you increase your hip range of motion, according to a study in the *Journal of Science and Medicine in Sport*.

THE BEST STRETCHES FOR YOUR CALVES

Straight-Leg Calf Stretch

Why it's good: It emphasizes your gastrocnemius.

Make the most of it: Hold this stretch for 30 seconds on each side, then repeat twice for a total of three sets. Perform this routine daily, and up to three times a day if you're really tight.

- Stand about 2 feet in front of a wall in a staggered stance.
- Place your hands on the wall and lean against it.
- Shift your weight to your back foot until you feel a stretch in your calf. Hold for the prescribed length of time.
- Switch leg positions and repeat.

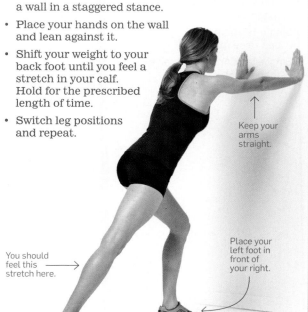

Keep your arms straight.

You should feel this stretch here.

Place your left foot in front of your right.

Bent-Leg Calf Stretch

Why it's good: It emphasizes your soleus.

Make the most of it: Hold this stretch for 30 seconds on each side, then repeat twice for a total of three sets. Perform this routine daily, and up to three times a day if you're really tight.

- Perform this the same as the straight-leg calf stretch, only move your back foot forward so the toes of that foot are even with the heel of your front foot.
- Bend both knees until you feel a comfortable stretch just above the ankle of your back leg.

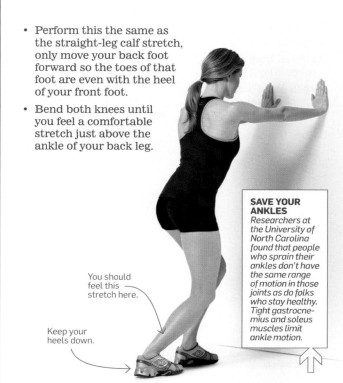

You should feel this stretch here.

Keep your heels down.

SAVE YOUR ANKLES
Researchers at the University of North Carolina found that people who sprain their ankles don't have the same range of motion in those joints as do folks who stay healthy. Tight gastrocnemius and soleus muscles limit ankle motion.

Quads & Calves

SCULPT PERFECT QUADS AND CALVES

Try these workouts from Kelly Baggett, performance coach and co-owner of Transformation Clinics in Springfield, Missouri. The quadriceps routine is a create-your-own workout that's designed to shape, firm, and strengthen your thighs. The calf workout is a personal favorite of Kelly's, since as he says, "You can do it anytime, anyplace." That includes your living room.

The Quad Workout

What to do: Choose one movement from Exercise Group A and one movement from Exercise Group B. For Exercise A, do four sets of 6 to 8 repetitions, resting for 3 minutes between sets. For Exercise B, do two sets of 10 to 12 repetitions for each leg, resting for 2 minutes between sets. Complete this workout once or twice a week.

EXERCISE GROUP A

Dumbbell squat (page 203)

Goblet squat (page 204)

Dumbbell front squat (page 204)

Barbell squat (page 198)

Barbell squat with heels raised (page 201)

Barbell front squat (page 199)

EXERCISE GROUP B

Reverse dumbbell lunge (page 217)

Reverse barbell lunge (page 213)

Dumbbell Bulgarian split squat (page 210)

Barbell Bulgarian split squat (page 208)

Single-leg squat (page 196)

Pistol squat (page 197)

The Calf Workout

What to do: Do one set of each exercise, in the order shown and without resting. For each exercise, complete as many repetitions as you can. One note: Perform the exercises as directed in this chapter, only skip the dumbbells—the routine is designed to be done with just your body weight. Complete the workout twice a week.

EXERCISES

Single-leg standing dumbbell calf raise (page 225)

Single-leg bent-knee calf raise (page 225)

Single-leg donkey calf raise (page 225)

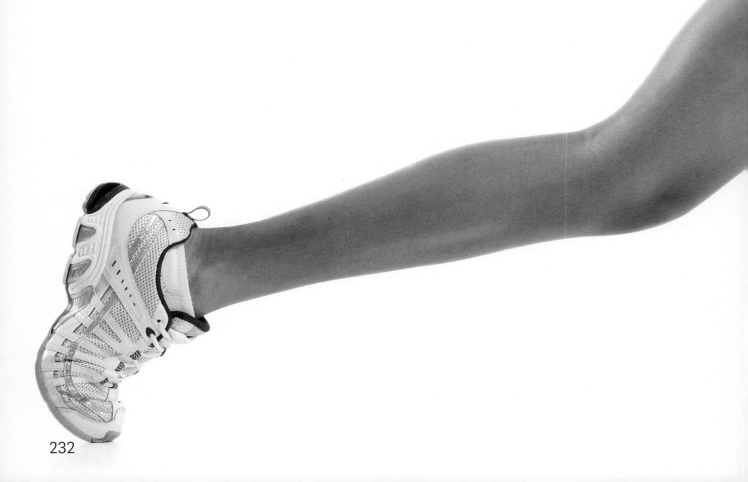

Chapter 9:
Glutes & Hamstrings
THE MUSCLES YOU CAN'T IGNORE

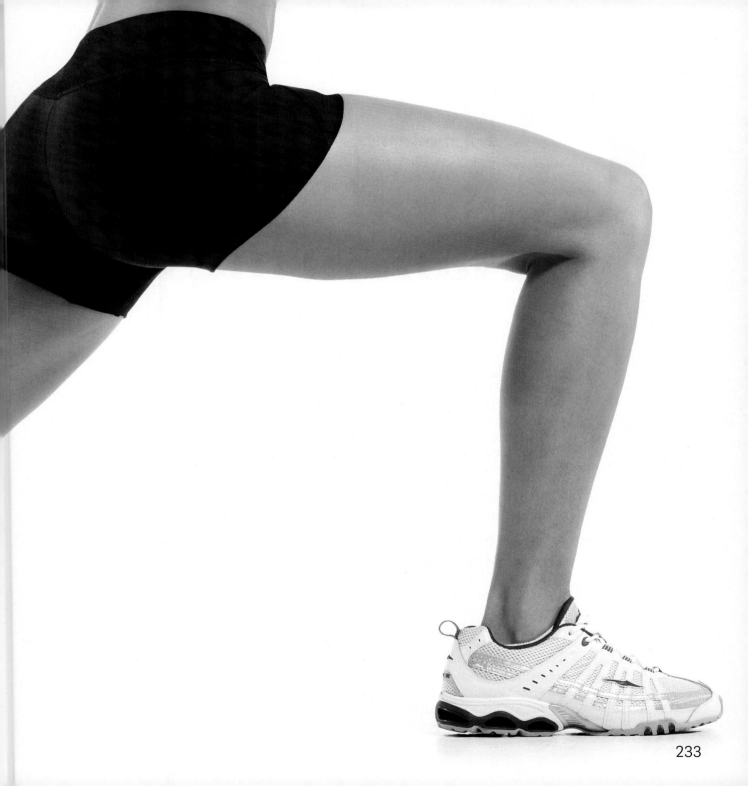

Glutes
& Hamstrings

Anytime you're standing, the muscles of your glutes and hamstrings are working. Trouble is, most of us are spending more and more of our days sitting—whether in front of a computer or 46-inch plasma. The impact of so much chair time: Our hip muscles not only become weak, they forget how to contract. This is especially true for your glutes. And that's a shame, since your glutes are your body's largest and perhaps most powerful muscle group.

What's more, when either your glutes or hamstrings are weak, it disrupts the muscular balance of your body, which can cause pain and injuries in your knees, hips, and lower back. The solution? Make working your glutes and hamstrings a top priority, using the exercises in this chapter.

Bonus Benefits

Greater calorie burn! Since the glutes are your biggest muscle group, they're also one of your top calorie burners.

No more pooch! Weak glutes can cause your hips to tilt forward. This puts more stress on your spine, which can lead to lower back discomfort. It also pushes your lower abdomen outward, making your tummy stick out. So to loose the pooch, strengthen your glutes!

Healthier knees! A strong set of hamstrings helps your anterior cruciate ligaments (ACLs) better stabilize your knees, lowering your risk of injury.

Meet Your Muscles

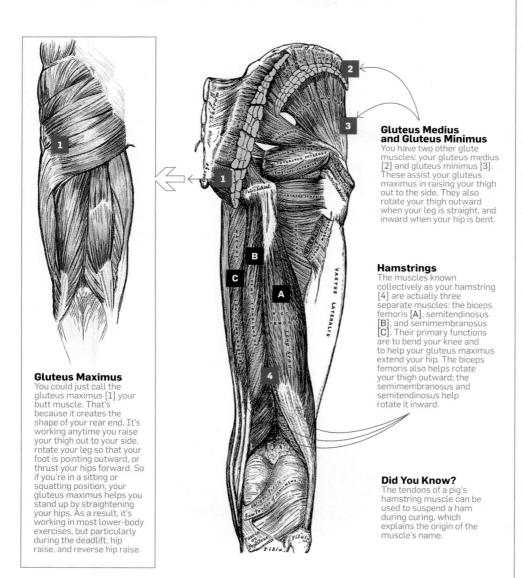

Gluteus Maximus

You could just call the gluteus maximus [1] your butt muscle. That's because it creates the shape of your rear end. It's working anytime you raise your thigh out to your side, rotate your leg so that your foot is pointing outward, or thrust your hips forward. So if you're in a sitting or squatting position, your gluteus maximus helps you stand up by straightening your hips. As a result, it's working in most lower-body exercises, but particularly during the deadlift, hip raise, and reverse hip raise.

Gluteus Medius and Gluteus Minimus

You have two other glute muscles: your gluteus medius [2] and gluteus minimus [3]. These assist your gluteus maximus in raising your thigh out to the side. They also rotate your thigh outward when your leg is straight, and inward when your hip is bent.

Hamstrings

The muscles known collectively as your hamstring [4] are actually three separate muscles: the biceps femoris [A], semitendinosus [B], and semimembranosus [C]. Their primary functions are to bend your knee and to help your gluteus maximus extend your hip. The biceps femoris also helps rotate your thigh outward; the semimembranosus and semitendinosus help rotate it inward.

Did You Know?

The tendons of a pig's hamstring muscle can be used to suspend a ham during curing, which explains the origin of the muscle's name.

MUSCLE MISTAKE
You Work Your Quads Harder Than Your Hamstrings

A study in the *American Journal of Sports Medicine* found that 70 percent of athletes with recurrent hamstring injuries suffered from muscle imbalances between their quadriceps and hamstrings. After correcting the imbalances by strengthening the hamstrings, every person in the study went injury-free for the entire 12-month follow-up. Now that's strong medicine.

Glutes & Hams | HIP RAISES

In this chapter, you'll find 62 exercises that target the muscles of your glutes and hamstrings. Throughout, you'll notice that certain exercises have been given the designation Main Move. Master this basic version of a movement, and you'll be able to do all of its variations with flawless form.

HIP RAISES

These exercises target the muscles of your glutes and hamstrings. What's more, they require you to activate your abdominal and lower-back muscles in order to keep your body stable—so they double as great core exercises.

MAIN MOVE
Hip Raises

- Lie faceup on the floor with your knees bent and your feet flat on the floor.

Make sure you're pushing with your heels. To make it easier, you can position your feet so that your toes rise off the floor.

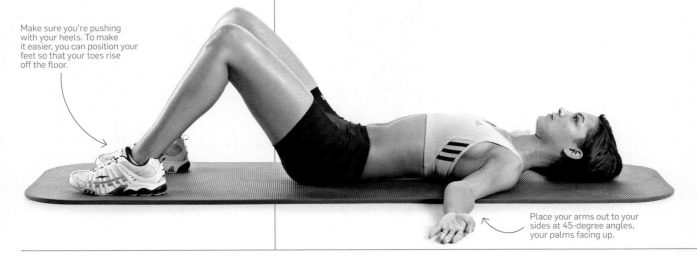

Place your arms out to your sides at 45-degree angles, your palms facing up.

GET YOUR BUTT IN GEAR
If your hamstrings cramp when you perform the hip raise, it's often a sign that your glutes are weak. That's because your hamstrings are having to work extra hard to keep your hips raised. For best results, raise your hips and hold them that way for 3 to 5 seconds per repetition. Twice a week, do two or three sets of 10 to 12 reps.

B

- Raise your hips so your body forms a straight line from your shoulders to your knees.
- Pause for up to 5 seconds in the up position, then lower your body back to the starting position.

15

Minutes of exercise it takes to improve your mood, according to a study in the *Journal of Sports and Exercise Psychology*.

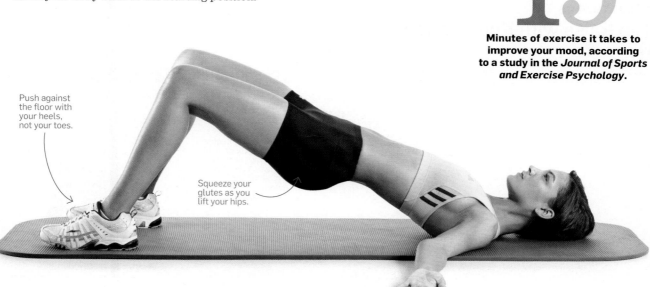

Push against the floor with your heels, not your toes.

Squeeze your glutes as you lift your hips.

Glutes & Hams | HIP RAISES

VARIATION #1
Weighted Hip Raise
- Place a weight plate on your hips and perform the exercise.

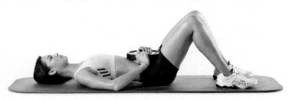

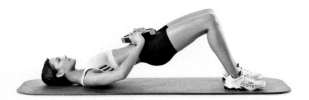

VARIATION #2
Hip Raise with Knee Press-Out
- Place a 20-inch mini-band just above your knees, and keep your knees from touching each other as you perform the movement.

Pushing outward against a band increases the activation of your gluteus maximus and gluteus medius.

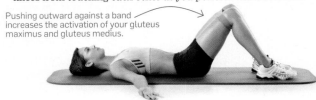

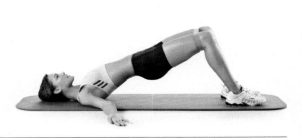

VARIATION #3
Hip Raise with Knee Squeeze

 A

- Place a rolled-up towel or an Airex pad between your knees, and hold it there as you perform the movement.

 B

- Don't allow the pad to slip as you raise your hips until your body forms a straight line from your shoulders to your knees.

TRAINER'S TIP
Pay attention as you raise your hips: If your knees tend to fall outward as you do the exercise, you probably have weak hip adductors, or groin muscles. Keeping a towel or cushion from falling to the floor as you do the exercise helps strengthen these inner-thigh muscles.

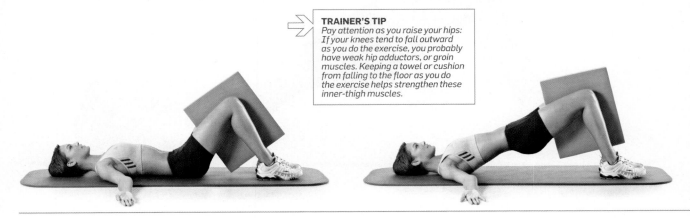

VARIATION #4
Marching Hip Raise
- Raise your hips and hold them that way.

- Lift one knee to your chest, lower back to the start, and lift your other knee to your chest. Continue to alternate back and forth.

VARIATION #5
Hip Raise with Feet on a Swiss Ball
- Perform the movement with your lower legs placed on a Swiss ball.

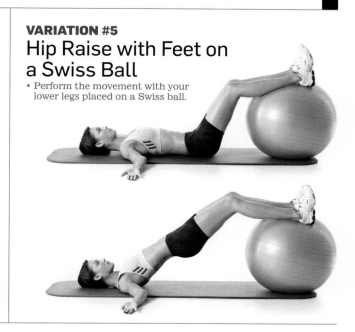

VARIATION #6
Marching Hip Raise with Feet on a Swiss Ball

A

- Place your feet flat on a Swiss ball.

B

- Lift one knee to your chest, lower back to the start, and lift your other knee to your chest. Continue to alternate back and forth.

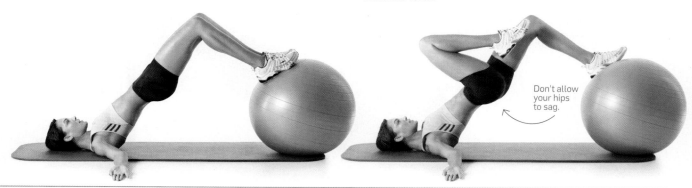

Don't allow your hips to sag.

Glutes & Hams | HIP RAISES

MAIN MOVE
Single-Leg Hip Raise

A

- Lie faceup on the floor with your left knee bent and your right leg straight.
- Raise your right leg until it's in line with your left thigh.

Place your arms out to your sides at 45-degree angles to your torso, your palms facing up.

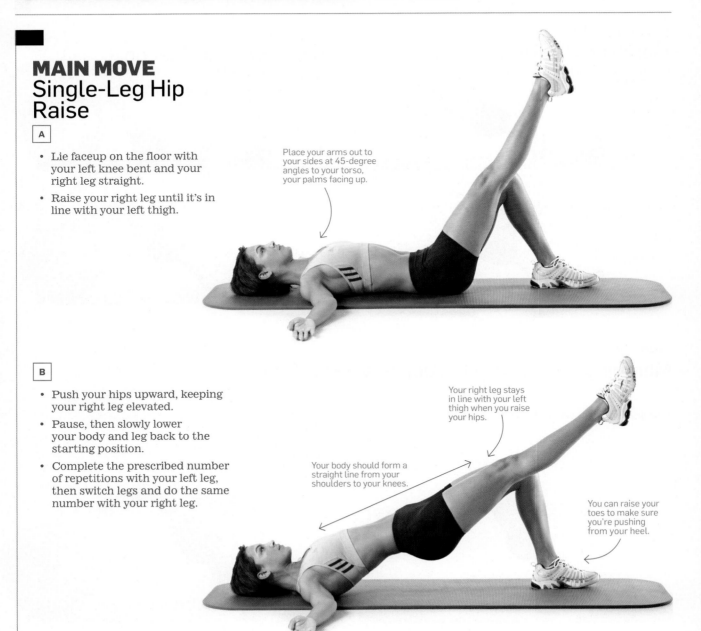

B

- Push your hips upward, keeping your right leg elevated.
- Pause, then slowly lower your body and leg back to the starting position.
- Complete the prescribed number of repetitions with your left leg, then switch legs and do the same number with your right leg.

Your right leg stays in line with your left thigh when you raise your hips.

Your body should form a straight line from your shoulders to your knees.

You can raise your toes to make sure you're pushing from your heel.

VARIATION #1
Single-Leg Hip Raise with Knee Hold

- Bring one knee toward your chest and hold it there as you perform the exercise.

TRAINER'S TIP
Holding one knee helps ensure you're using your glutes to raise your hips—and not your lower back muscles.

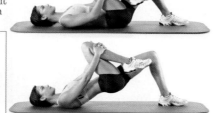

VARIATION #2
Single-Leg Hip Raise with Foot on a Bosu Ball

- Place your left foot on a Bosu ball.
- Raise your hips, lower, and repeat.

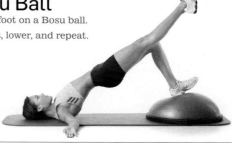

VARIATION #3
Single-Leg Hip Raise with Foot on Step

- Position your butt against a 6-inch step.
- Place your left foot on the step.
- Raise your hips, lower, and repeat.

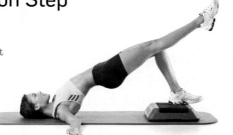
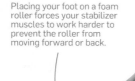

VARIATION #4
Single-Leg Hip Raise with Foot on Bench

- Place your left heel on a bench, with your butt on the floor.
- Raise your hips, lower, and repeat.

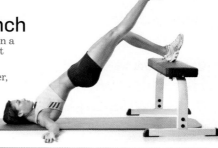

VARIATION #5
Single-Leg Hip Raise with Foot on a Foam Roller

Placing your foot on a foam roller forces your stabilizer muscles to work harder to prevent the roller from moving forward or back.

- Place your left foot on a foam roller.
- Raise your hips, lower, and repeat.

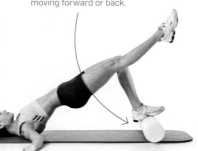

VARIATION #6
Single-Leg Hip Raise with Foot on a Medicine Ball

Placing your foot on a medicine ball forces your stabilizer muscles to work harder to prevent the ball from moving forward or back, or from side to side.

- Place your left foot on a medicine ball.
- Raise your hips, lower, and repeat.

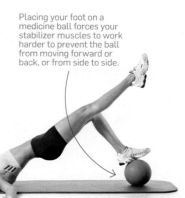

Glutes & Hams | HIP RAISES

VARIATION #7
Hip Raise with Head on a Bosu Ball
• Place your head and upper back on a Bosu ball.

Elevating your upper body increases the demand on your glutes.

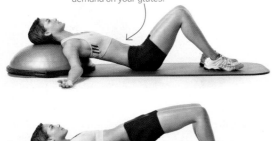

VARIATION #8
Single-Leg Hip Raise with Head on a Bosu Ball
• Place your head and upper back on a Bosu ball, and hold your left leg in the air so that it's in line with your right thigh.

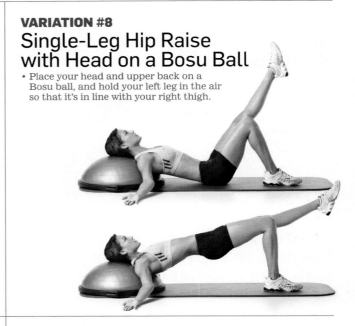

VARIATION #9
Hip Raise with Head on a Swiss Ball
• Place your head and upper back on a Swiss ball.

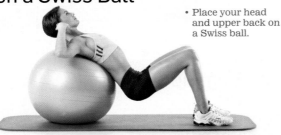

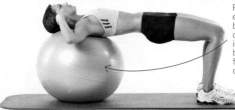

Performing this exercise on a Swiss ball forces your core to work harder in order to keep the ball from moving forward and back, or from side to side.

VARIATION #10
Single-Leg Hip Raise with Head on a Swiss Ball
• Place your head and upper back on a Swiss ball, and lift right leg in the air so that it's in line with your left thigh.

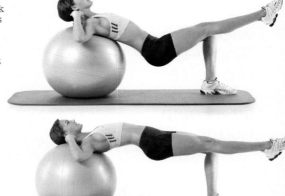

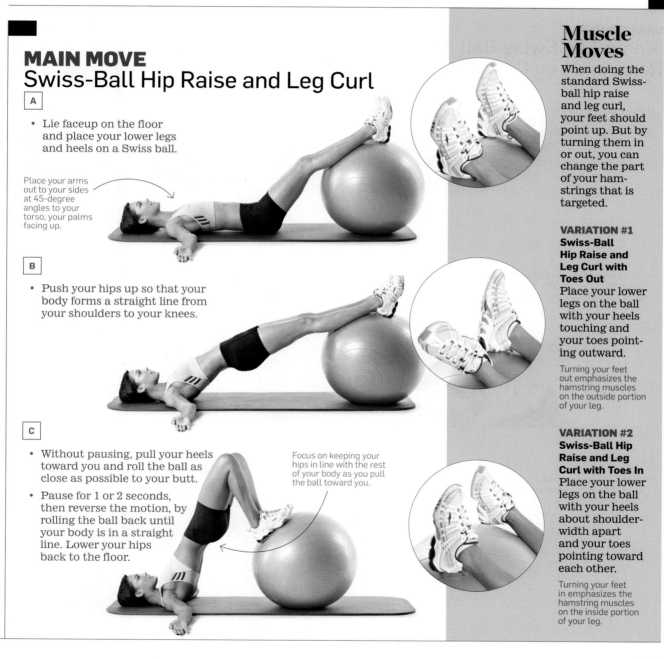

MAIN MOVE
Swiss-Ball Hip Raise and Leg Curl

A

- Lie faceup on the floor and place your lower legs and heels on a Swiss ball.

Place your arms out to your sides at 45-degree angles to your torso, your palms facing up.

B

- Push your hips up so that your body forms a straight line from your shoulders to your knees.

C

- Without pausing, pull your heels toward you and roll the ball as close as possible to your butt.

- Pause for 1 or 2 seconds, then reverse the motion, by rolling the ball back until your body is in a straight line. Lower your hips back to the floor.

Focus on keeping your hips in line with the rest of your body as you pull the ball toward you.

Muscle Moves

When doing the standard Swiss-ball hip raise and leg curl, your feet should point up. But by turning them in or out, you can change the part of your hamstrings that is targeted.

VARIATION #1
Swiss-Ball Hip Raise and Leg Curl with Toes Out
Place your lower legs on the ball with your heels touching and your toes pointing outward.

Turning your feet out emphasizes the hamstring muscles on the outside portion of your leg.

VARIATION #2
Swiss-Ball Hip Raise and Leg Curl with Toes In
Place your lower legs on the ball with your heels about shoulder-width apart and your toes pointing toward each other.

Turning your feet in emphasizes the hamstring muscles on the inside portion of your leg.

Glutes & Hams | HIP RAISES

VARIATION #3
Single-Leg Swiss-Ball Hip Raise and Leg Curl

A

- Raise your right leg in the air so that it's a few inches off the ball, nearly in line with your left thigh.

Place your arms out to your sides at 45-degree angles to your torso, your palms facing up.

B

- Push your hips up so that your body forms a straight line from your shoulders to your knees.

Squeeze your glutes as you lift your hips.

Brace your core.

C

- Without pausing, pull your left heel toward you and roll the ball as close as possible to your butt.

You should really feel this in your left hamstring.

MAIN MOVE
Sliding Leg Curl

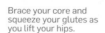

- Lie faceup on the floor and place each heel on a Valslide with your knees bent and your heels near your butt.

Brace your core and squeeze your glutes as you lift your hips.

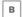

- Keeping your hips in line with your torso, slide your heels out until your legs are straight.
- Reverse the movement back to the starting position.

Your body should form a straight line from your shoulders to your knees.

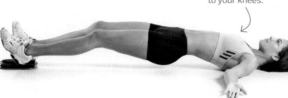

VARIATION
Single-Leg Sliding Leg Curl

- Raise your right leg in the air so that it's in line with your left thigh, and hold it that way as you perform the exercise.

- Keeping your hips in line with your torso, slide your heel out until your leg is straight.

Your body should form a straight line from your shoulders to your knees.

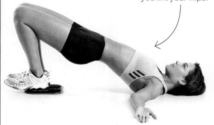

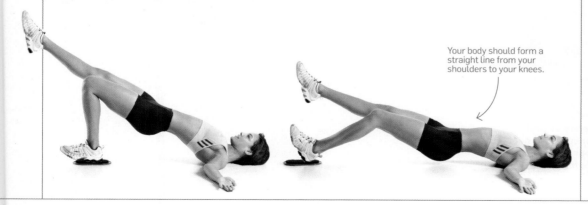

MAIN MOVE
Reverse Hip Raise

A

- Lie chest down on the edge of a bench or Roman chair so that your torso is on the bench but your hips aren't.

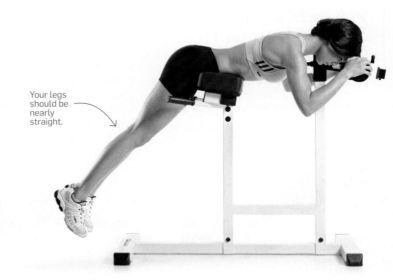

Your legs should be nearly straight.

B

- Lift your legs until your thighs are in line with your torso.
- Pause, then lower to the starting position.

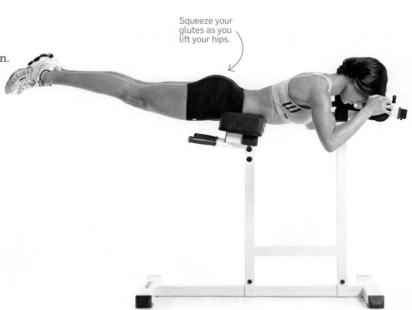

Squeeze your glutes as you lift your hips.

25

Minutes of weight training that actually improved the effectiveness of a subsequent flu shot, according to a study in *Brain, Behavior, and Immunity*. Scheduled to get pricked? Do your workout 6 to 12 hours beforehand.

VARIATION #1
Bent-Knee Reverse Hip Raise

- Start with your knees bent 90 degrees, and then straighten them as you raise your hips.

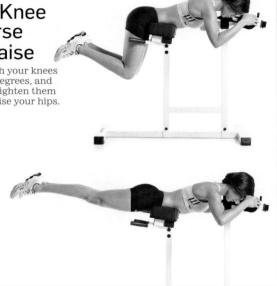

VARIATION #2
Swiss-Ball Reverse Hip Raise

- Instead of lying on a bench, lie on a Swiss ball and place your hands flat on the floor.

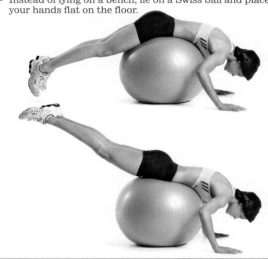

VARIATION #3
Bent-Knee Swiss-Ball Reverse Hip Raise

 A

- Instead of lying on a bench, lie on a Swiss ball and place your hands flat on the floor.

B

- Straighten your legs as you raise your hips.

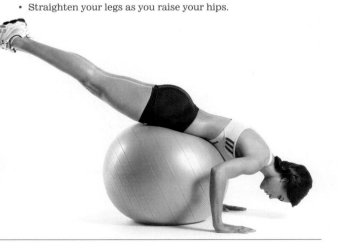

BENT-KNEE DEADLIFTS
These exercises target the muscles of your glutes and hamstrings, along with scores of others. In fact, because deadlifts strongly activate your quadriceps, core, back, and shoulder muscles, too, they're among the best total-body exercises you can do.

MAIN MOVE
Barbell Deadlift

A

- Load the barbell and roll it against your shins.
- Bend at your hips and knees and grab the bar with an overhand grip, your hands just beyond shoulder width.

B

- Without allowing your lower back to round, pull your torso back and up, thrust your hips forward, and stand up with the barbell.
- Squeeze your glutes as you perform the movement.
- Lower the bar to the floor, keeping it as close to your body as possible.

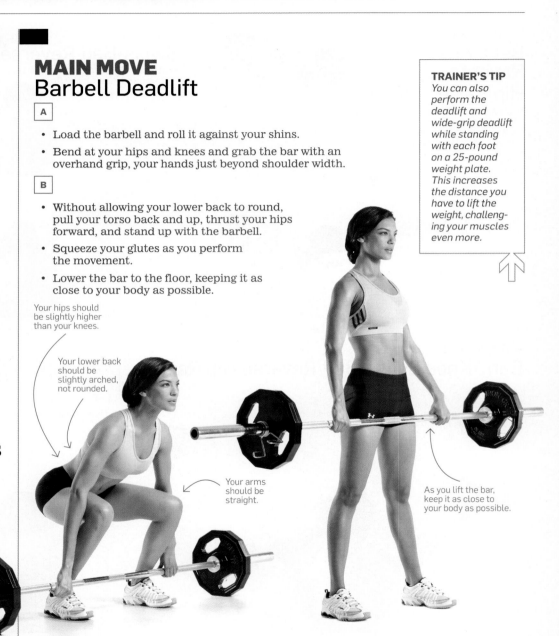

Your hips should be slightly higher than your knees.

Your lower back should be slightly arched, not rounded.

Your arms should be straight.

As you lift the bar, keep it as close to your body as possible.

TRAINER'S TIP
You can also perform the deadlift and wide-grip deadlift while standing with each foot on a 25-pound weight plate. This increases the distance you have to lift the weight, challenging your muscles even more.

VARIATION #1
Wide-Grip Barbell Deadlift

 A

- Use an overhand grip that's about twice shoulder width.

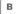 **B**

- Once standing, reverse the movement and slowly lower the bar back to the floor.

THE ULTIMATE DEADLIFT?
Using a wider grip provides three bonus benefits: (1) It increases the demand on your upper-back muscles, (2) forces your forearm and hand muscles to work harder, and (3) boosts your range of motion.

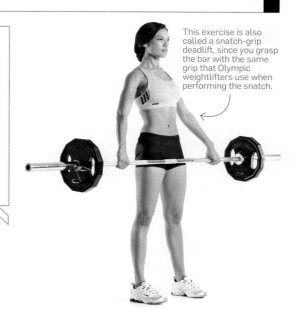

This exercise is also called a snatch-grip deadlift, since you grasp the bar with the same grip that Olympic weightlifters use when performing the snatch.

VARIATION #2
Single-Leg Barbell Deadlift

- Place the instep of one foot on a bench that's about 2 feet behind you.
- Complete the prescribed number of reps with your right foot on the bench, then do the same number with your left foot on the bench.

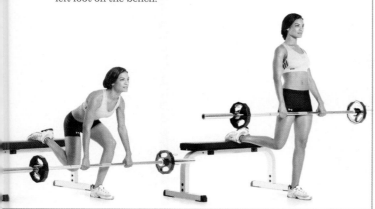

VARIATION #3
Sumo Deadlift

- Stand with your feet about twice shoulder-width apart and your toes pointed out at an angle.
- Grasp the center of the bar with your hands 12 inches apart and palms facing you.

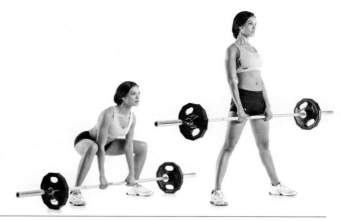

MAIN MOVE
Dumbbell Deadlift

A

- Set a pair of dumbbells on the floor in front of you.
- Bend at your hips and knees, and grab the dumbbells with an overhand grip.

B

- Without allowing your lower back to round, stand up with the dumbbells.
- Lower the dumbbells to the floor.

490

Most weight, in pounds, ever deadlifted by a woman weighing 123 pounds or less.

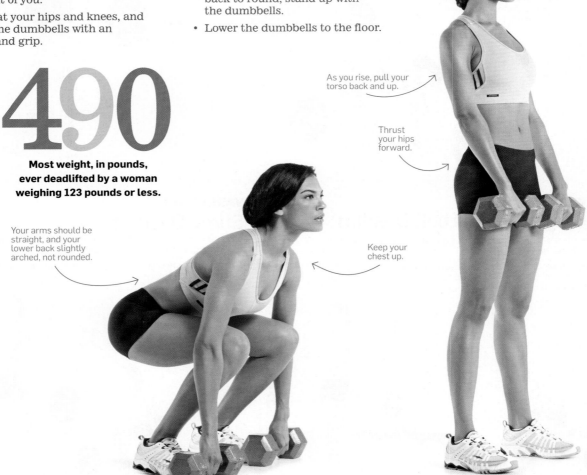

Your arms should be straight, and your lower back slightly arched, not rounded.

As you rise, pull your torso back and up.

Thrust your hips forward.

Keep your chest up.

VARIATION #1
Single-Arm Deadlift

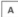

- Use just one dumbbell for this version of the exercise. Place the dumbbell on the floor next to your right ankle.

- Complete the prescribed number of repetitions with the weight in your right hand, then do the same number with it in your left.

This exercise is also called the suitcase deadlift, since it's the same movement you use to pick up luggage.

VARIATION #2
Single-Leg Deadlift

- Grab a pair of light dumbbells and stand on your left foot. (If dumbbells make this too hard, just use your bodyweight as shown.)
- Lift your right foot behind you and bend your knee so your right lower leg is parallel to the floor.

B

- Bend forward at your hips, and slowly lower your body as far as you can, or until your right lower leg almost touches the floor.
- Pause, then push your body back to the starting position.
- If this exercise is too difficult, perform the move as directed, but instead of raising the foot of your non-working leg, let the toes of your shoe rest on the floor for balance.

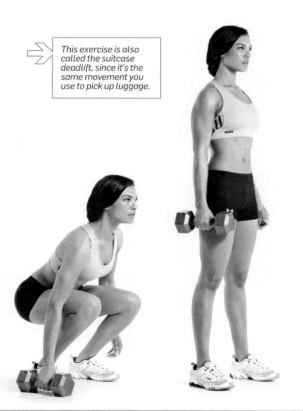

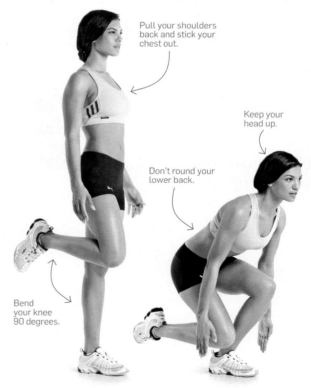

Pull your shoulders back and stick your chest out.

Keep your head up.

Don't round your lower back.

Bend your knee 90 degrees.

STRAIGHT-LEG DEADLIFTS

These exercises target the muscles of your glutes and hamstrings. They also work your core, especially the muscles of your lower back. One other benefit: They can help improve the flexibility of your hamstrings, since they stretch those muscles every time you lower the weight.

MAIN MOVE
Barbell Straight-Leg Deadlift

A

- Grab a barbell with an overhand grip that's just beyond shoulder width, and hold it at arm's length in front of your hips.

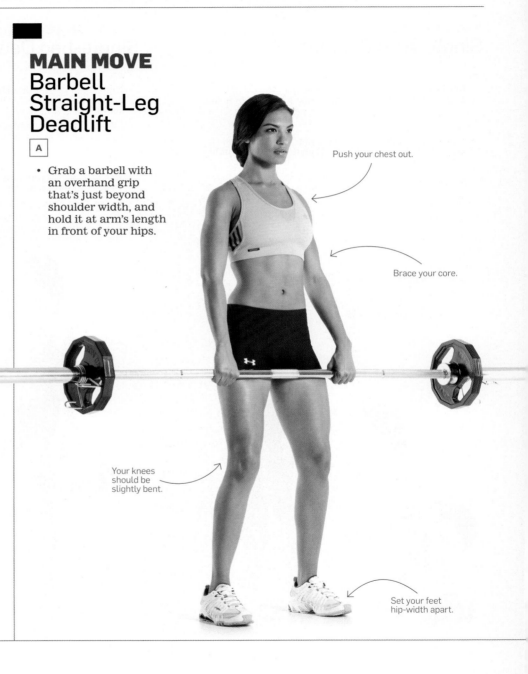

Push your chest out.

Brace your core.

Your knees should be slightly bent.

Set your feet hip-width apart.

TRAINER'S TIP
To lift your torso back to the starting position, squeeze your glutes and thrust your hips forward. This ensures you're engaging your hip muscles, instead of relying more on your lower back.

B

- Without changing the bend in your knees, bend at your hips and lower your torso until it's almost parallel to the floor.
- Pause, then raise your torso back to the starting position.

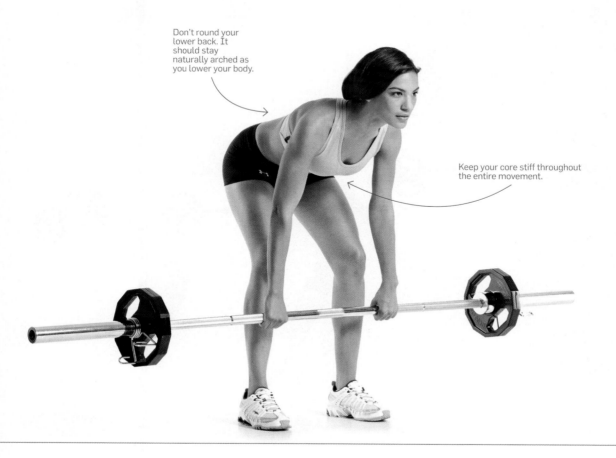

Don't round your lower back. It should stay naturally arched as you lower your body.

Keep your core stiff throughout the entire movement.

Glutes & Hams

VARIATION #1
Single-Leg Barbell Straight-Leg Deadlift

- Perform the movement while balanced on one leg, instead of two.
- Complete the prescribed number of repetitions with the same leg, then do the same number on your other leg.

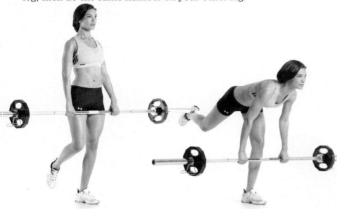

VARIATION #2
Barbell Good Morning

- Instead of holding the barbell at arm's length in front your body, position it across your upper back and hold it with an overhand grip.

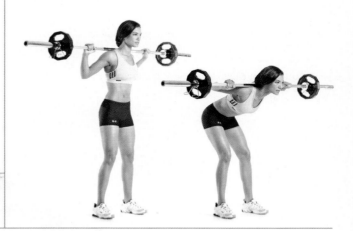

VARIATION #3
Split Barbell Good Morning

 A

- Position the barbell across your upper back and hold it with an overhand grip.
- Stand about a foot in front of a 6-inch step, and place your left heel on it.

 B

- Keeping your lower back naturally arched, bend forward at your hips as far as you comfortably can.
- Pause, then raise your torso back to the starting position.

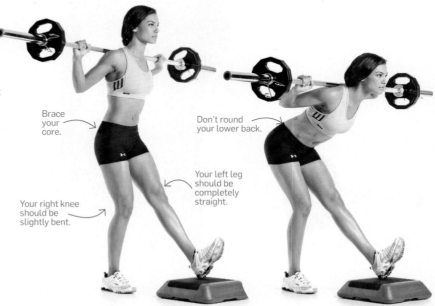

Brace your core.

Don't round your lower back.

Your left leg should be completely straight.

Your right knee should be slightly bent.

VARIATION #4
Single-Leg Barbell Good Morning

- Position the barbell across your upper back and hold it with an overhand grip.
- Perform the movement while balanced on one leg, instead of two.

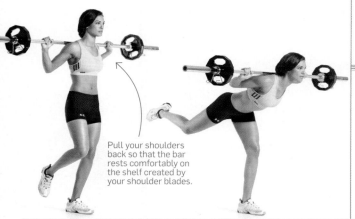

Pull your shoulders back so that the bar rests comfortably on the shelf created by your shoulder blades.

VARIATION #5
Zercher Good Morning

- Position the barbell in the crooks of your arms, and hold it tightly against your body as you do the movement.

You can also wrap a towel around the bar or use a bar pad for cushioning.

To secure the bar, squeeze your forearms to your upper arms.

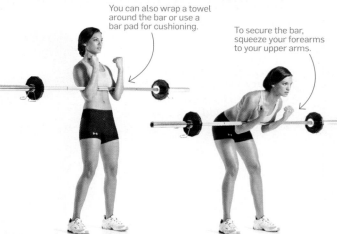

VARIATION #6
Seated Barbell Good Morning

 A

- Sit upright on a bench and hold a barbell across your upper back.

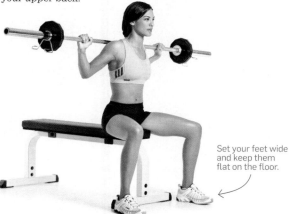

Set your feet wide and keep them flat on the floor.

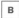 **B**

- Keeping the natural arch in your lower back, bend forward at your hips and lower your torso as far as you comfortably can.
- Pause, then raise your torso back to the starting position.

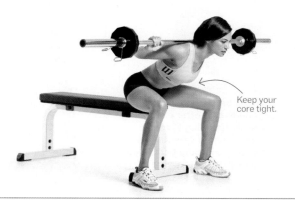

Keep your core tight.

255

MAIN MOVE
Dumbbell Straight-Leg Deadlift

A

- Grab a pair of dumbbells with an overhand grip, and hold them at arm's length in front of your thighs.
- Stand with your feet hip-width apart and your knees slightly bent.

B

- Without changing the bend in your knees, bend at your hips, and lower your torso until it's almost parallel to the floor.
- Pause, then raise your torso back to the starting position.

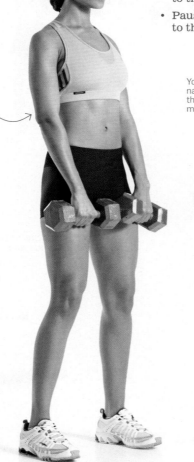

Brace your core.

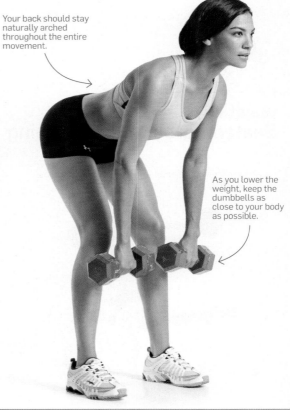

Your back should stay naturally arched throughout the entire movement.

As you lower the weight, keep the dumbbells as close to your body as possible.

2

Times better people did on cognitive tests after exercising while listening to music compared to sweating in silence, according to an Ohio State University study.

VARIATION #1
Single-Leg Dumbbell Straight-Leg Deadlift

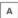

- Perform a dumbbell straight-leg deadlift while balanced on one leg, instead of two.

- Complete the prescribed number of repetitions with the same leg, then do the same number on your other leg.

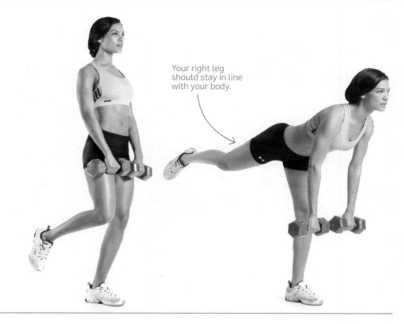

Your right leg should stay in line with your body.

VARIATION #2
Rotational Dumbbell Straight-Leg Deadlift

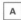

- Grab a light dumbbell in your right hand and stand on your left foot with your knee slightly bent.
- Lift your right foot off the floor and bend your knee slightly.

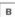

- Without changing the bend in your left knee, bend at your hips and lower your torso as you rotate it to the left and touch the dumbbell to your left foot.
- Pause, then raise your torso back to the starting position.
- Complete the prescribed number of repetitions standing on your left foot, with the weight in your right hand. Then do the same number on your right foot, with the weight in your left hand.

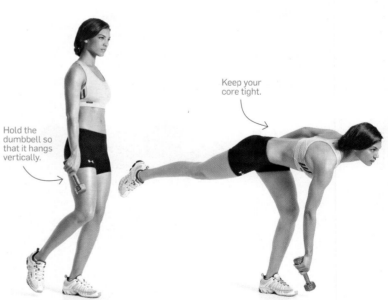

Hold the dumbbell so that it hangs vertically.

Keep your core tight.

Glutes & Hams

MAIN MOVE
Back Extension

- Position yourself in the back-extension station and hook your feet under the leg anchors.
- Keeping your back naturally arched, lower your upper body as far as you comfortably can.

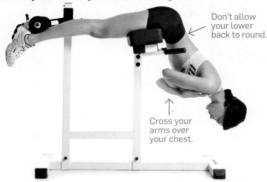

Don't allow your lower back to round.

Cross your arms over your chest.

B

- Squeeze your glutes and raise your torso until it's in line with your lower body.
- Pause, then slowly lower your torso back to the starting position.

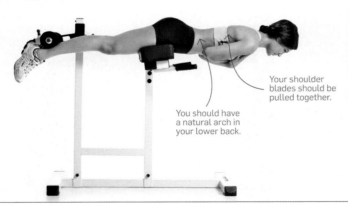

Your shoulder blades should be pulled together.

You should have a natural arch in your lower back.

VARIATION
Single-Leg Back Extension

- Position yourself in the back-extension station with just one foot hooked under the leg anchors.

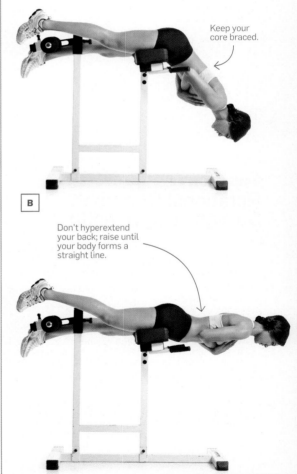

Keep your core braced.

Don't hyperextend your back; raise until your body forms a straight line.

MAIN MOVE
Cable Pull Through

A

- Attach a rope handle to the low pulley of a cable machine.
- Grab an end of the rope in each hand and stand with your back to the weight stack.
- Bend at your hips and knees and lower your torso until it's at about a 45-degree angle to the floor.

B

- Thrust your hips forward and raise your torso back to the starting position.

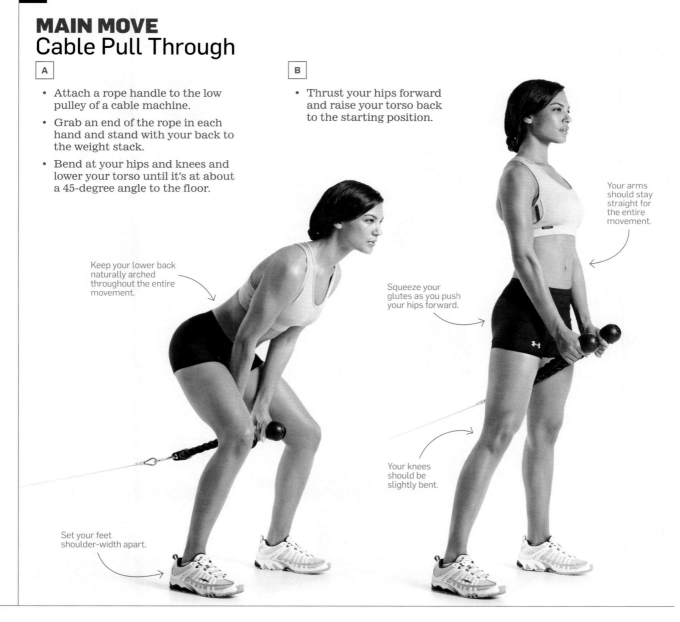

Your arms should stay straight for the entire movement.

Keep your lower back naturally arched throughout the entire movement.

Squeeze your glutes as you push your hips forward.

Your knees should be slightly bent.

Set your feet shoulder-width apart.

Glutes & Hams |

STEPUPS

These exercises target the muscles of your glutes and hamstrings. That's because you have to push your hips forward forcefully to perform the movements. Stepups also work your quadriceps, since they require you to straighten your knee against resistance.

MAIN MOVE
Barbell Stepup

A

- Stand in front of a bench or step, and place your left foot firmly on the step.

B

- Press your left heel into the step and push your body up until your left leg is straight.
- Then lower your body back down until your right foot touches the floor, and repeat.
- Complete the prescribed number of repetitions with your left leg, then do the same number with your right leg.

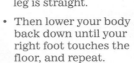

Pull your shoulders back so that the bar rests comfortably on the shelf created by your shoulder blades.

The step should be high enough that your knee is bent at least 90 degrees.

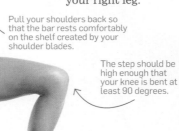

Your left foot stays in this position for the entire exercise.

Keep your right foot elevated.

VARIATION
Barbell Lateral Stepup

- Stand with your left side next to a step, and place your left foot on the step.

- Push your body up as you would for a standard barbell stepup. Then lower yourself back down. Complete the prescribed number of reps with your left leg, then do the same number with your right leg.

Keep your torso upright as you lift your body.

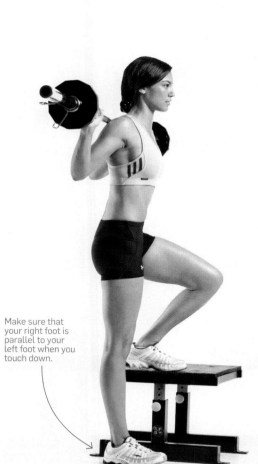

Make sure that your right foot is parallel to your left foot when you touch down.

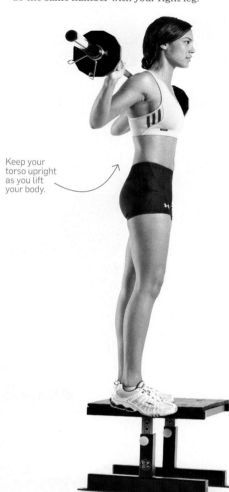

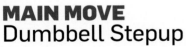

MAIN MOVE
Dumbbell Stepup

A

- Grab a pair of dumbbells and hold them at arm's length at your sides. Stand in front of a bench or step, and place your left foot firmly on the step.

- The step should be high enough that your knee is bent 90 degrees.

B

- Press your left heel into the step and push your body up until your left leg is straight and you're standing on one leg on the bench, keeping your right foot elevated.

- Lower your body back down until your right foot touches the floor. That's one repetition.

- Complete the prescribed number of repetitions with your left leg, then do the same number with your right leg.

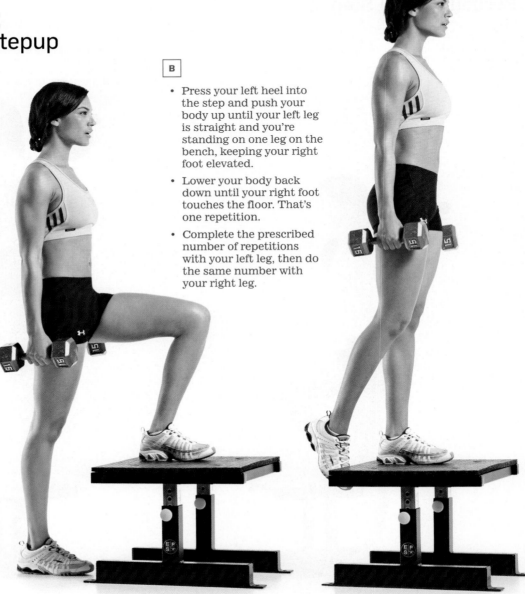

VARIATION #1
Lateral Dumbbell Stepup

A

- Grab a pair of dumbbells and stand with your left side next to a step.
- Place your left foot on the step.

B

- Press your left foot into the bench and push your body up until both legs are straight.
- Lower back down to the starting position.
- Complete the prescribed number of reps with your left leg, then do the same number with your right leg.

VARIATION #2
Crossover Dumbbell Stepup

A

- Grab a pair of dumbbells and stand with your left side next to a step.
- Place your right foot on the step.

B

- Press your right foot into the bench and push your body up until both legs are straight.
- Lower your body back down to the starting position.
- Complete the prescribed number of reps with your right leg, then do the same number with your left leg.

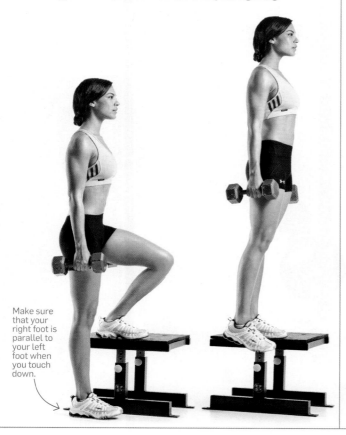

Make sure that your right foot is parallel to your left foot when you touch down.

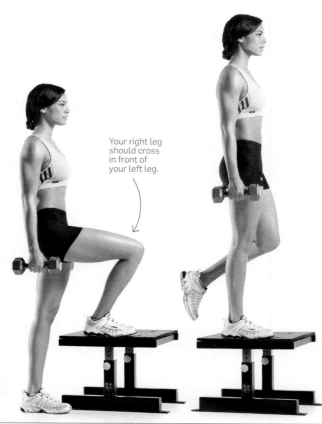

Your right leg should cross in front of your left leg.

Glutes & Hams |

HIP ABDUCTION
These exercises target your hip abductors, primarily a hip muscle called the *gluteus medius*.

MAIN MOVE
Standing Cable Hip Abduction

A

- Attach an ankle strap to the low pulley of a cable station, and then place the strap around your left ankle.

- Stand with your right side facing the weight stack.

- Let your left leg cross in front of your right leg. (You should be standing far enough away from the machine that the cable remains taut.)

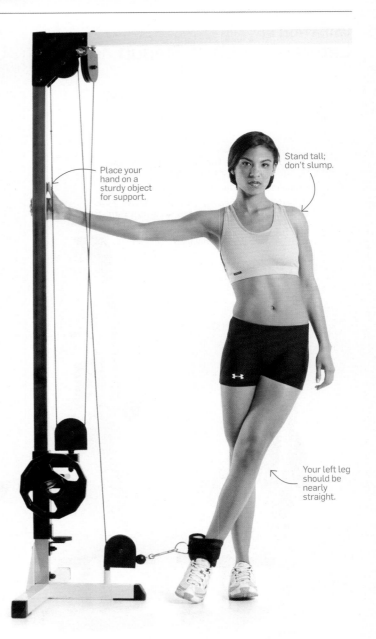

Place your hand on a sturdy object for support.

Stand tall; don't slump.

Your left leg should be nearly straight.

B

- Without changing the bend in your knee, raise your left leg out to your left side as far as you can.
- Pause, then slowly return to the starting position.
- Complete the prescribed number of repetitions with your left leg, then turn around and do the same number with your right leg.

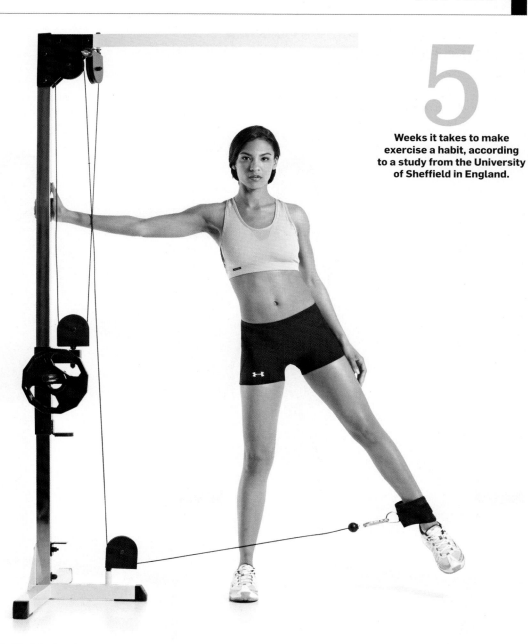

5

Weeks it takes to make exercise a habit, according to a study from the University of Sheffield in England.

Glutes & Hams | HIP ABDUCTIONS

STANDING CABLE HIP ABDUCTION VARIATION
Standing Resistance-Band Hip Abduction

A

- Instead of using a cable station, simply secure a mini-band to a sturdy object, then loop it around your ankle.

B

- Raise your leg straight out to the side, as far as you can.

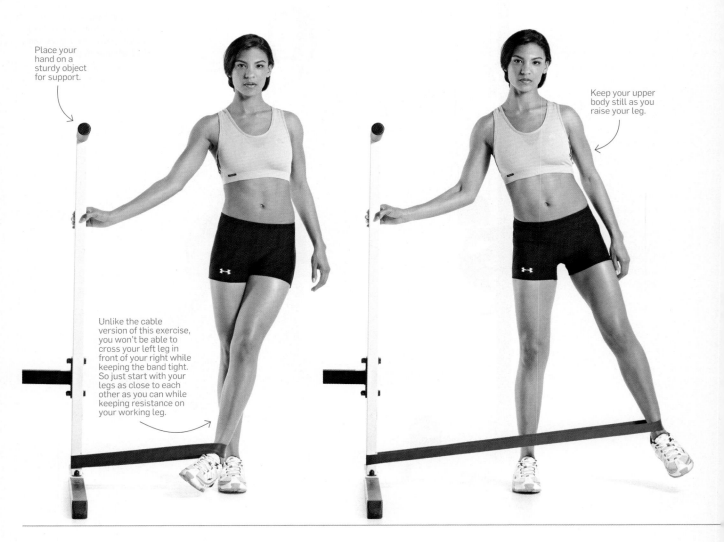

Place your hand on a sturdy object for support.

Keep your upper body still as you raise your leg.

Unlike the cable version of this exercise, you won't be able to cross your left leg in front of your right while keeping the band tight. So just start with your legs as close to each other as you can while keeping resistance on your working leg.

Band Side Leg Raise

- Lie on your left side on the floor.
- Loop a mini-band around both ankles.
- Rest your head on your left arm.
- Brace your right hand on the floor in front of your chest.
- Without moving any other part of your body, raise your right leg as high as you can.
- Pause, then return to the starting position.

Your legs should be straight, with your right leg on top of, but just behind, your left leg.

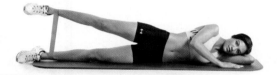

Clamshell

- Lie on your left side on the floor, with your hips and knees bent 45 degrees.
- Your right leg should be on top of your left leg, your heels together.
- Keeping your feet in contact with each other, raise your right knee as high as you can without moving your pelvis.
- Pause, then return to the starting position.
- Don't allow your left leg to move off the floor.

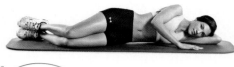

As the name suggests, think of a clamshell opening as you do the exercise.

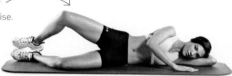

Lateral Band Walks

 A

- Place both legs between a mini-band, and position the band just below your knees.

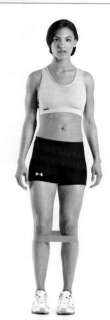

TRAINER'S TIP
This exercise is great to use as a warmup before any lower body exercise, and just about any sport—especially those that require you to move laterally, such as basketball, tennis, and racquetball. Do one set before you hit the court.

 B

- Take small steps to your right for 20 feet. Then sidestep back to your left for 20 feet. That's one set.

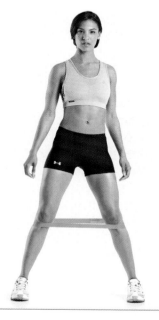

Glutes & Hams

THE BEST EXERCISE YOU'VE NEVER DONE
Single-Arm Dumbbell Swing

This movement works your hamstrings and glutes explosively. That means you'll target your very important fast-twitch muscle fibers. These are the fibers that atrophy fastest with age and that are crucial in almost every activity you do—even simply raising yourself out of a chair. So you might say this exercise will help keep your body young. It also works your core, quadriceps, and shoulder muscles, making it a great move for anyone who's short on training time.

A

- Grab a dumbbell with an overhand grip and hold it in front of your waist at arm's length. (You can also do the exercise two handed, holding the dumbbell with both hands.)
- Bend at your hips and knees and lower your torso until it forms a 45-degree angle to the floor.
- Swing the dumbbell between your legs.

B

- Keeping your arm straight, thrust your hips forward, straighten your knees, and swing the dumbbell up to chest level as you rise to standing position.
- Now squat back down as you swing the dumbbell between your legs again.
- Swing the weight back and forth forcefully.

BONUS EXERCISE!
Kettlebell Swing
- Perform the same movement while grasping a kettlebell instead of a dumbbell.

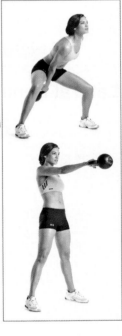

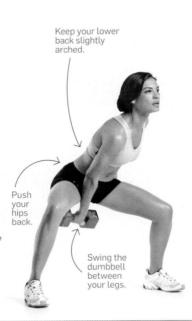

Keep your lower back slightly arched.

Push your hips back.

Swing the dumbbell between your legs.

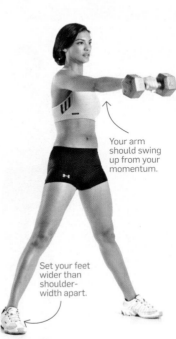

Your arm should swing up from your momentum.

Set your feet wider than shoulder-width apart.

THE BEST STRETCH FOR YOUR HAMSTRINGS
Standing Hamstring Stretch

Why it's good:
It stretches your hamstrings from both your hip and your knee. Bending your knee more increases the stretch near your hip; keeping it straight increases the stretch at your knee.

Make the most of it: Hold this stretch for 30 seconds on each side, then repeat two times. Do the routine daily, and up to three times a day if you're really tight.

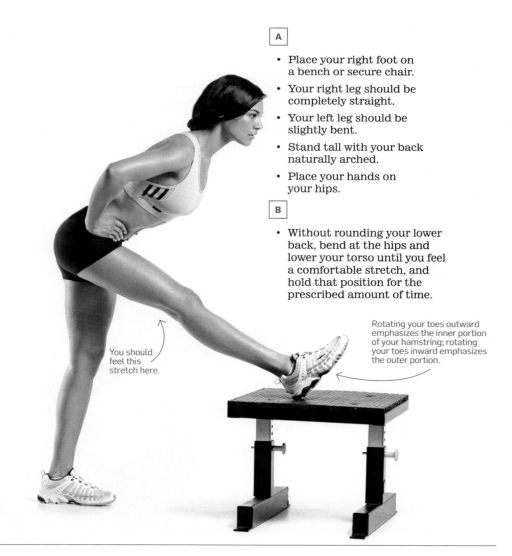

A
- Place your right foot on a bench or secure chair.
- Your right leg should be completely straight.
- Your left leg should be slightly bent.
- Stand tall with your back naturally arched.
- Place your hands on your hips.

B
- Without rounding your lower back, bend at the hips and lower your torso until you feel a comfortable stretch, and hold that position for the prescribed amount of time.

Rotating your toes outward emphasizes the inner portion of your hamstring; rotating your toes inward emphasizes the outer portion.

You should feel this stretch here.

Glutes & Hams

THE BEST STRETCH FOR YOUR GLUTES
Lying Glute Stretch

Why it's good: It loosens your glutes. When these muscles are tight, you may be more likely to experience lower back pain.

Make the most of it: Hold this stretch for 30 seconds on each side, then repeat twice for a total of three sets. Perform this routine daily, and up to three times a day if you're really tight.

- Lie faceup on the floor with your knees and hips bent.
- Cross your left leg over your right so that your left ankle sits across your right thigh.

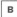

- Grab your left knee with both hands and pull it toward the middle of your chest until you feel a comfortable stretch in your glutes.

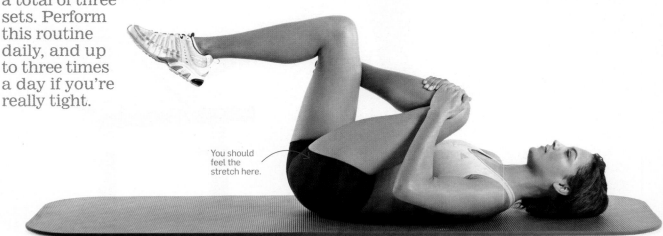

You should feel the stretch here.

Turn the page to learn how to
SCULPT THE PERFECT BACKSIDE

Turn the page to learn how to
SCULPT THE PERFECT BACKSIDE

Glutes & Hams

SCULPT THE PERFECT BACKSIDE

Sculpt your glutes and hamstrings with this 4-week workout program from Mike Robertson, CSCS, co-owner of Indianapolis Fitness and Sports Training.

While this routine is designed to work your entire lower body—including your quadriceps—as well as your core, its main focus is on the muscles on the backs of your thighs. This helps to shore up the long-time weaknesses that contribute to poor posture and, as a result, often lead to back pain and a less-attractive physique. And, of course, because you're working your big lower-body muscles, you'll burn a ton of calories. So as a bonus, this workout will help melt your middle, too.

What to do: Do each workout once a week, resting for at least 2 days between sessions. So you might do Workout A on Tuesday and Workout B on Friday. Perform the warmup before each workout. It's designed to help improve your flexibility and also prepare your muscles for the work that's about to come. Note that in each workout, the number of repetitions you perform increases each week. This helps ensure that you're continually challenging your muscles.

Warmup

Alternate back and forth between these movements without resting. Hold each exercise for 30 seconds before moving on to the other. Complete a total of three sets of each.

Kneeling hip flexor stretch (page 228)

Hip raises (page 236)

Workout A

EXERCISE	WEEK 1			WEEK 2			WEEK 3			WEEK 4		
	SETS	REPS	REST	SETS	REPS	REST	SETS	REPS	REST	SETS	REPS	REST
Barbell straight-leg deadlift (page 252)	2	8	90	3	8	90	3	10	90	3	12	90
Dumbbell split squat (page 209)	2	8	90	3	8	90	3	10	90	3	12	90
Single-leg barbell straight-leg deadlift (page 254)	2	8	90	3	8	90	3	10	90	3	12	90
Back extension (page 258)	2	8	60	3	8	60	3	10	60	3	12	60
Barbell rollout (page 292)	2	8	60	3	8	60	3	10	60	3	12	60

Workout B

EXERCISE	WEEK 1			WEEK 2			WEEK 3			WEEK 4		
	SETS	REPS	REST	SETS	REPS	REST	SETS	REPS	REST	SETS	REPS	REST
Braced squat (page 194)	2	8	90	3	8	90	3	10	90	3	12	90
Cable pull through (page 259)	2	8	90	3	8	90	3	10	90	3	12	90
Dumbbell stepup (page 262)	2	8	90	3	8	90	3	10	90	3	12	90
Swiss-ball hip raise and leg curl (page 243)	2	8	60	3	8	60	3	10	60	3	12	60
Plank (page 278)	2	8	60	3	8	60	3	10	60	3	12	60

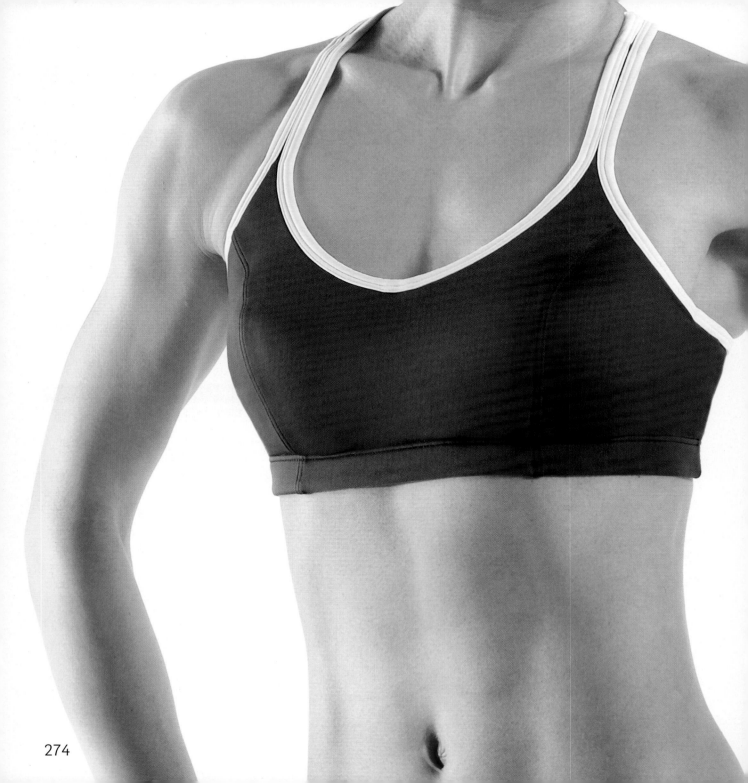

Chapter 10: Core
YOUR CENTER OF ATTRACTION

Core

If the number of infomercial products is any indication, people spend more money on their abs than on any other muscle group. And why wouldn't they? Your abs—or more specifically, your core, which also includes the muscles of your lower back and hips—are involved in every single movement you do. And not just in the gym. If it weren't for your core muscles, you wouldn't even be able to stand or sit upright.

Of course, all of this usually has little to do with most women's desire for tight tummy. It's likely your true motivation is the visual appeal of a firm midriff.

Perhaps that's because a flat stomach is an outward sign of a healthy, fit body. The take-home message: Sculpting toned abs makes your body not only look better, but work better, too.

Bonus Benefits

Live longer! A Canadian study of more than 8,000 people over 13 years found that those with the weakest abdominal muscles had a death rate more than twice that of the people with the strongest midsections.

Lift more! A stronger core supports your spine, making your entire body more structurally sound. That allows you to use heavier weights on every exercise.

A pain-free back! California State University researchers found that when people followed a 10-week core workout program, they experienced 30 percent less back pain.

Meet Your Muscles

Abdominals

There's no doubt that the most popular abs muscle is the rectus abdominis [1], also known as the six-pack. Despite its nickname, this muscle actually consists of eight segments that are separated by a dense connective tissue called fascia [A]. This muscle is one of those that counteract the pull of the muscles that extend your lower back, helping to keep your spine stable. Its other main duty is to pull your torso toward your hips. That's why you can work this muscle by doing situps and crunches. However, the best way to train your rectus abdominis—and your core as a whole—is with spinal stability exercises, such as the plank and side plank.

The abs muscles on the sides of your torso are the external obliques [2] and internal obliques [3]. These muscles help bend your torso to your side, help rotate your torso to your left and right, and perhaps most important, actually act to resist your torso from rotating. So rotational exercises such as the kneeling rotational chop train these muscles, as do antirotation exercises like the kneeling stability chop.

A long strip of fascia—the linea alba—creates the separation line down the middle of your abs and helps prevent your abs from being ripped apart by your obliques.

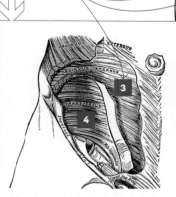

Your deepest abdominal muscle is the transverse abdominis [4]. This muscle lies beneath your rectus abdominis and obliques, and its job is to pull your abdominal wall inward—as when you're sucking in your gut.

YOUR CORE, DEFINED

While it's common to use the words *core* and *abs* interchangeably, it's not entirely accurate. That's because the term *core* actually describes the more than two dozen abdominal, lower-back, and hip muscles that stabilize your spine to keep your torso upright. What's more, your core muscles allow you to bend your torso forward, back, and from side to side, as well as rotate. As a result, your core is critical in everything you do—except, perhaps, sleeping.

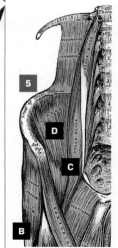

Hips

A group of muscles on the fronts of your hips, known as your hip flexors [5], also play a valuable role in core strength. The reason: They originate on either your spine or pelvis, an area that you might call the ground floor of your core. A number of muscles qualify as hip flexors, but the main ones are the tensor fascia latae [B], psoas [C], and iliacus [D]. As the name suggests, these muscles allow you to flex your hips. To visualize, imagine raising your upper legs toward your chest. You can target these muscles with exercises such as the reverse crunch and the hanging leg raise.

Lower Back

There are many lower-back muscles that contribute to your core strength, but for simplicity's sake, the main ones are your erector spinae (shown as sacropsinalis) [6], multifidus [7], and quadratus lumborum [8]. Collectively, these muscles help keep your spine stable and also allow it to bend backward and to the side. They're best trained with stability exercises such as the plank, side plank, and the prone cobra, and also with any exercise that requires you to bend or pull.

What's more, even though your gluteus maximus is technically a hip muscle—and was covered in depth in Chapter 9—it's also worth mentioning here. That's because it's attached to your lower back by connective tissue and, therefore, works in conjunction with your other core muscles.

Core | STABILITY EXERCISES

In this chapter, you'll find more than 100 exercises that target the muscles of your core. You'll notice that certain exercises have been designated as a Main Move. Master this basic version of an exercise, and you'll be able to do all its variations with flawless form.

STABILITY EXERCISES

These exercises improve your ability to stabilize your spine. This is essential for lower-back health and peak performance in any sport. But don't worry: Stability exercises are also highly effective at working the abdominal muscles that are most visible—including the ones that make up your six-pack.

MAIN MOVE
Plank

- Start to get into a pushup position, but bend your elbows and rest your weight on your forearms instead of on your hands.

- Your body should form a straight line from your shoulders to your ankles.

- Brace your core by contracting your abs as if you were about to be punched in the gut.

- Hold this position for 30 seconds—or as directed—while breathing deeply.

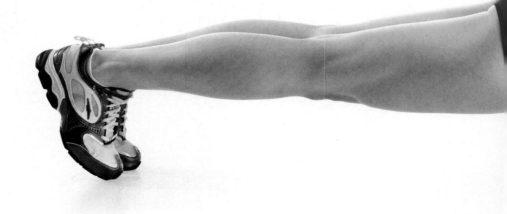

IF YOU CAN'T HOLD THE PLANK POSITION FOR 30 SECONDS, *hold for 5 to 10 seconds, rest for 5 seconds, and repeat as many times as needed to total 30 seconds. Each time you perform the exercise, try to hold each repetition a little longer so that you reach your 30-second goal with fewer repetitions. Want more options? Try the 45-degree plank, the kneeling plank, or the quadruped, and work your way up to the plank.*

MUSCLE MISTAKE
You Think Crunches Make You Thin

Researchers at the University of Virginia found that it takes 250,000 crunches to burn 1 pound of fat—that's 100 crunches a day for 7 years. So simply working the muscles buried beneath your gut won't give you a six-pack. Your best strategy for fat loss is to work all of the muscles of your body, spending most of your time training the big muscles of your lower body and back. That's because the more muscles you work, the more calories you burn.

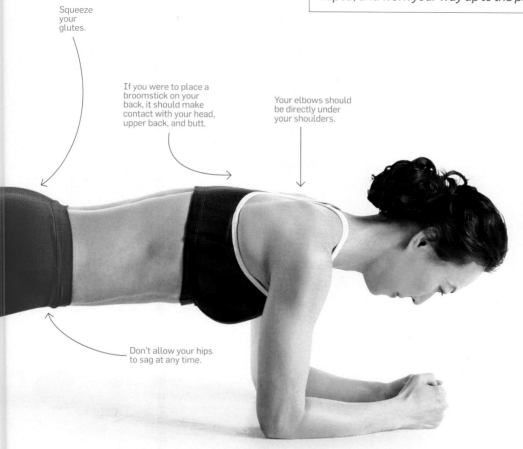

Squeeze your glutes.

If you were to place a broomstick on your back, it should make contact with your head, upper back, and butt.

Your elbows should be directly under your shoulders.

Don't allow your hips to sag at any time.

Core | STABILITY EXERCISES

VARIATION #1
45-Degree Plank
• Place your forearms on a bench instead of on the floor.

The plank is easier when you place your elbows on a bench, since you don't have to support as much of your body weight.

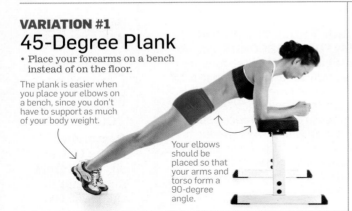

Your elbows should be placed so that your arms and torso form a 90-degree angle.

VARIATION #2
Kneeling Plank
• Instead of performing the exercise with your legs straight, bend your knees so that they help support your body weight.

Your body should form a straight line from your shoulders to your knees.

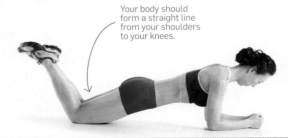

VARIATION #3
Elevated-Feet Plank
• Place both feet on a bench.

Elevating your feet increases the difficulty of the exercise.

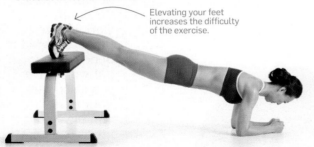

VARIATION #4
Single-Leg Elevated-Feet Plank
• Place one foot on a bench and hold your other foot a couple of inches above it. Switch legs each set.

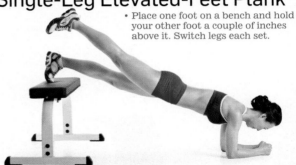

VARIATION #5
Extended Plank
• Place your weight on your hands (as you would for a pushup). Move your hands forward for a greater challenge.

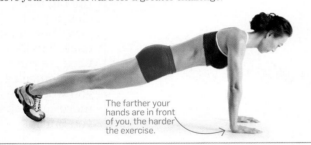

The farther your hands are in front of you, the harder the exercise.

VARIATION #6
Wide-Stance Plank with Leg Lift
• Move your feet out wider than your shoulders, and hold one foot a few inches off the floor. Switch legs each set.

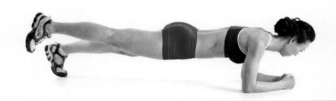

VARIATION #7
Wide-Stance Plank with Diagonal Arm Lift

- Move your feet out wider than your shoulders, instead of placing them close together.
- Raise and straighten your right arm—with your thumb pointing up—and hold it diagonally in relation to your torso.
- Hold for 5 to 10 seconds and switch arms. That's one rep.

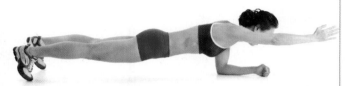

VARIATION #8
Wide-Stance Plank with Opposite Arm and Leg Lift

- Move your feet out wider than your shoulders.
- Hold your left foot and your right arm off the floor for 5 to 10 seconds, then switch arms and legs and repeat. That's one rep.

When you raise your arm and leg, focus on holding your hips and torso in place.

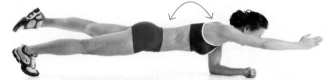

VARIATION #9
Swiss-Ball Plank

- Place your feet and shins on a Swiss ball.

VARIATION #10
Swiss-Ball Plank with Feet on Bench

- Place your forearms on a Swiss ball and your feet on a bench.

Putting your feet in on the bench raises your feet to the same level as your elbows, similar to how you would be on the floor—only the instability of the Swiss ball makes it harder to hold your position.

TWICE THE ABS WORKOUT
Canadian researchers determined that your abs work nearly twice as hard when you do a plank on a Swiss ball instead of on the floor.

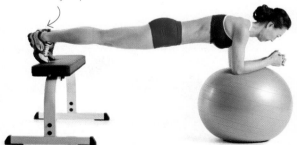

Core | STABILITY EXERCISES

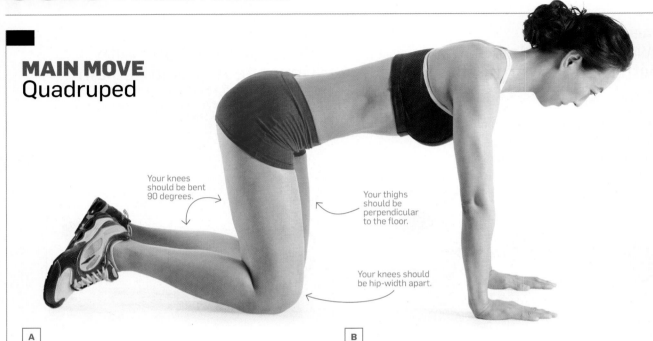

MAIN MOVE
Quadruped

Your knees should be bent 90 degrees.

Your thighs should be perpendicular to the floor.

Your knees should be hip-width apart.

 A

- Get down on your hands and knees with your palms flat on the floor and shoulder-width apart.
- Relax your core so that your lower back and abdomen are in their natural positions.

 B

- Without allowing your lower back to rise or round, brace your abs as if you were about to be punched in the gut. Hold your abs tight for 5 to 10 seconds, breathing deeply throughout the exercise. That's one repetition.

VARIATION #1
Fire Hydrant In-Out

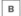 **A**

- Without allowing your lower-back posture to change, raise your right knee as close as you can to your chest. (Your knee may not move forward much.)

B

- Keeping your right knee bent, raise your thigh out to the side without moving your hips.

C

- Kick your raised right leg straight back until it's in line with your torso. That's one rep.

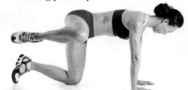

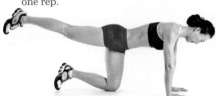

VARIATION #2
Quadruped with Leg Lift

- Without allowing your lower-back posture to change, raise and straighten your left leg until it's in line with your body. Hold for 5 to 10 seconds.

- Return to the starting position. Repeat with your right leg. Continue to alternate back and forth.

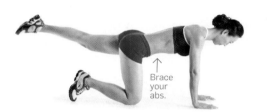

Brace your abs.

VARIATION #3
Bird Dog

- Brace your abs, and raise your right arm and left leg until they're in line with your body. Hold for 5 to 10 seconds.

- Return to the starting position. Repeat with your left arm and right leg. Continue to alternate back and forth.

Try to keep your hips and lower back still, even as you switch arms and legs.

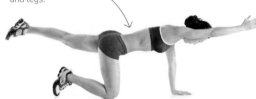

Swiss-Ball Opposite Arm and Leg Lift

- Lie belly-side down with your navel over the center of a Swiss ball.

- You should be on the balls of both feet, with your hands placed flat on the floor.

- Brace your abs, and raise your right arm and left leg until they're in line with your body and hold that position for a few seconds.

- Return to the starting position. Repeat with your left arm and right leg. Continue to alternate back and forth.

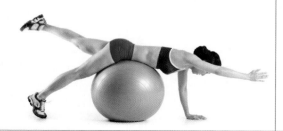

Cat Camel

- Position yourself on your hands and knees.

- Gently arch your lower back—don't push—then lower your head between your shoulders and raise your upper back toward the ceiling, rounding your spine. That's one repetition.

- Move back and forth slowly, without pushing at either end of the movement.

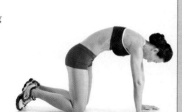

Floss Away Back Pain

The cat camel may look funny, but slowly flexing and extending your spine in small ranges of motion is a great way to prepare your core for any activity. What's more, this movement can help prevent back pain because it "flosses" the nerves of your lower back as they exit your spinal canal. This helps keep the nerves from becoming pinched, lowering your risk of painful conditions such as sciatica. It can also help free a nerve that's already impinged. A good routine: Do 5 to 10 reps.

MAIN MOVE
Side Plank

A

- Lie on your left side with your knees straight.
- Prop your upper body up on your left elbow and forearm.

B

- Brace your core by contracting your abs forcefully as if you were about to be punched in the gut.
- Raise your hips until your body forms a straight line from your ankles to your shoulders.
- Breathe deeply for the duration of the exercise.
- Hold this position for 30 seconds (or as directed). That's one set.
- Turn around so that you're lying on your right side and repeat.

IF YOU CAN'T HOLD THE SIDE PLANK FOR 30 SECONDS, *hold for 5 to 10 seconds, rest for 5 seconds, and repeat as many times as needed to total 30 seconds. Each time you perform the exercise, try to hold each repetition a little longer, so that you reach your 30-second goal with fewer repetitions.*

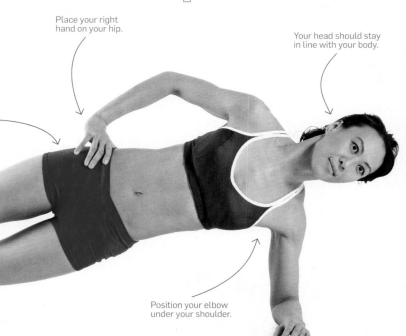

Place your right hand on your hip.

Your head should stay in line with your body.

Keep your hips raised and pushed forward.

Position your elbow under your shoulder.

VARIATION #1
Modified Side Plank
• Bend your knees 90 degrees.

Bending your knees reduces the amount of your body weight that you have to lift.

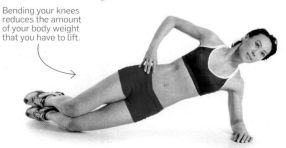

VARIATION #2
Rolling Side Plank
• Start by performing a side plank with your right side down. Hold for 1 second or 2 seconds, then roll your body over onto both elbows—into a plank—and hold for a second. Next, roll all the way up onto your left elbow so that you're performing a side plank facing the opposite direction. Hold for another second or two. That's one repetition. Make sure to move your entire body as a single unit each time you roll.

VARIATION #3
Side Plank with Feet on Bench
• Place both feet on a bench.

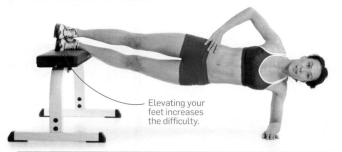

Elevating your feet increases the difficulty.

VARIATION #4
Side Plank with Elbow on Swiss Ball
• Place your forearm on a Swiss ball.

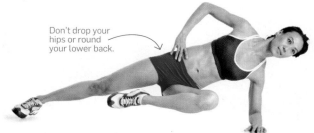

The instability of the Swiss ball forces your core to work even harder.

VARIATION #5
Single-Leg Side Plank
• Raise your top leg as high as you can and hold it that way for the duration of the exercise.

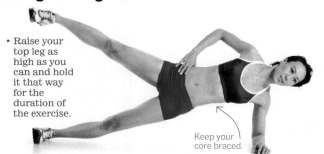

Keep your core braced.

VARIATION #6
Side Plank with Knee Tuck
• Lift your bottom leg toward your chest and hold it that way for the duration of the exercise.

Don't drop your hips or round your lower back.

Core | STABILITY EXERCISES

VARIATION #7
Side Plank with Reach Under

- Lift your body into a side plank, and start with your right arm raised straight above you so that it's perpendicular to the floor.

- Reach under and behind your torso with your right hand, then lift your arm back up to the starting position. That's one rep.

Keeping your abs braced, rotate your torso to your right as you reach behind you with your right arm.

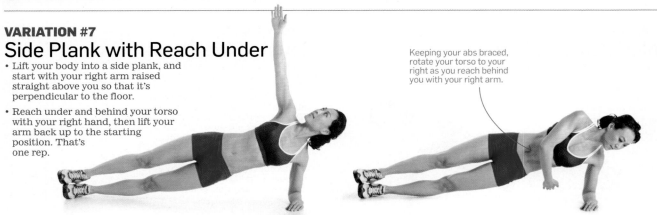

VARIATION #8
Plyometric Side Plank

- Raise your top leg slightly, and move it forward and back at an even tempo.

Moving your leg back and forth increases the challenge to your core by forcing you to stabilize your weight under conditions of varying force and movements.

Before attempting this exercise, you should be able to hold the side plank for 60 seconds.

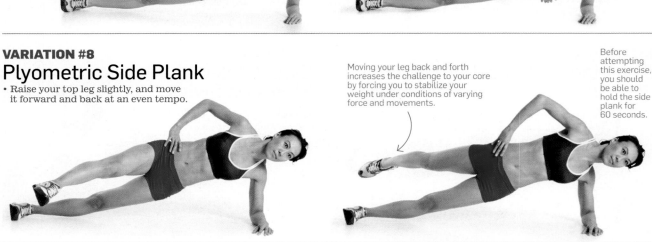

VARIATION #9
Side Plank and Row

- Attach a handle to the low pulley of a cable machine and grab it with your right hand.

- Brace your core and raise your body into a side plank.

Your arm should be straight.

- Bend your elbow and pull the handle to your rib cage, keeping your hips pushed up and forward.

- Slowly straighten your arm back out in front of you. That's one repetition.

Resist the urge to rotate at the hips or shoulders.

The cable should be taut.

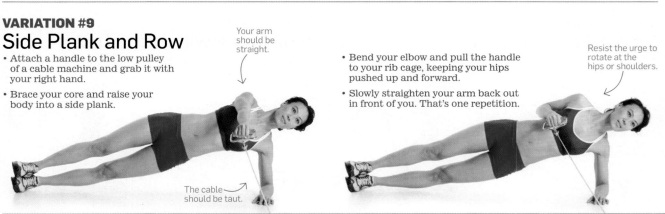

T-Stabilization

A

- Assume a pushup position.
- Your body should form a straight line from your head to your ankles.

Brace your core.

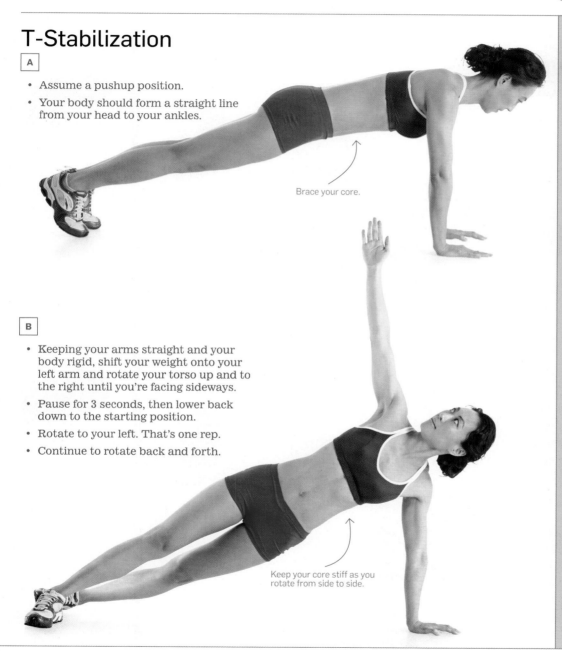

B

- Keeping your arms straight and your body rigid, shift your weight onto your left arm and rotate your torso up and to the right until you're facing sideways.
- Pause for 3 seconds, then lower back down to the starting position.
- Rotate to your left. That's one rep.
- Continue to rotate back and forth.

Keep your core stiff as you rotate from side to side.

Do You Measure Up?

Researchers in Finland found that people with poor muscular endurance in their lower backs are 3.4 times more likely to develop lower-back problems than those who have fair or good endurance. And turns out, a side-plank test is one of the best ways to gauge this endurance. Simply perform a side plank for as long as you can without allowing your hips to drop or drift backward. A good score: 60 seconds. If you don't meet this standard, start focusing more on your core.

Core | STABILITY EXERCISES

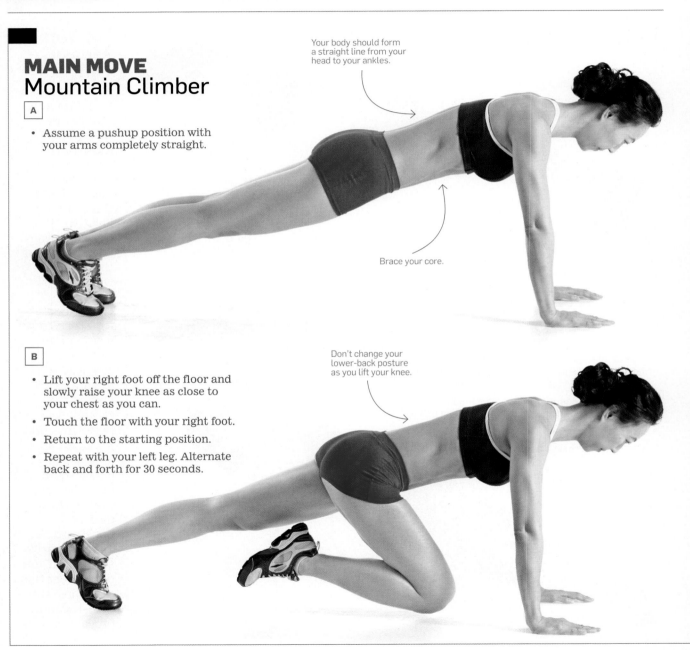

MAIN MOVE
Mountain Climber

A

- Assume a pushup position with your arms completely straight.

Your body should form a straight line from your head to your ankles.

Brace your core.

B

- Lift your right foot off the floor and slowly raise your knee as close to your chest as you can.
- Touch the floor with your right foot.
- Return to the starting position.
- Repeat with your left leg. Alternate back and forth for 30 seconds.

Don't change your lower-back posture as you lift your knee.

VARIATION #1
Mountain Climber with Hands on Bench

- Place your hands on a bench, then alternate raising each knee.

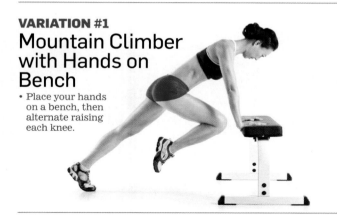

VARIATION #2
Mountain Climber with Hands on Medicine Ball

- Place your hands on a medicine ball, then alternate raising each knee.

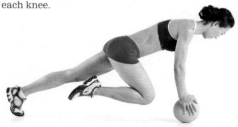

VARIATION #3
Mountain Climber with Hands on Swiss Ball

- Place your hands on a Swiss ball, then alternate raising each knee.

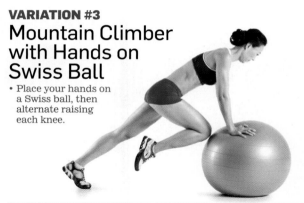

VARIATION #4
Mountain Climber with Feet on Valslides

- Place each foot on a Valslide and bring one knee toward your chest by sliding your foot forward.

As in the standard mountain climber, you can also perform this move with your hands on a bench, Swiss ball, or medicine ball.

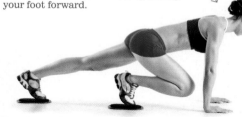

VARIATION #5
Cross-Body Mountain Climber

- Raise your right knee toward your left elbow, lower, and then raise your left knee to your right elbow.

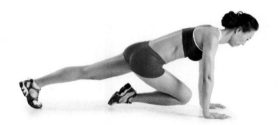

VARIATION #6
Cross-Body Mountain Climber with Feet on Swiss Ball

- With your feet on a Swiss ball, raise one knee toward your left elbow, lower, then raise the other knee.

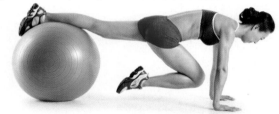

Core | STABILITY EXERCISES

MAIN MOVE
Swiss-Ball Jackknife

A

- Assume a pushup position with your arms completely straight.
- Rest your shins on a Swiss ball.
- Your body should form a straight line from your head to your ankles.

B

- Without changing your lower-back posture, roll the Swiss ball toward your chest by pulling it forward with your feet.
- Pause, then return the ball to the starting position by lowering your hips and rolling the ball backward.

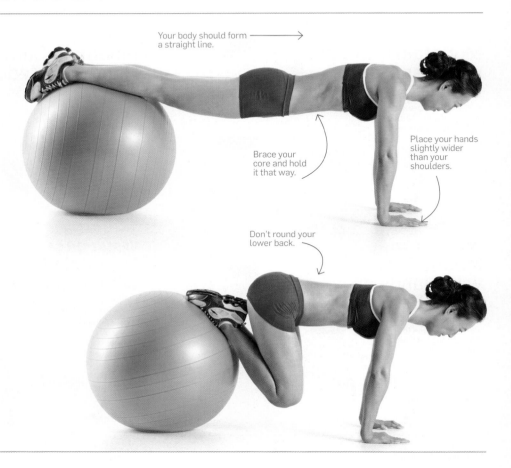

Your body should form a straight line.

Brace your core and hold it that way.

Place your hands slightly wider than your shoulders.

Don't round your lower back.

VARIATION
Single-Leg Swiss-Ball Jackknife

A

- Perform the exercise with just one leg, lifting one in the air as you pull the ball forward.

Don't round your lower back.

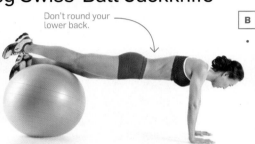

B

- Complete the prescribed number of repetitions with the same leg raised, and then do the same number with your other leg raised.

Keep your free leg elevated.

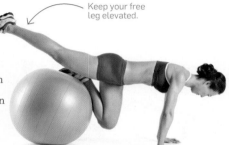

MAIN MOVE
McGill Curlup

 A

- Lie faceup on the floor with your right leg straight and flat on the floor. Your left knee should be bent, and your left foot flat.

- Place your palms on the floor underneath the natural arch in your lower back. (Don't flatten your back.)

B

- Slowly raise your head and shoulders off the floor without bending your lower back, and hold this position for 7 or 8 seconds, breathing deeply the entire time. That's one repetition.

- Complete the prescribed number of reps, then do the same number with your left leg straight and your right bent.

This McGill curlup forces you to work your entire abdominal muscle complex while keeping your lower back in its naturally arched position. So it minimizes stress on your spine while increasing the endurance of the muscles. That makes it a valuable exercise for helping to prevent future lower-back pain.

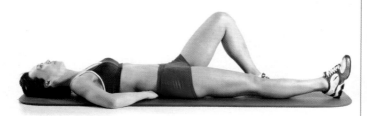

Don't tuck your chin.

Don't flatten your lower back as you curl your torso up.

VARIATION
Curlup with Raised Elbows

- Raise your elbows off the floor as you curl up.

Raising your elbows makes the exercise even harder.

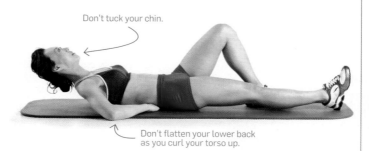

MUSCLE MISTAKE
You Don't Do Stability Exercises

For years, scientists thought that the main function of the abdominal muscles was to flex the spine. This is what you do when you round your lower back during a situp.

But the reality is that your abs' top job is to *stabilize* your spine, actually preventing it from flexing. In fact, these muscles are the reason your torso stays upright instead of falling forward due to gravity. So stability exercises—like the ones seen here—are likely the best way to train your core.

Swiss-Ball Rollout

A

- Sit on your knees in front of a Swiss ball and place your forearms and fists on the ball.

Keep your core braced.

Your lower back should be naturally arched.

Your elbows should be bent about 90 degrees.

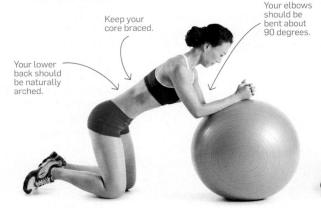

B

- Slowly roll the ball forward, straightening your arms and extending your body as far as you can without allowing your lower back to "collapse."
- Use your abdominal muscles to pull the ball back to your knees.

Don't let your hips sag.

Keep your core braced.

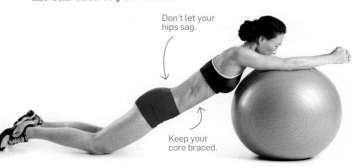

Barbell Rollout

A

- Load a barbell with a 10-pound plate on each side and affix collars.
- Kneel on the floor and grab the bar with an overhand, shoulder-width grip.
- Your shoulders should start over the barbell.

B

- Slowly roll the bar forward, extending your body as far as you can without allowing your hips to sag.
- Use your abdominal muscles to pull the bar back to your knees.

Your shoulders should start over the barbell.

Stiffen your core and squeeze your glutes to keep your lower back from collapsing.

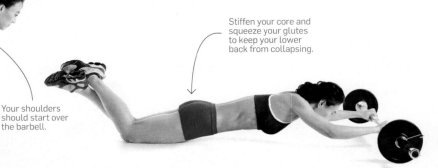

MAIN MOVE
Slide Out

- Kneel on the floor and place both hands on a Valslide.

Keep your body rigid.

Your hands should be under your shoulders.

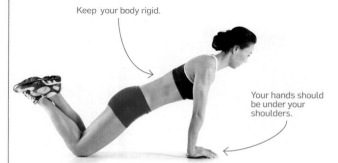

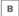

- Slowly push the Valslide forward, extending your body as far as you can without allowing your hips to sag.
- Use your abdominal muscles to pull your hands back to below your shoulders.

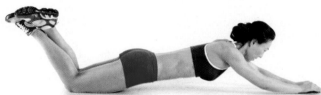

VARIATION
Alternating Slide Out

- Place each hand on a Valslide and assume a pushup position with your arms completely straight and your legs extended.

Your body should form a straight line from your head to your ankles.

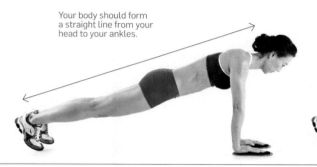

- Keeping your body rigid and your arms straight, slide your right hand out in front of you as far as you comfortably can.
- Reverse the movement back to the starting position by pulling the Valslide back.
- Your body should remain rigid for the entire movement.
- Repeat, only push your left hand out this time. Alternate back and forth each repetition.

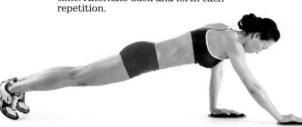

Core |

Lateral Roll

A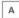

- Lie with your upper back placed firmly on a Swiss ball.
- Raise your hips so that your body forms a straight line from your knees to your shoulders.
- Hold a pole or broomstick, with your arms straight out from your sides.

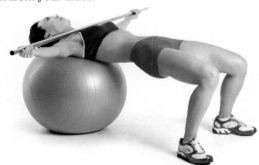

B

- Without allowing your hips or arms to sag, roll across the Swiss ball as far as you can, taking tiny steps with your feet.
- Reverse directions and roll as far as you can to the other side.

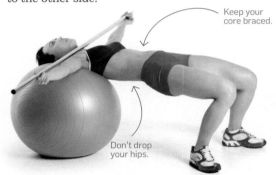

Keep your core braced.

Don't drop your hips.

Static Back Extension

- Position yourself in the back-extension station and hook your feet under the leg anchors.
- Raise your torso until it's in line with your lower body.
- Hold this position for 60 seconds, or until you can't maintain perfect form.

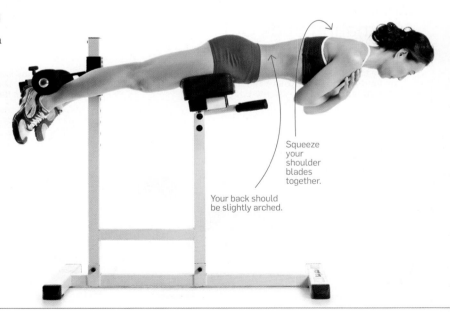

Squeeze your shoulder blades together.

Your back should be slightly arched.

Prone Cobra

- Lie facedown on the floor with your legs straight and your arms next to your sides, palms down.

B

- Contract your glutes and the muscles of your lower back, and raise your head, chest, arms, and legs off the floor.

- Simultaneously rotate your arms so that your thumbs point toward the ceiling. At this time, your hips should be the only parts of your body touching the floor. Hold this position for 60 seconds.

IF YOU CAN'T HOLD THE PRONE COBRA FOR 60 SECONDS, *hold for 5 to 10 seconds, rest for 5 seconds, and repeat as many times as needed to total 60 seconds. Each time you perform the exercise, try to hold each repetition a little longer so that you reach your 60-second goal with fewer repetitions. If the exercise is too easy, you can hold light dumbbells in your hands when you do it.*

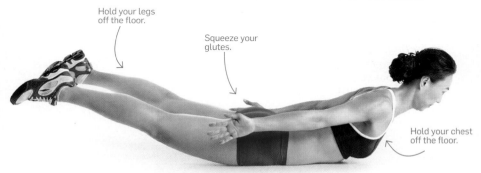

Hold your legs off the floor.

Squeeze your glutes.

Hold your chest off the floor.

Cable Core Press

A

- With a hand-over-hand grip, grab a handle attached to the mid pulley of a cable station.

- Stand with your right side facing the weight stack and spread your feet about shoulder-width apart, your knees slightly bent.

- Step away from the stack so the cable is taut. Hold the handle against your chest and brace your abs.

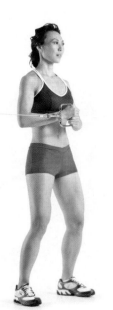

B

- Slowly press your arms in front of you until they're completely straight, pause for a second, and bring them back.

- Do all your reps, then turn around and work your other side.

THE OBJECTIVE OF THIS EXERCISE IS TO AVOID ROTATION. *So if you're hiking up your hip or rotating your shoulders, you're using too much weight. Squeeze your abs, keep your chest up and shoulders back, and move your arms at a slow and steady pace.*

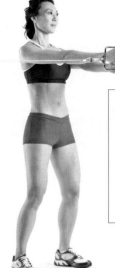

Core | STABILITY EXERCISES

MAIN MOVE
Kneeling Stability Chop

A

- Attach a rope handle to the high pulley of a cable station. Kneel down next to the handle so that your right side faces the weight stack.
- With both hands, grasp the rope with an overhand grip.
- Your shoulders should be turned toward the rope, but your belly button should be pointing forward.

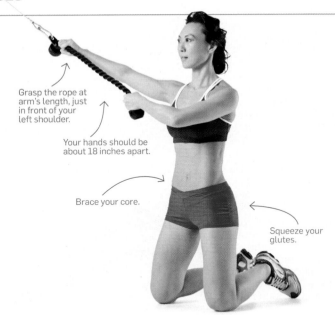

Grasp the rope at arm's length, just in front of your left shoulder.

Your hands should be about 18 inches apart.

Brace your core.

Squeeze your glutes.

B

- Keep your torso upright for the entire movement.
- Without moving your torso, pull the rope past your left hip.
- Reverse the movement to return to the starting position.
- Complete the prescribed number of repetitions toward your left side, then kneel with your left side facing the weight stack and do the same number of reps toward your right side.

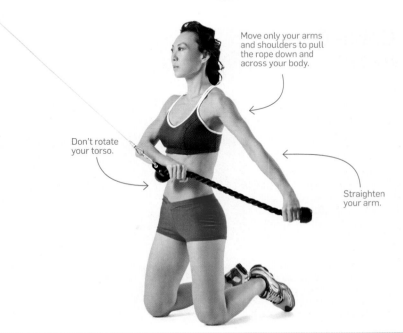

Move only your arms and shoulders to pull the rope down and across your body.

Don't rotate your torso.

Straighten your arm.

VARIATION #1
Half-Kneeling Stability Chop

A

- Kneel down so that your outside knee is on the floor but your inside knee is bent 90 degrees, with your inside foot flat on the floor.

Your torso should be upright.

Inside knee

Outside knee

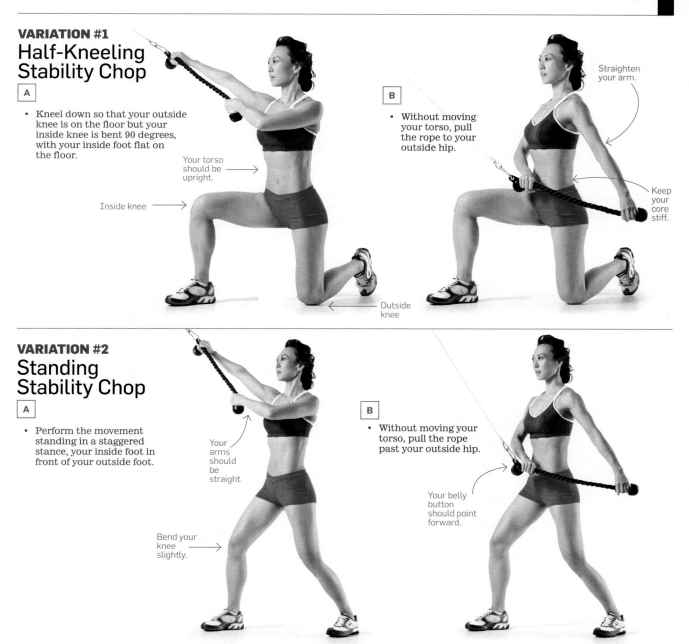

B

- Without moving your torso, pull the rope to your outside hip.

Straighten your arm.

Keep your core stiff.

VARIATION #2
Standing Stability Chop

A

- Perform the movement standing in a staggered stance, your inside foot in front of your outside foot.

Your arms should be straight.

Bend your knee slightly.

B

- Without moving your torso, pull the rope past your outside hip.

Your belly button should point forward.

MAIN MOVE
Kneeling Stability Reverse Chop

A

- Attach a rope handle to the low pulley of a cable station. Kneel down next to the handle so that your right side faces the weight stack.

- With both hands, grasp the rope with an overhand grip.

- Your shoulders should be turned toward the rope, but your belly button should be pointing forward.

B

- Keep your torso upright for the entire movement.

- Without moving your torso, pull the rope past your left shoulder.

- Reverse the movement to return to the starting position.

- Complete the prescribed number of repetitions toward your left side, then kneel with your left side facing the weight stack and do the same number of reps toward your right side.

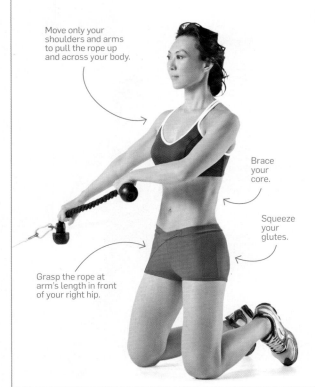

Move only your shoulders and arms to pull the rope up and across your body.

Brace your core.

Squeeze your glutes.

Grasp the rope at arm's length in front of your right hip.

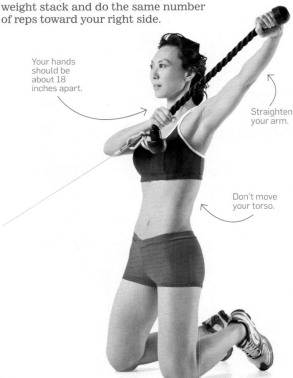

Your hands should be about 18 inches apart.

Straighten your arm.

Don't move your torso.

VARIATION #1
Half-Kneeling Stability Reverse Chop

A

- Kneel down so that your inside knee is on the floor but your outside knee is bent 90 degrees, with your outside foot flat on the floor.

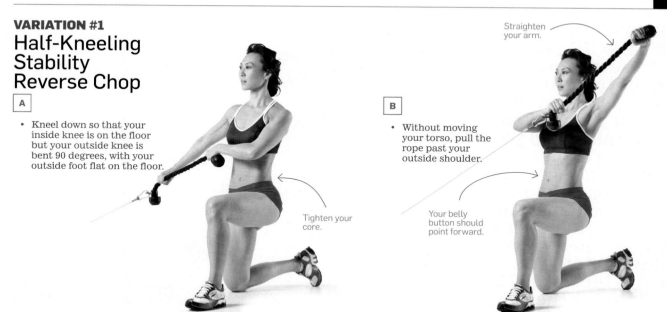

Tighten your core.

B

- Without moving your torso, pull the rope past your outside shoulder.

Straighten your arm.

Your belly button should point forward.

VARIATION #2
Standing Stability Reverse Chop

A

- Perform the movement standing in a staggered stance, your outside foot in front of your inside foot.

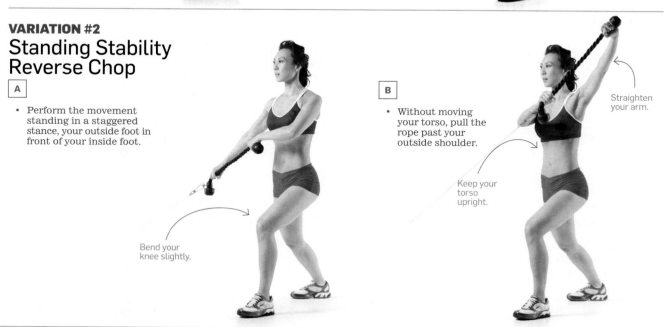

Bend your knee slightly.

B

- Without moving your torso, pull the rope past your outside shoulder.

Straighten your arm.

Keep your torso upright.

ROTATIONAL EXERCISES

These exercises target all of your abdominal muscles, with an emphasis on your obliques. They also help your abs work in conjunction with the muscles of your lower back and hips so that you can rotate your body with more power. These movements are ideal for anyone who plays tennis, softball, or golf, since they improve your ability to throw and swing explosively.

10

Number of additional reps people could complete while listening to their favorite music on an MP3 player, according to a study from the College of Charleston.

MAIN MOVE
Russian Twist

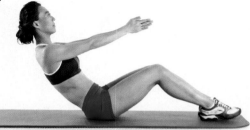

- Sit on the floor with your knees bent and your feet flat.
- Hold your arms straight out in front of your chest with your palms together.
- Lean back so your torso is at a 45-degree angle to the floor.

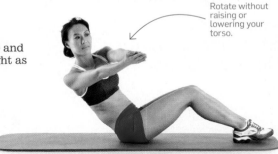

Rotate without raising or lowering your torso.

- Brace your core and rotate to the right as far as you can.

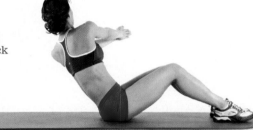

- Pause, then reverse your movement and twist all the way back to the left as far as you can.

VARIATION #1
Weighted Russian Twist

 A

- With both hands, hold the ends of a dumb-bell, the sides of a weight plate, or a medicine ball as you perform the movement.

Your arms should be straight.

Hold your torso at a 45-degree angle for the entire movement.

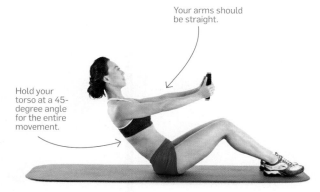

B

- Brace your core, and rotate your torso to the right as far as you can.

Keep your feet flat on the floor.

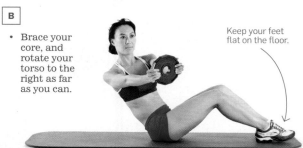

C

- Rotate to the left as far as you can.

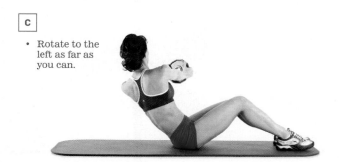

VARIATION #2
Elevated-Feet Russian Twist

 A

- Raise your feet a few inches off the floor and hold them there as you perform the movement

Brace your core.

Your knees should be bent.

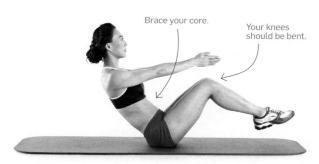

B

- Rotate your torso to the right.

Don't drop your feet.

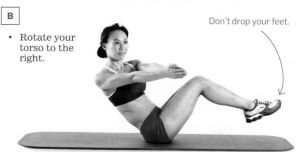

C

- Rotate your torso to the left.

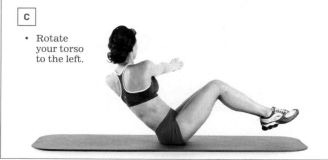

Core | ROTATIONAL EXERCISES

VARIATION #3
Cycling Russian Twist

- Lift your legs so they're elevated but parallel with the floor.
- Extend your left leg and twist to the right as you pull your right knee to your chest. Don't let your legs touch the floor at any point during the move.

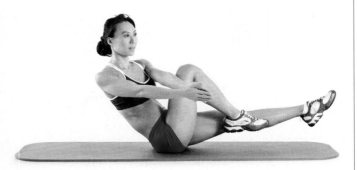

B

- Rotate to the left as you raise your left knee and straighten your right leg.

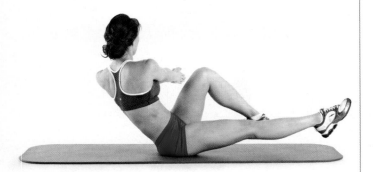

VARIATION #4
Swiss-Ball Russian Twist

A

- Lie with your middle and upper back placed firmly on a Swiss ball.
- Raise your hips so that your body forms a straight line from your knees to your shoulders.
- Hold your arms straight out in front of your chest with your palms together.

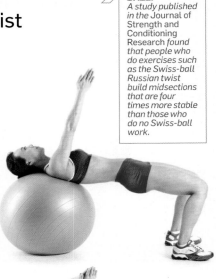

GET ON THE BALL!
A study published in the Journal of Strength and Conditioning Research found that people who do exercises such as the Swiss-ball Russian twist build midsections that are four times more stable than those who do no Swiss-ball work.

B

- Brace your core and roll your upper body to the right as far as you can.

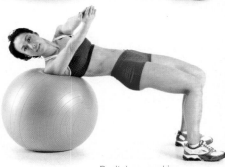

Don't drop your hips, but allow them to rotate naturally.

C

- Reverse your movement and roll all the way back to the left as far as you can.

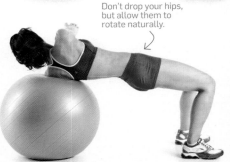

MAIN MOVE
Hip Crossover

 A

- Lie faceup on the floor with your arms straight out from your sides, palms facing up.
- Raise your legs off the floor so that your hips and knees are bent 90 degrees.

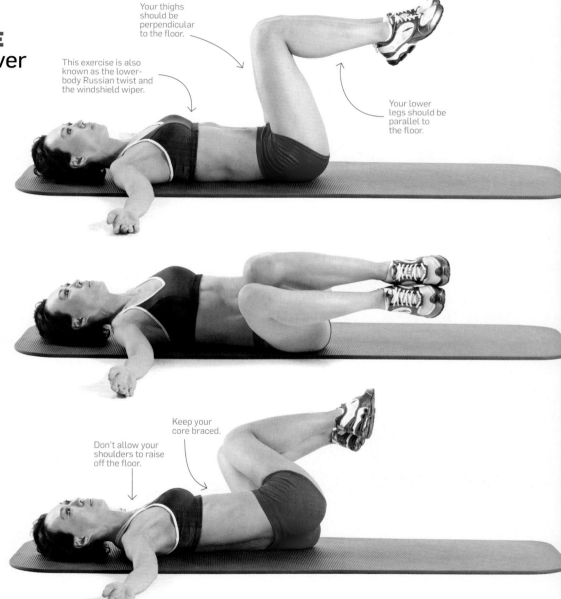

Your thighs should be perpendicular to the floor.

This exercise is also known as the lower-body Russian twist and the windshield wiper.

Your lower legs should be parallel to the floor.

B

- Brace your abs and lower your legs to the right as far as you comfortably can without lifting your shoulders off the floor.

 C

- Reverse the movement all the way to the left. Continue to alternate back and forth.

Don't allow your shoulders to raise off the floor.

Keep your core braced.

Core | ROTATIONAL EXERCISES

VARIATION
Swiss-Ball Hip Crossover

A

- Hold a Swiss ball between your lower legs and the backs of your thighs.

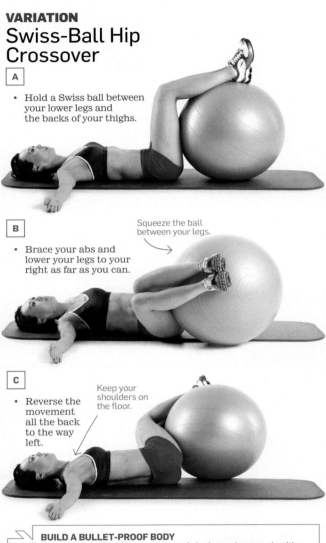

B

- Brace your abs and lower your legs to your right as far as you can.

Squeeze the ball between your legs.

C

- Reverse the movement all the back to the way left.

Keep your shoulders on the floor.

> **BUILD A BULLET-PROOF BODY**
> *Core exercises like hip crossovers and planks can keep you healthy. Medicine & Science in Sports & Exercise reports that researchers tracked college basketball and track athletes before their seasons and found that those who suffered lower-body injuries had 32 percent less core strength than those who avoided such injuries. Strong stabilizing muscles in the hips, lower back, and abdominal areas provided safe foundations for the injury-free players.*

Dumbbell Chop

A

- Grab a dumbbell and hold it with both hands above your right shoulder.
- Rotate your torso to your right.

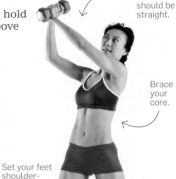

Your arm should be straight.

Brace your core.

B

- Swing the dumbbell down and to the outside of your left knee by rotating to the left and bending at your hips.
- Reverse the movement to return to the start.
- Complete the prescribed number of reps toward your left side, then do the same number on your right side, holding the dumbbell over your left shoulder.

Set your feet shoulder-width apart.

Don't round your lower back.

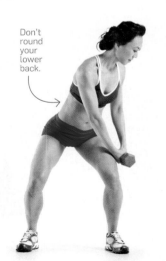

Medicine-Ball Side Throw

A

- Grab a medicine ball and stand sideways about 3 feet from a brick or concrete wall, your left side closer to the wall.
- Hold the ball at chest level with your arms straight, and rotate your torso to your right.

B

- Quickly switch directions and throw as hard as you can against the wall to your left.
- As the ball rebounds off the wall, catch it and repeat the movement.
- Complete the prescribed number of repetitions, then do the same number with your right side facing the wall, throwing from your left.

30

Percentage more control that golfers had on the putting green after an 11-week workout plan that included rotational medicine-ball exercises.

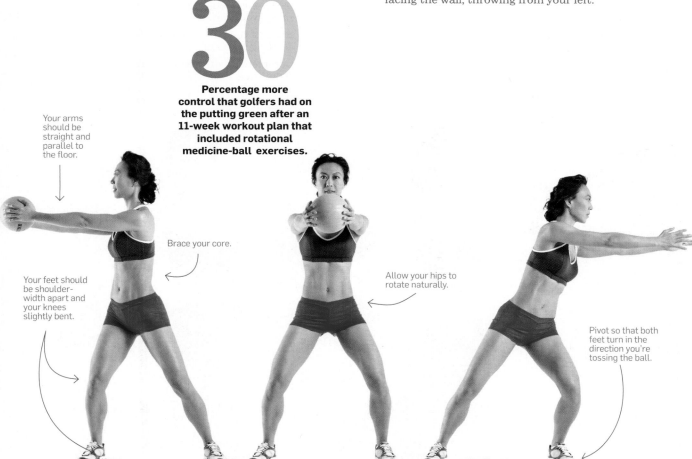

Your arms should be straight and parallel to the floor.

Brace your core.

Your feet should be shoulder-width apart and your knees slightly bent.

Allow your hips to rotate naturally.

Pivot so that both feet turn in the direction you're tossing the ball.

MAIN MOVE
Kneeling Rotational Chop

A

- Attach a rope handle to the high pulley of a cable station. Kneel down next to the handle so that your right side faces the weight stack.
- Rotate your body to grip the rope with both hands.
- Your torso should be turned toward the cable machine.

B

- Keep your torso upright for the entire movement.
- In one movement, pull the rope down and past your left hip as you simultaneously rotate your torso.
- Reverse the movement to return to the starting position.
- Complete the prescribed number of repetitions to your left side, then do the same number with your left side facing the stack, pulling toward your right.

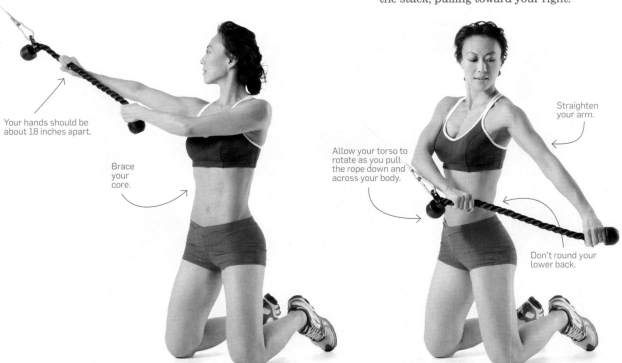

Your hands should be about 18 inches apart.

Brace your core.

Allow your torso to rotate as you pull the rope down and across your body.

Straighten your arm.

Don't round your lower back.

VARIATION #1
Standing Split Rotational Chop
• Perform the movement standing in a staggered stance, your inside foot in front of your outside foot.

Stiffen your core.

Your knees should be bent.

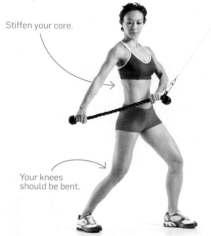

VARIATION #2
Standing Rotational Chop
• Perform the movement while standing with your feet shoulder-width apart.

Bend your knees slightly.

Your feet should be angled toward the weight stack.

Pivot to your left as you pull the cable down and to your left.

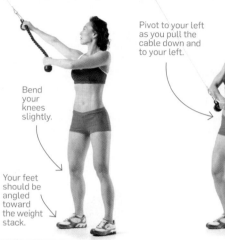
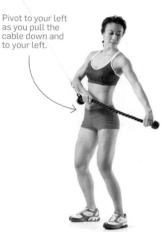

VARIATION #3
Half-Kneeling Rotational Chop

 A

• Kneel down so that your outside knee is on the floor but your inside knee is bent 90 degrees with your inside foot flat on the floor.

Bend your left arm and straighten your right arm as you pull the rope down.

B

• Pull the rope past your outside hip.

Keep your core braced.

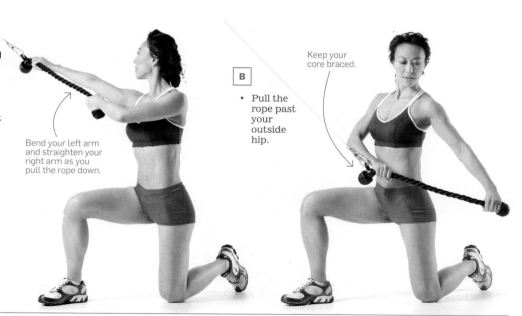

MAIN MOVE
Kneeling Rotational Reverse Chop

- Attach a rope handle to the low pulley of a cable station. Kneel down next to the handle so that your right side faces the weight stack.
- Brace your core and rotate your body to grip the rope with both hands.
- Your shoulders should be turned toward the cable machine.

B

- Keep your torso upright for the entire movement.
- In one movement, pull the rope past your left shoulder as you simultaneously rotate your torso to the left.
- Reverse the movement to return to the starting position.
- Complete the prescribed number of reps to your left side, then do the same number with your left side facing the stack, rotating to your right.

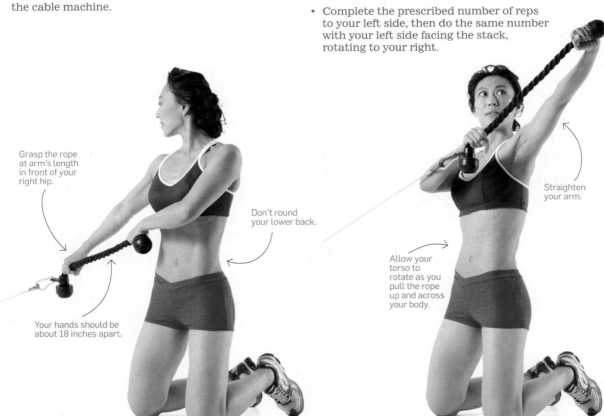

Grasp the rope at arm's length in front of your right hip.

Don't round your lower back.

Your hands should be about 18 inches apart.

Straighten your arm.

Allow your torso to rotate as you pull the rope up and across your body.

VARIATION #1
Standing Split Rotational Reverse Chop

- Perform the movement standing in a staggered stance, your outside foot in front of your inside foot.

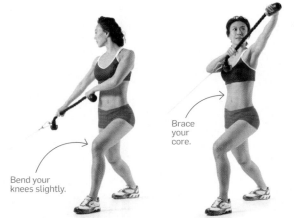

Bend your knees slightly.

Brace your core.

VARIATION #2
Standing Rotational Reverse Chop

- Perform the movement while standing with your feet shoulder-width apart.

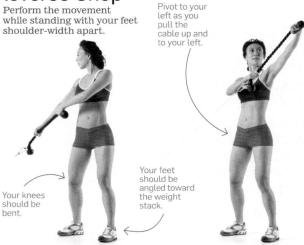

Pivot to your left as you pull the cable up and to your left.

Your knees should be bent.

Your feet should be angled toward the weight stack.

VARIATION #3
Half-Kneeling Rotational Reverse Chop

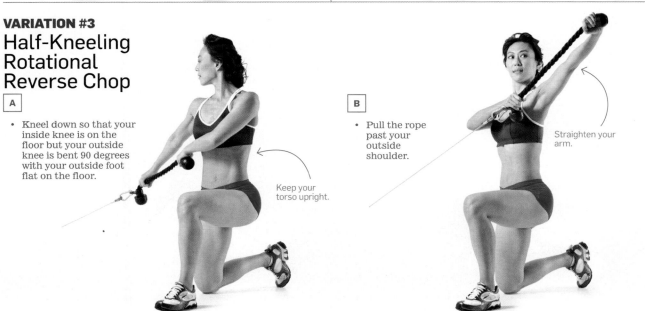

A

- Kneel down so that your inside knee is on the floor but your outside knee is bent 90 degrees with your outside foot flat on the floor.

Keep your torso upright.

B

- Pull the rope past your outside shoulder.

Straighten your arm.

TRUNK FLEXION EXERCISES

These exercises target your rectus abdominis, a.k.a. your six-pack muscles. They also work your internal and external obliques.

MAIN MOVE
Situp

A

- Lie faceup on the floor with your knees bent and feet flat.

Place your fingertips behind your ears.

Your elbows should be in line with your body.

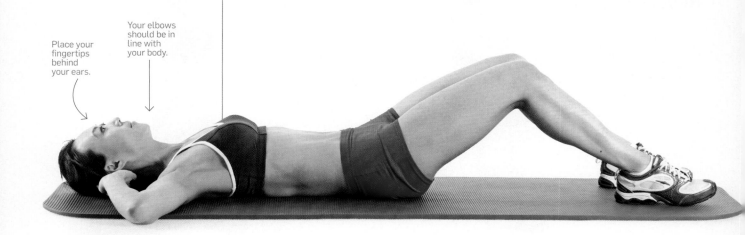

B

- Raise your torso to a sitting position.
- The movement should be fluid, not jerky—if it's the latter, you need to use a variation that's easier.
- Slowly lower your torso back to the starting position.

23

Percent reduction in heart disease risk linked to doing just 30 minutes of weight training a week, according to a Harvard University study.

MUSCLE MISTAKE
You Do Situps to Protect Your Back

While these exercises work well for targeting your ab muscles, they require you to round your lower back repeatedly. This can actually contribute to lower-back problems in some people, as well as aggravate pre-existing damage. So if you already have back pain, you should avoid these exercises. And as a general rule, make stability exercises the backbone of your core workout, since they've been shown to be beneficial to spinal health.

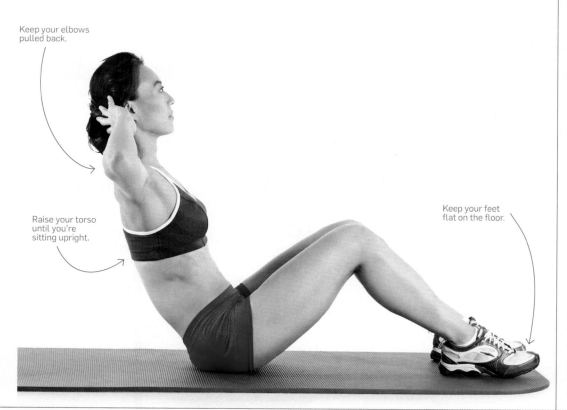

Keep your elbows pulled back.

Raise your torso until you're sitting upright.

Keep your feet flat on the floor.

Core | TRUNK FLEXION EXERCISES

VARIATION #1
Negative Situp

- Sit with your feet flat on the floor and your legs bent—as if you had just performed a situp—and slowly lower your body.

> During a negative situp, try to lower your torso at the same rate from start to finish. If you can't control your speed, identify the point at which you start to collapse and hold just above that point for 5 seconds on each repetition.

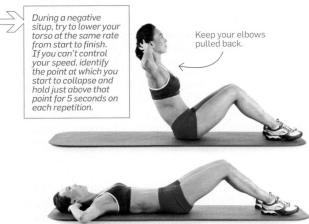

Keep your elbows pulled back.

VARIATION #2
Modified Situp

- Hold your arms completely straight next to your body, raised just a bit so that they're parallel to the floor.

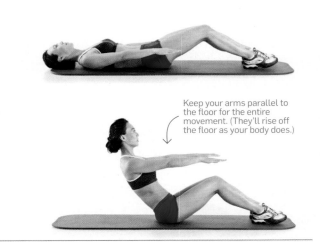

Keep your arms parallel to the floor for the entire movement. (They'll rise off the floor as your body does.)

VARIATION #3
Crossed-Arms Situp

A

- Perform the situp with your arms crossed in front of your chest.

B

- Contract your abs and curl your torso upward.

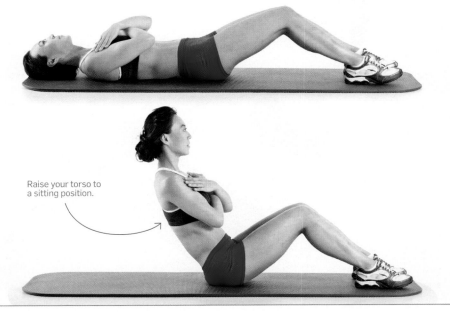

Raise your torso to a sitting position.

VARIATION #4
Weighted Situp
• Perform the situp while holding a weight plate across your chest.

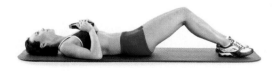

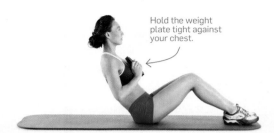

Hold the weight plate tight against your chest.

VARIATION #5
Alternating Situp
• As you raise your torso, rotate it to the left so that your left elbow touches your left knee. Lower, and on the next situp, rotate to the other side so that your right elbow touches your right knee.

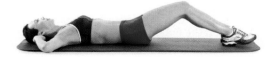

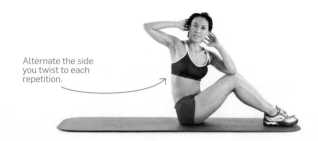

Alternate the side you twist to each repetition.

VARIATION #6
Decline Situp

A

• Position your feet under the leg anchors of a decline bench, and lie flat on your back.

B

• Raise your torso to a sitting position.

Don't pull your head forward as you raise your body. If you can't help it, the exercise is too hard for you.

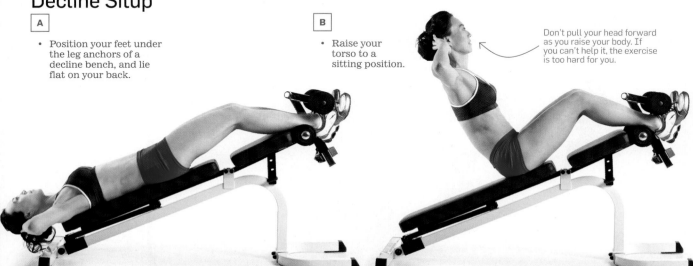

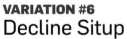

MAIN MOVE
Crunch

 A

- Sit on the floor with your knees bent and your feet flat on the floor.
- Place your fingertips behind your ears, and pull your elbows back so that they're in line with your body.

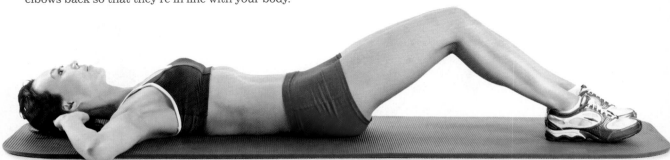

 B

- Raise your head and shoulders and crunch your rib cage toward your pelvis.
- Pause, then slowly return to the starting position.

Don't pull your head forward.

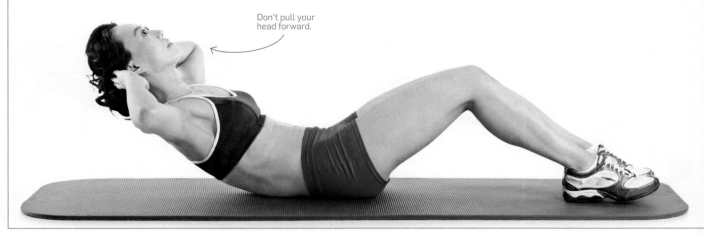

VARIATION #1
Crossed-Arms Crunch
* Perform the crunch with your arms crossed in front of your chest.

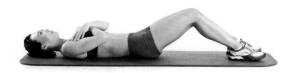

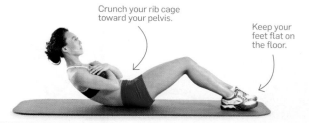

Crunch your rib cage toward your pelvis.

Keep your feet flat on the floor.

VARIATION #2
Weighted Crunch
* Perform the crunch while holding a weight plate across your chest.

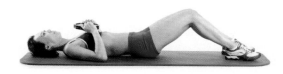

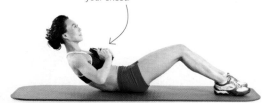

Hold the weight plate tight against your chest.

VARIATION #3
Elbow-to-Knee Crunch
* Lie faceup with your hips and knees bent 90 degrees so that your lower legs are parallel to the floor.

* Place your fingers on the sides of your forehead.

* Lift your shoulders off the floor and hold them there.

* Twist your upper body to the right as you pull your right knee in as fast as you can until it touches your left elbow. Simultaneously straighten your left leg.

* Return to the starting position and repeat to the right.

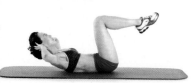

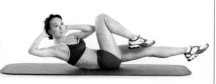

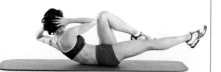

VARIATION #4
Raised-Legs Crunch
* Lie on your back with your hips bent 90 degrees and your legs straight.

* Hold your arms straight above your chest.

* Reach for your toes by crunching your head and shoulders off the floor.

* Lower your head and shoulders to the starting position.

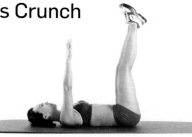

Your legs should point toward the ceiling.

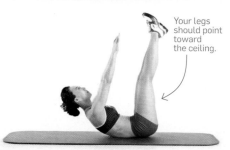

Core | TRUNK FLEXION EXERCISES

MAIN MOVE
V-Up

A

- Lie faceup on the floor with your legs and arms straight.
- Hold your arms straight above the top of your head.

Your arms should be in line with your body.

B

- In one movement, simultaneously lift your torso and legs as if you're trying to touch your toes.
- Lower your body back to the starting position.

Your torso and legs should form a V.

Keep your head in line with your body; don't crane your neck forward.

Your legs should be straight.

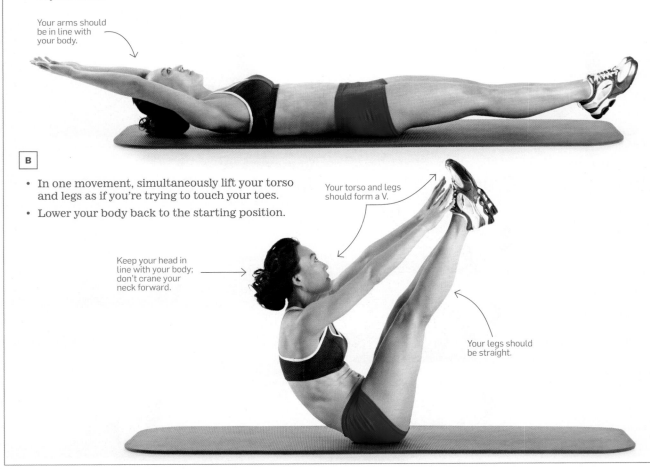

VARIATION #1
Medicine-Ball V-Up

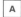

- Hold a medicine ball as you do the exercise.

- In one movement, lift your torso and legs as your bring the ball toward your feet.

Your arms should be straight.

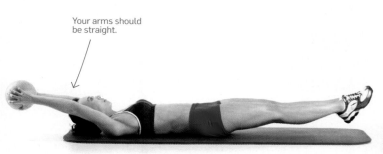

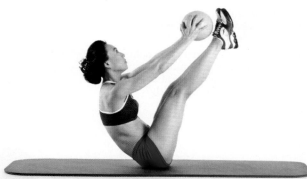

VARIATION #2
Modified V-Up

- Lie faceup on the floor with your legs straight and your arms at your sides.

- In one movement, quickly lift your torso into an upright position as you pull your knees to your chest.
- Lower your body back to the starting position.

Hold your arms slightly off the floor, your palms facing down.

Keep your arms parallel to the floor.

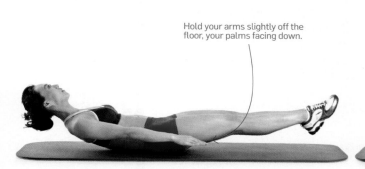

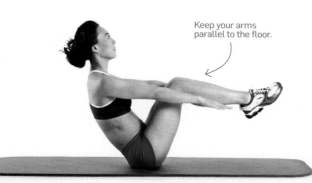

Core | TRUNK FLEXION EXERCISES

MAIN MOVE
Swiss-Ball
Crunch

 A

- Lie with your hips, lower back, and shoulders in contact with a Swiss ball.

- Place your fingertips behind your ears, and pull your elbows back so that they're in line with your body.

B

- Raise your head and shoulders and crunch your rib cage toward your pelvis.

- Pause, then slowly return to the starting position.

- Don't allow your hips to drop as you crunch up.

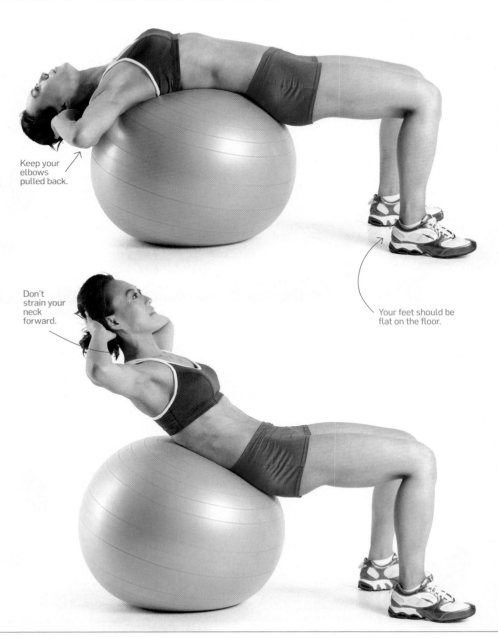

Keep your elbows pulled back.

Your feet should be flat on the floor.

Don't strain your neck forward.

318

VARIATION #1
Weighted Swiss-Ball Crunch

- Hold a weight plate across your chest.

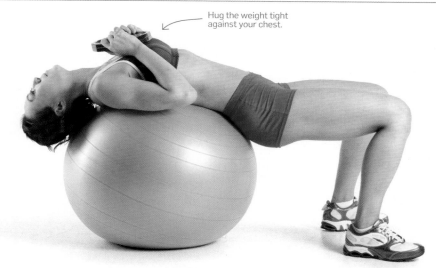

Hug the weight tight against your chest.

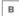

- Raise your head and shoulders off the ball.

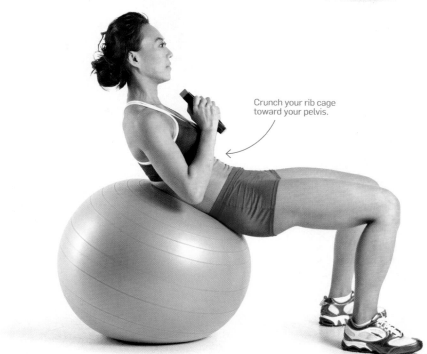

Crunch your rib cage toward your pelvis.

Core | TRUNK FLEXION EXERCISES

MAIN MOVE
Medicine-Ball Slam

A

- Grab a medicine ball and hold it above your head.

B **C**

- Reach back as far as you can, then slam the ball to the floor in front of you.

VARIATION
Single-Leg Medicine-Ball Slam

- Stand on one leg as you perform the exercise.

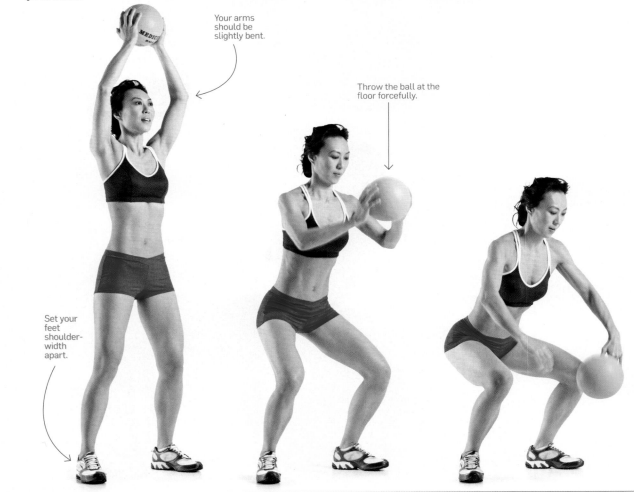

Your arms should be slightly bent.

Throw the ball at the floor forcefully.

Set your feet shoulder-width apart.

Kneeling Cable Crunch

- Attach a rope handle to the high pulley of a cable station, and kneel with your back to the weight stack.
- Drape the rope around your neck and hold an end against your chest with each hand.

- Crunch your rib cage toward your pelvis.
- Pause, then slowly return to the starting position.

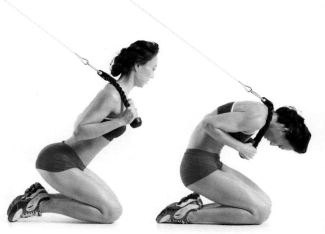

Standing Cable Crunch

- Attach a rope handle to the high pulley of a cable station, and stand with your back to the weight stack.
- Drape the rope around your neck and hold an end against your chest with each hand.
- Your elbows should be pointing straight down to the floor.

- Crunch your rib cage toward your pelvis.
- Pause, then slowly return to the starting position.

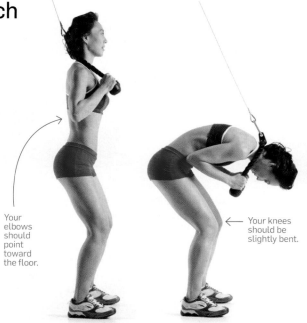

Your elbows should point toward the floor.

Your knees should be slightly bent.

Train Your Abs—Fast

Scientists in Spain found that performing abdominal exercises at a fast tempo activates more muscle than doing them slowly. That's because to increase your rate of movement, your muscles have to generate higher amounts of force, say the researchers. Their recommendation: Do as many reps as you can in 20 seconds. You'll target your fast-twitch muscle fibers, which are the ones with the greatest potential for size and strength.

HIP FLEXION EXERCISES

These exercises target your hip flexors and your external obliques. They also work many of your other core muscles, including your rectus abdominis.

MAIN MOVE
Reverse Crunch

A

- Lie faceup on the floor with your palms facing down.
- Bend your hips and knees 90 degrees.

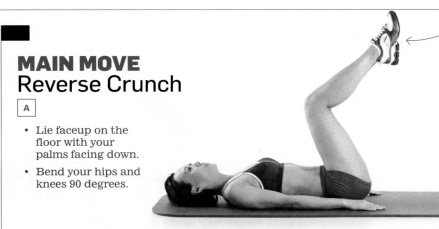

Hold your feet together.

B

- Raise your hips off the floor and crunch them inward.

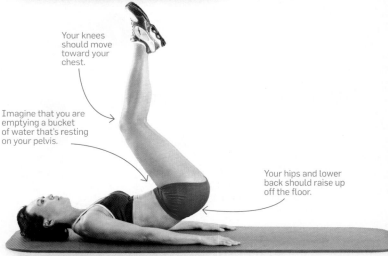

Your knees should move toward your chest.

Imagine that you are emptying a bucket of water that's resting on your pelvis.

Your hips and lower back should raise up off the floor.

C

- Pause, then slowly lower your legs until your heels nearly touch the floor.

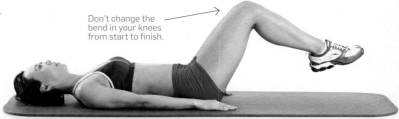

Don't change the bend in your knees from start to finish.

VARIATION #1
Swiss-Ball Reverse Crunch

A

- Lie faceup on a Swiss ball with your legs bent.

B

- Lift your hips up and in, pause, then lower them back to the starting position.

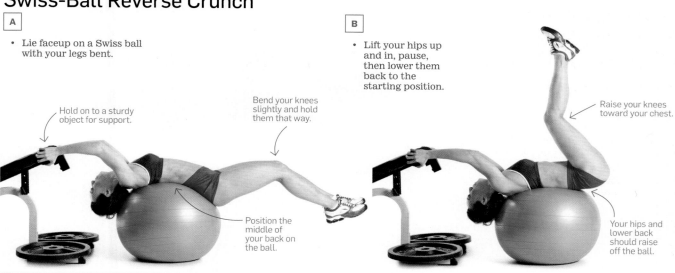

Hold on to a sturdy object for support.

Bend your knees slightly and hold them that way.

Position the middle of your back on the ball.

Raise your knees toward your chest.

Your hips and lower back should raise off the ball.

VARIATION #2
Incline Reverse Crunch

A

- Lie faceup on a slant board with your hips lower than your head. Grab the bar behind your head for support, or simply grasp the sides of the bench.

B

- Lift your knees toward your chest.

C

- Slowly lower your feet toward the floor.

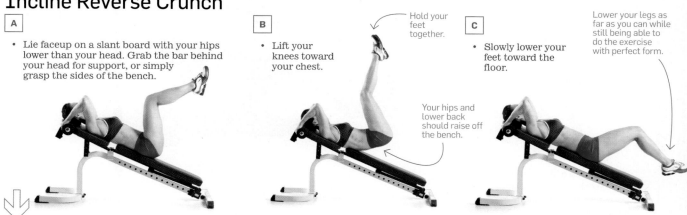

Hold your feet together.

Your hips and lower back should raise off the bench.

Lower your legs as far as you can while still being able to do the exercise with perfect form.

To make the incline reverse crunch even harder, hold a dumbbell between the inside edges of your shoes (as shown) as you perform the exercise. Keep your feet together, and the dumbbell won't fall.

Core | HIP FLEXION EXERCISES

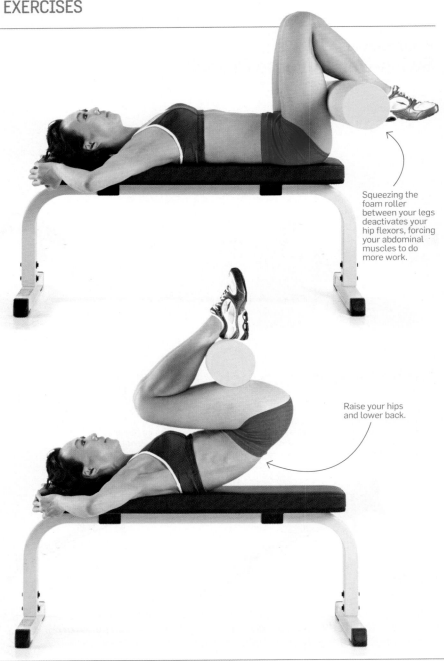

MAIN MOVE
Foam-Roller Reverse Crunch on Bench

A

- Lie faceup on a bench and hold a foam roller between the backs of your ankles and thighs.
- The fronts of your thighs should be facing your chest.
- Grasp the sides of the bench, next to your head.

B

- Raise your hips and bring your knees toward your shoulders without releasing the roller.
- Pause, then lower.

70

Percent more likely people who don't work out are to experience age-related macular degeneration—the leading cause of adult blindness—compared to those who exercise 3 times a week, according to a University of Wisconsin study.

Squeezing the foam roller between your legs deactivates your hip flexors, forcing your abdominal muscles to do more work.

Raise your hips and lower back.

VARIATION #1
Foam-Roller Reverse Crunch with Dumbbell

A

- Lie on the floor instead of on a bench, and grasp a heavy dumbbell that's set on the floor behind you.

B

- Raise your hips and bring your knees to your chest.

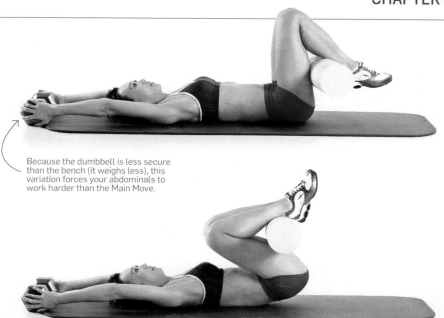

Because the dumbbell is less secure than the bench (it weighs less), this variation forces your abdominals to work harder than the Main Move.

VARIATION #2
Foam-Roller Reverse Crunch with Medicine Ball

A

- Lie on the floor instead of on a bench, and grasp a medicine ball that's set on the floor behind you.

B

- Raise your hips and bring your knees to your chest.

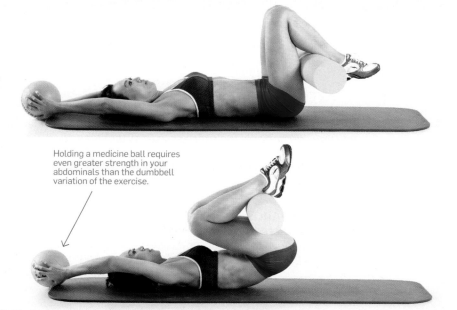

Holding a medicine ball requires even greater strength in your abdominals than the dumbbell variation of the exercise.

Core | HIP FLEXION EXERCISES

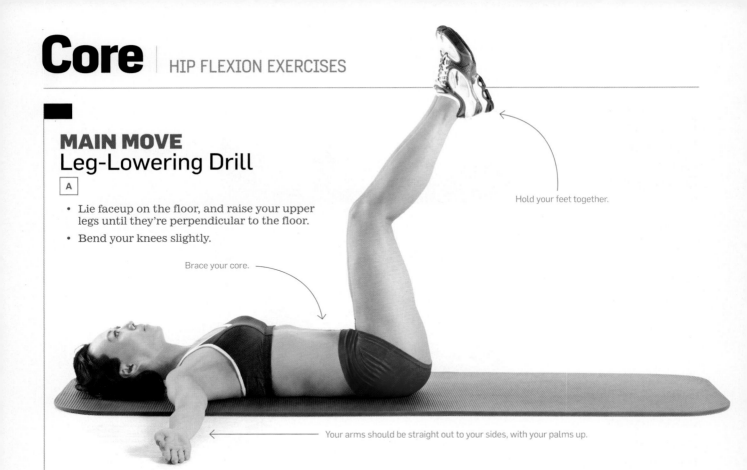

Hold your feet together.

MAIN MOVE
Leg-Lowering Drill

A

- Lie faceup on the floor, and raise your upper legs until they're perpendicular to the floor.
- Bend your knees slightly.

Brace your core.

Your arms should be straight out to your sides, with your palms up.

IF THE LEG-LOWERING DRILL IS TOO EASY:
Straighten your legs a little more. And keep doing so as it becomes easier, until you can perform the exercise with straight legs and without allowing the arch in your lower back to increase. You can also perform this on an incline bench, in a position similar to that of the incline reverse crunch.

IF IT'S TOO HARD:
Determine where the arch in your lower back starts to increase, and pause just above that point for a two-count each repetition. Then return to the starting position. You can also try the single-leg-lowering drill.

B

- Without changing the arch in your lower back or the angle of your knees, brace your core and try to take 3 to 5 seconds to lower your feet as close to the floor as you can. One trick: Press your lower back toward the floor as you perform the movement.
- Once your feet touch the floor, raise them back to the starting position and repeat.

Keep the same bend in your knees from start to finish.

When you can't stop the arch in your lower back from increasing, raise your legs back up to the start.

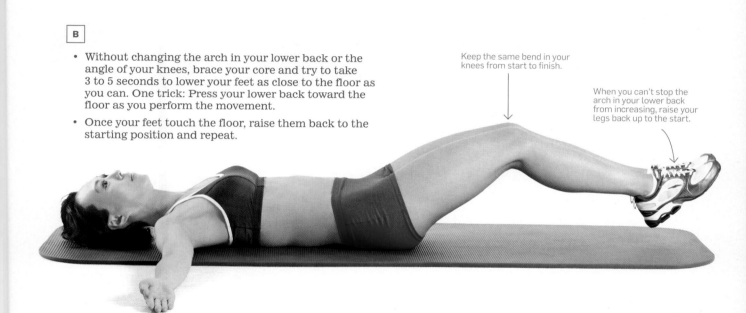

VARIATION
Single-Leg-Lowering Drill

- Hold one leg to your torso with both hands. Do all your reps, then switch legs and repeat.

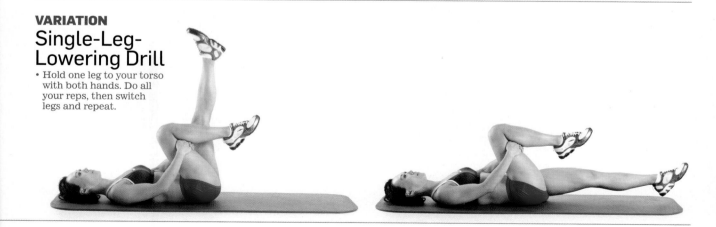

Swiss-Ball Pike

A

- Assume a pushup position with your arms completely straight.
- Position your hands slightly wider than and in line with your shoulders.
- Rest your shins on a Swiss ball.
- Your body should form a straight line from your head to your ankles.

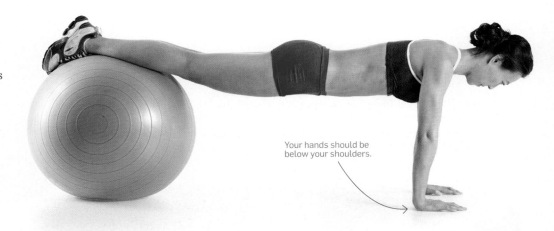

Your hands should be below your shoulders.

B

- Without bending your knees, roll the Swiss ball toward your body by raising your hips as high as you can.
- Pause, then return the ball to the starting position by lowering your hips and rolling the ball backward.

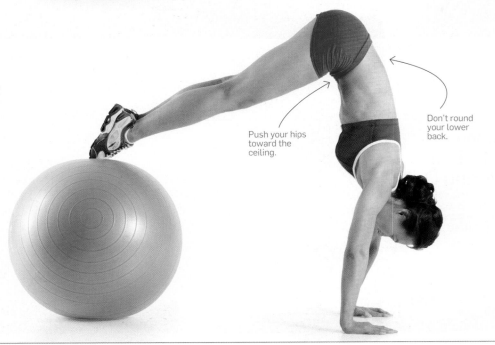

Push your hips toward the ceiling.

Don't round your lower back.

MAIN MOVE
Hanging Leg Raise

A

- Grab a chinup bar with an overhand, shoulder-width grip, and hang from the bar with your knees slightly bent and feet together. (If you have access to elbow supports—sling-like devices that hang from the bar—you may prefer to use those.)

B

- Simultaneously bend your knees, raise your hips, and curl your lower back underneath you as you lift your thighs toward your chest.
- Pause when the fronts of your thighs reach your chest, then slowly lower your legs back to the starting position.

VARIATION
Hanging Single-Leg Raise

- Maintain an upright torso, and simply raise one leg as far as you can without allowing your other leg to pull forward. Pause, then slowly lower back to the starting position and repeat with your other leg. Alternate back and forth.

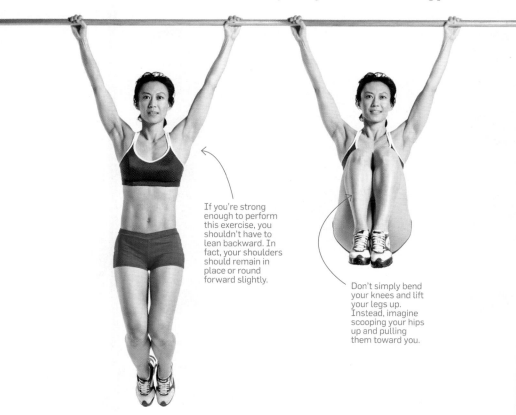

If you're strong enough to perform this exercise, you shouldn't have to lean backward. In fact, your shoulders should remain in place or round forward slightly.

Don't simply bend your knees and lift your legs up. Instead, imagine scooping your hips up and pulling them toward you.

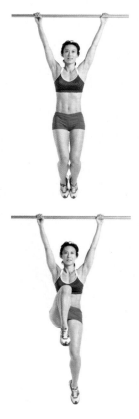

Core | HIP FLEXION EXERCISES

Hanging Hurdle

A

- Place a bench under and perpendicular to a chinup bar.
- Hang from the bar with your legs to one side of the bench, feet together and knees slightly bent.

B

- Without changing the bends in your knees or elbows, lift your legs over the bench to the opposite side.
- Repeat back and forth for 10 to 15 seconds.

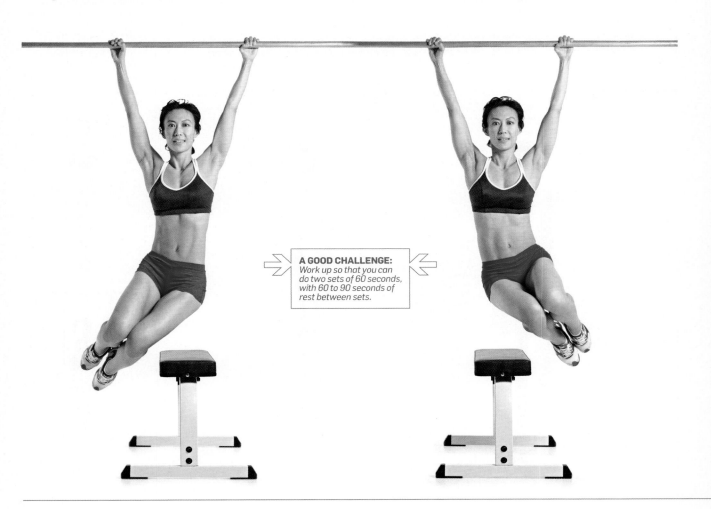

A GOOD CHALLENGE:
Work up so that you can do two sets of 60 seconds, with 60 to 90 seconds of rest between sets.

Medicine-Ball Leg Drops

A

- Lie faceup on the floor and squeeze a light medicine ball between your ankles.
- Keep your legs nearly straight and hold them directly above your hips.

B

- Allow your legs to drop straight down as far as possible without touching the floor. (It should feel like you're "throwing on the brakes.")
- In the same motion, return your legs to the starting position as fast as possible. That's one rep.

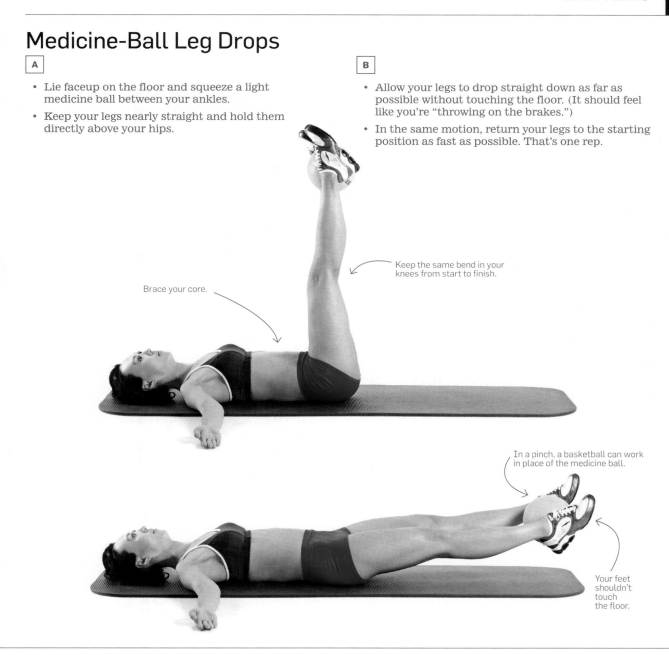

Keep the same bend in your knees from start to finish.

Brace your core.

In a pinch, a basketball can work in place of the medicine ball.

Your feet shouldn't touch the floor.

SIDE FLEXION EXERCISES These exercises target your internal and external obliques, the muscles on the sides of your torso. They also hit your quadratus lumborum, a lower-back muscle that helps you bend to the side.

Side Crunch

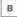

- Lie faceup with your knees together and bent 90 degrees.
- Without moving your upper body, lower your knees to the right so that they're touching the floor.
- Place your fingers behind your ears.

- Raise your shoulders toward your hips.
- Pause for 1 second, then take 2 seconds to lower your upper body back to the starting position.

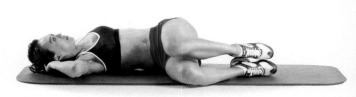

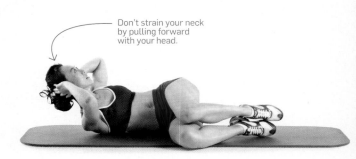

Don't strain your neck by pulling forward with your head.

Overhead Dumbbell Side Bend

- Hold a pair of dumbbells over your head, in line with your shoulders, with your arms straight.

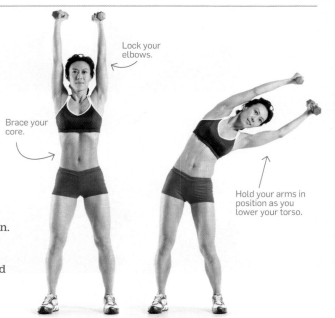

- Without twisting your upper body, slowly bend directly to your left side as far as you can.
- Pause, return to an upright position, then bend to your right side. Alternate back and forth with each repetition.

Lock your elbows.

Brace your core.

Hold your arms in position as you lower your torso.

Hanging Oblique Raise

A

- Grasp a chinup bar with an overhand grip and hang from it at arm's length.
- Lift your legs until your hips and knees are bent at 90-degree angles.

B

- Raise your right hip toward your right armpit.
- Pause, then return to the starting position and lift your left hip toward your left armpit. Alternate back and forth with each repetition.

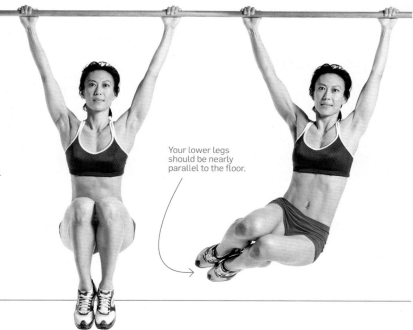

Your lower legs should be nearly parallel to the floor.

Swiss-Ball Side Crunch

A

- Lie sideways on a Swiss ball and brace your right foot against a wall or against a heavy object. Place your fingers behind your ears.

B

- Lift your shoulders and crunch sideways toward your hip.
- Pause, then return to the starting position.
- Complete the prescribed number of reps on that side, then do the same number on your other side.

Keep your left foot flat on the floor for balance and stability.

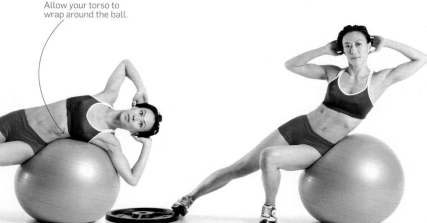

Allow your torso to wrap around the ball.

Core

THE BEST CORE EXERCISE YOU'VE NEVER DONE
Core Stabilization

Instead of rotating your core to move a weight, this exercise moves the weight around your core. Constantly shifting the location of the load forces your core muscles to perpetually adjust in order to keep your body stable. This not only builds your abs, but also more closely mimics the way your core muscles have to fire when you're playing sports—giving you an edge anytime you step on the court.

A

- Sit on the floor with your knees bent.
- Hold a weight plate straight out in front of your chest.
- Lean back so your torso is at a 45-degree angle to the floor, and brace your core.

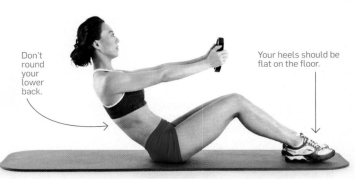

Don't round your lower back.

Your heels should be flat on the floor.

B

- Without moving your torso, slowly (take 2 seconds) rotate your arms to the right as far as you can. Pause for 3 seconds.

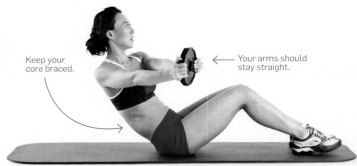

Keep your core braced.

Your arms should stay straight.

C

- Slowly rotate your arms to the left as far as you can.
- Pause again, then continue to alternate back and forth for the allotted time. A good goal: 30 seconds.

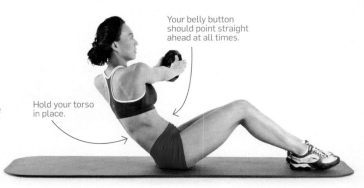

Your belly button should point straight ahead at all times.

Hold your torso in place.

THE BEST STRETCH FOR YOUR CORE
Half-Kneeling Rotation

Why it's good: Long hours of sitting at a desk or in front of a steering wheel can reduce the ability of your upper spine to rotate and bend to the side. This can lead to rounded shoulders and a hunched posture. This stretch increases the mobility of your upper spine, improving your posture as well as enhancing your rotation for sports such as golf, tennis, and softball.

Make the most of it: Hold this stretch for 5 seconds per repetition, and do 15 repetitions. Do a total of three sets. Perform this routine daily, and up to three times a day if you're really tight.

A

- Hold a broomstick across your upper back.
- Kneel down on your left knee and bend your right knee 90 degrees, with your right foot flat on the floor.
- Brace your abs and hold them that way.

Your torso should be upright.

B

- Keeping your back naturally arched, rotate your left shoulder toward your right knee. Hold that position for the prescribed amount of time.
- Return to the starting position. That's one repetition.
- Complete the prescribed number of reps toward your right side, then switch knee positions and do the same number to your left side.

Keep your core braced.

335

Core

BUILD PERFECT ABS

Work your abs like never before, with these cutting-edge core routines from Tony Gentilcore, CSCS. Tony is the cofounder of Cressey Performance in Hudson, Massachusetts, and a frequent guest host of an always informative Internet podcast called The Fit-Cast. (Check it out at http://fitcast.com.) Each of the three workouts he's provided sculpts your six-pack by forcing your abs to resist rotation and work double time to keep your spine stable.

How to do the workouts: Choose one of the three routines and perform the exercises in the order shown, using the prescribed sets, reps, and rest periods. Do the exercises as a circuit, completing one set of each in succession. Once you've done one set of each exercise, repeat the entire circuit two more times. For best results, complete this workout twice a week. After 4 weeks, try one of the other routines.

Workout A

EXERCISE 1: Cable core press (page 295)
Do 10 repetitions for each side, then rest for 30 to 45 seconds and move on to the next exercise.

EXERCISE 2: Reverse crunch (page 322)
Do 12 repetitions, then rest for 30 to 45 seconds and move on to the next exercise.

EXERCISE 3: Barbell rollout (page 292)
Do 8 repetitions, then rest for 60 seconds and repeat the entire circuit two times.

Workout B

EXERCISE 1: Kneeling stability chop (page 296)
Do 8 repetitions for each side, then rest for 30 to 45 seconds and move on to the next exercise.

EXERCISE 2: Swiss-ball plank (page 281)
Hold for 30 seconds, then rest for 30 to 45 seconds and move on to the next exercise.

EXERCISE 3: Swiss-ball rollout (page 292)
Do 8 repetitions, then rest for 60 seconds and repeat the entire circuit two times.

Workout C

EXERCISE 1: Single-arm cable chest press (page 58)
Do 10 repetitions for each side, then rest for 30 to 45 seconds and move on to the next exercise.

EXERCISE 2: Standing stability chop (page 297)
Do 10 repetitions for each side, then rest for 30 to 45 seconds and move on to the next exercise.

EXERCISE 3: Rolling side plank (page 285)
Hold each position for 5 seconds, then rest for 60 seconds and repeat the entire circuit two times.

BONUS ABS WORKOUT!

For each routine, perform the exercises in the order shown, using the prescribed sets, reps, and rest periods. The Level 1 routine is the easiest, and a good place for beginners to start; the Level 3 routine is the most difficult. For best results, complete this workout twice a week. If you start with the Level 1 workout, do it for 3 or 4 weeks, then progress to Level 2, and so forth.

LEVEL 1

1. Plank (page 278)
Hold the plank for 30 seconds. Rest for 30 seconds and repeat once.

2. Mountain climber with hands on bench (page 287)
Each time your raise your knee toward your chest, pause for 2 seconds, and then slowly lower your leg back to the start. Alternate your legs back and forth for 30 seconds. Rest for 30 seconds and repeat once.

3. Side plank (page 284)
Hold the plank for 30 seconds. Rest for 30 seconds and repeat once.

LEVEL 2

1. Elevated-feet plank (page 280)
Hold the plank for 30 seconds. Rest for 30 seconds and repeat once.

2. Mountain climber with hands on Swiss ball (page 289)
Each time your raise your knee toward your chest, pause for 2 seconds, and then slowly lower your leg back to the start. Alternate your legs back and forth for 30 seconds. Rest for 30 seconds and repeat once.

3. Side plank with feet on bench (page 285)
Hold the plank for 30 seconds. Rest for 30 seconds and repeat once.

LEVEL 3

1. Extended plank (page 280)
Hold the plank for 30 seconds. Rest for 30 seconds and repeat once.

2. Swiss-ball jackknife (page 290)
Do two sets of 15 reps, resting for 30 seconds between sets.

3. Single-leg side plank (page 285)
Hold the plank for 30 seconds. Rest for 30 seconds and repeat once.

BONUS WORKOUT: SAVE YOUR BACK IN 7 MINUTES

To reduce your chances of a back attack, try this workout from Stuart McGill, PhD, professor of spine biomechanics at the University of Waterloo, and author of *Low Back Disorders*. This 7-minute (or less) workout increases the endurance of your deep back and abdominal muscles, to improve spine stability and ultimately reduce lower-back stress. Do this routine once a day, every day. Simply perform the exercises as a circuit, doing one set of each movement without rest in between.

Cat camel (page 283)
Do five to eight repetitions.

McGill curlup (page 291)
Hold the curlup position for 7 or 8 seconds, then lower momentarily. That's one repetition. Do four repetitions, then switch legs and repeat.

Side plank (page 284)
Hold the side-plank position for 7 or 8 seconds, then lower your hips for a moment. That's one repetition. Do four or five repetitions, then switch sides and repeat.

Bird dog (page 283)
Hold the bird-dog position for 7 or 8 seconds, then lower your arm and leg momentarily. That's one rep. Do four repetitions, then switch arms and legs and repeat.

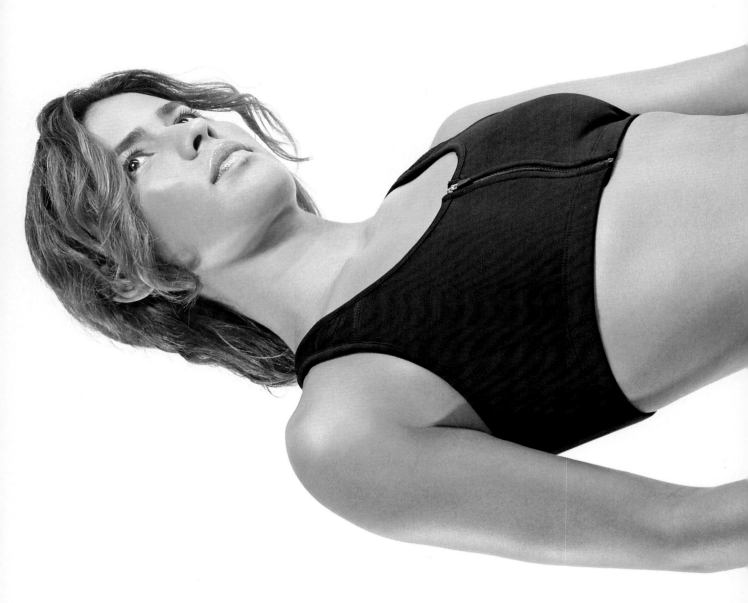

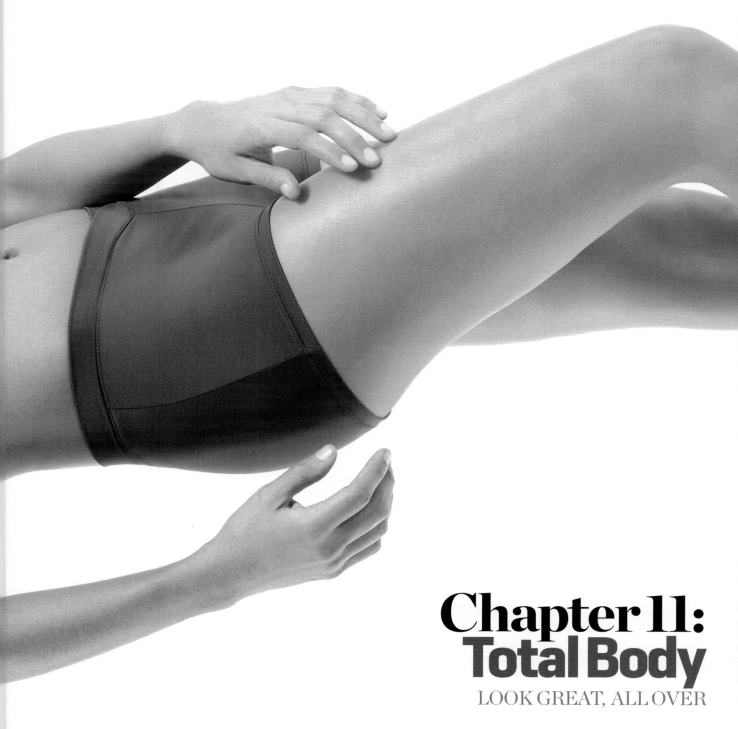

Chapter 11:
Total Body
LOOK GREAT, ALL OVER

Total Body

You might say exercises that work your total body are ideal for anyone who doesn't like to work out. Why? Because they target several large muscle groups at once, so you can accomplish an intense heart- and lung-pumping workout—that torches calories and stokes your metabolism—with fewer exercises and in less time than ever before. Of course, for those same exact reasons, total-body moves are also great for those who *do* love to work out.

In this chapter, you'll find 18 total-body exercises. Some will look familiar, since they're combinations of exercises from previous sections. Others will seem novel. But there's one trait they all share: These movements are among the fastest ways to burn fat and build total-body muscle.

Bonus Benefits

An athletic body! Total-body exercises improve your coordination and balance. So you'll be more graceful in every activity—from tennis to running to beach volleyball.

A healthier heart! The combination exercises will convince you that the term *cardio* doesn't just apply to aerobic exercise.

Greater strength! Full-body exercises require muscles all over your body to fire simultaneously. This enhances your strength from head to toe, helping eliminate the weaknesses that may be holding you back.

COMBINATION EXERCISES

Most of these exercises are combinations of movements that appear in other chapters. Each exercise works the muscles of your upper body, lower body, and core, and is a great addition to any fat-loss workout.

Barbell Front Squat to Push Press

A
- Hold the bar with an overhand grip that's just beyond shoulder width.
- Raise your upper arms until they're parallel to the floor.
- Set your feet shoulder-width apart.

B
- Keeping your upper arms parallel to the floor, push your hips back, bend your knees, and lower your body as far as you can.

C
- Simultaneously push your body back to the start as you press the bar over your head.

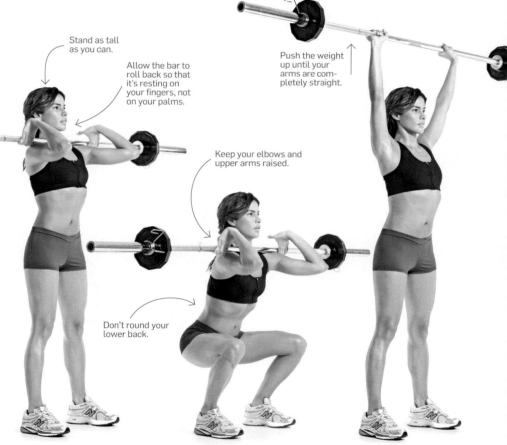

Stand as tall as you can.

Allow the bar to roll back so that it's resting on your fingers, not on your palms.

Push the weight up until your arms are completely straight.

Keep your elbows and upper arms raised.

Don't round your lower back.

Total Body |

Barbell Straight-Leg Deadlift to Row

A
- Grab a barbell with an overhand grip and hold it at arm's length in front your thighs.
- Stand with your feet shoulder-width apart and your knees slightly bent.

B
- Keeping your back naturally arched, bend at your hips and lower torso until it's nearly parallel to the floor.

C
- Pull the bar to your upper abs.
- Pause, then reverse through each step of the movement to return to the starting position.

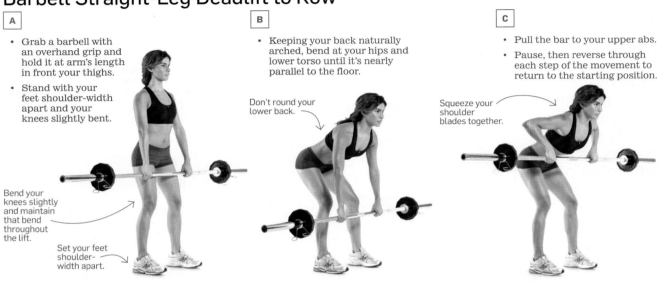

Bend your knees slightly and maintain that bend throughout the lift.

Set your feet shoulder-width apart.

Don't round your lower back.

Squeeze your shoulder blades together.

Dumbbell Straight-Leg Deadlift to Row

A
- Let a pair of dumbbells hang at arm's length in front of your hips.

B
- Bend at your hips and lower your torso into a bent-over position.

C
- Pull the dumbbells to the sides of your torso.

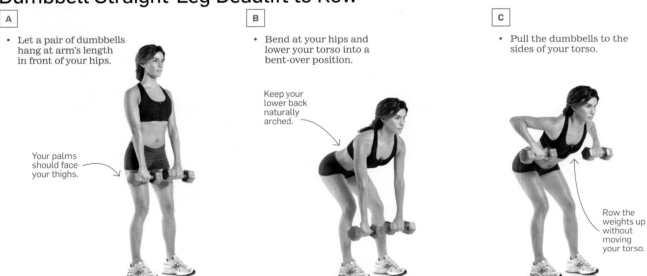

Your palms should face your thighs.

Keep your lower back naturally arched.

Row the weights up without moving your torso.

Thrusters

A

- Grab a pair of dumbbells and hold them next to your shoulders, your palms facing each other.
- Stand tall with your feet shoulder-width apart.

TRAINER'S TIP
Initiate the movement by pushing your hips backward, then bend your knees and lower your body as far as possible. (The deeper you squat, the better.)

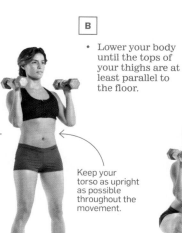

B

- Lower your body until the tops of your thighs are at least parallel to the floor.

Keep your torso as upright as possible throughout the movement.

C

- Push your body back to a standing position as you press the dumbbells directly over your shoulders.
- Lower the dumbbells back to the starting position.

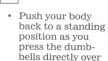
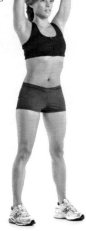

Dumbbell Hammer Curl to Lunge to Press

A

- Grab a pair of dumbbells and hold them at arm's length next to your sides, your palms facing each other.
- Stand tall with your feet hip-width apart.

Keep your torso upright for the entire movement.

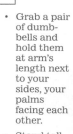

B

- Step forward with your right leg and lower your body until your front knee is bent at least 90 degrees.
- As you lunge, curl the dumbbells.

Your back knee should nearly touch the floor.

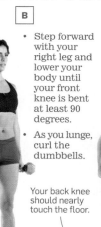

C

- Press the dumbbells directly above your shoulders.

Your arms should be straight.

D

- Push yourself back to the start, then lower the weights and repeat.

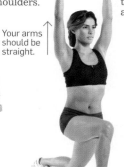

MUSCLE MISTAKE

You Don't Use Total-Body Moves to Tone Your Muscles

Big mistake. Whether a muscle is visible or not primarily depends on how much fat is covering it. And because total-body exercises burn more calories than isolation exercises such as biceps curls and triceps extensions, multi-muscle movements are far more valuable for helping to define your arms. The reason: You simply can't choose the location of the fat you burn, no matter what exercise you do.

Total Body | COMBINATION EXERCISES

Single-Arm Stepup and Press

 A

- Grab a dumbbell and hold it in your right hand, just outside your shoulder, your palm facing your shoulder.

- Place your left foot on box or a step that's about knee height.

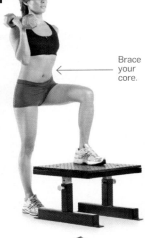

Brace your core.

B

- Push down with your left heel, and step up onto the box as you push the dumbbell straight above your right shoulder.

- To return to the starting position, lower your right foot back to the floor.

- Complete the prescribed number of repetitions with your left foot on the box and the weight in your right hand, then switch arms and legs and do the same number of reps.

Straighten your arm completely.

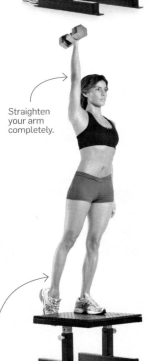

Your right leg should be held in the air.

Single-Arm Reverse Lunge and Press

A

- Grab a dumbbell with your right hand, and hold it next to your right shoulder, your palm facing in.

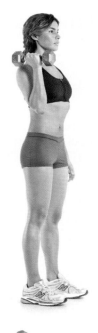

2

Times more fat people lost when they trained their entire body 3 days a week, compared to working each muscle group only once a week, according to University of Alabama scientists.

B

- Step backward with your right leg and lower your body into a reverse lunge as you simultaneously press the dumbbell straight above your shoulder.

- To return to the starting position, lower the dumbbell as you push yourself back up. That's one rep.

- Complete all your reps, then switch arms and legs and repeat.

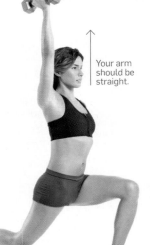

Your arm should be straight.

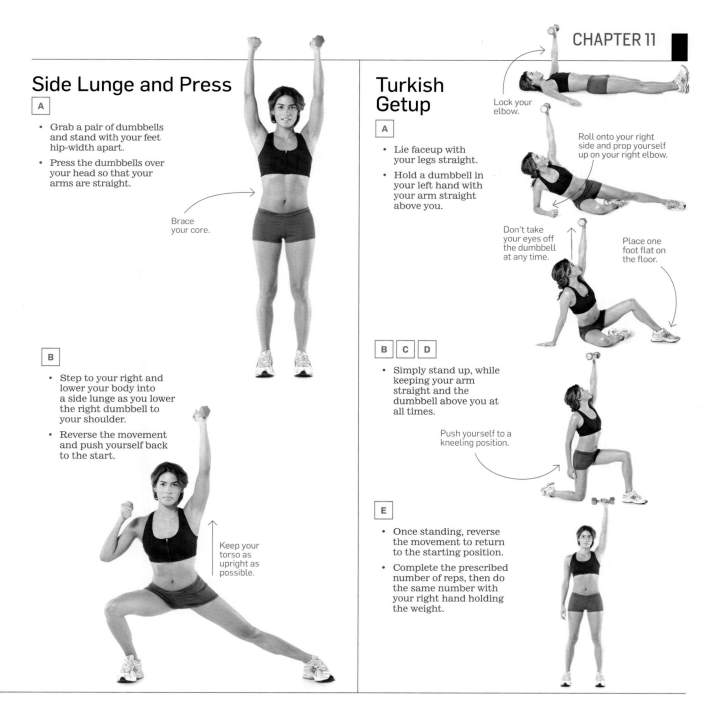

Side Lunge and Press

A

- Grab a pair of dumbbells and stand with your feet hip-width apart.
- Press the dumbbells over your head so that your arms are straight.

Brace your core.

B

- Step to your right and lower your body into a side lunge as you lower the right dumbbell to your shoulder.
- Reverse the movement and push yourself back to the start.

Keep your torso as upright as possible.

Turkish Getup

A

- Lie faceup with your legs straight.
- Hold a dumbbell in your left hand with your arm straight above you.

Lock your elbow.

Roll onto your right side and prop yourself up on your right elbow.

Don't take your eyes off the dumbbell at any time.

Place one foot flat on the floor.

B **C** **D**

- Simply stand up, while keeping your arm straight and the dumbbell above you at all times.

Push yourself to a kneeling position.

E

- Once standing, reverse the movement to return to the starting position.
- Complete the prescribed number of reps, then do the same number with your right hand holding the weight.

POWER EXERCISES

These exercises target your fast-twitch muscle fibers, the ones with the greatest potential for size and strength. Your goal should be to perform each of these movements as quickly as possible, while maintaining control of the weight at all times. If you play sports, these exercises are ideal for enhancing your ability to produce power, a combination of strength and speed that's the key to jumping higher, sprinting faster, and throwing farther.

Barbell High Pull

A

- Load the barbell with a light weight and roll it against your shins. If adding weight makes the exercise too difficult, perform it with just barbell (as shown).
- Grab the bar with an overhand grip that's just beyond shoulder width.
- Bend at your hips and knees to squat down.
- Raise your chest and hips until your arms are straight.

B

- Pull the bar as high as you can by explosively standing up as you bend your elbows and raise your upper arms.
- You should rise up on your toes.
- Reverse the movement to return to the starting position.

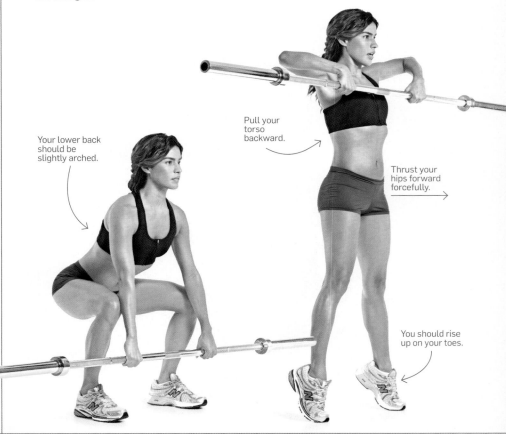

Your lower back should be slightly arched.

Pull your torso backward.

Thrust your hips forward forcefully.

You should rise up on your toes.

Barbell Hang Pull

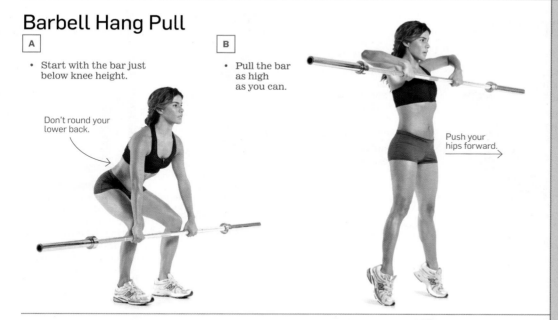

A
- Start with the bar just below knee height.

Don't round your lower back.

B
- Pull the bar as high as you can.

Push your hips forward.

Dumbbell Hang Pull

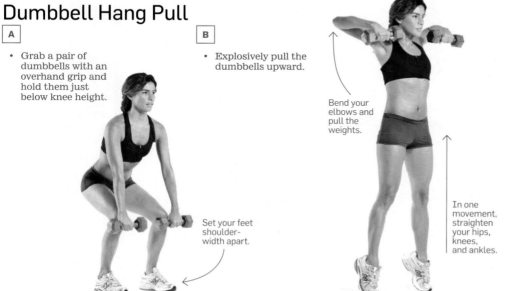

A
- Grab a pair of dumbbells with an overhand grip and hold them just below knee height.

Set your feet shoulder-width apart.

B
- Explosively pull the dumbbells upward.

Bend your elbows and pull the weights.

In one movement, straighten your hips, knees, and ankles.

Olympic Lifts for Everyone

Consider the barbell high pull and the other power exercises in this chapter to be simplified versions of the Olympic lifts used in the weight-lifting competitions you see at the Summer Games. While the Olympic lifts are quite technical and hard to learn, the high pull and jump shrug provide similar benefits with a much lower degree of difficulty. The reason: They require the same basic pulling movements but eliminate the "catch" phase, which yields little in terms of muscle work and is what makes these exercises so complicated.

Total Body | POWER EXERCISES

Barbell Jump Shrug

A

- Grab a barbell with an overhand grip that's just beyond shoulder width.
- Bend at your hips and knees until the barbell hangs just below your knees.

B

- Simultaneously thrust your hips forward, shrug your shoulders forcefully, and jump as high as you can.
- Land as softly as you can, and reset.

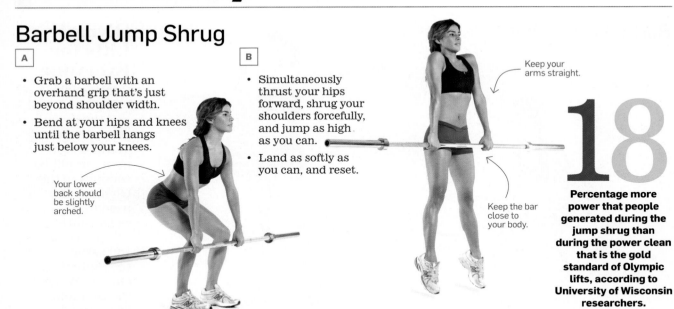

Your lower back should be slightly arched.

Keep your arms straight.

Keep the bar close to your body.

18

Percentage more power that people generated during the jump shrug than during the power clean that is the gold standard of Olympic lifts, according to University of Wisconsin researchers.

Wide-Grip Jump Shrug

- Use an overhand grip that's about twice shoulder width.

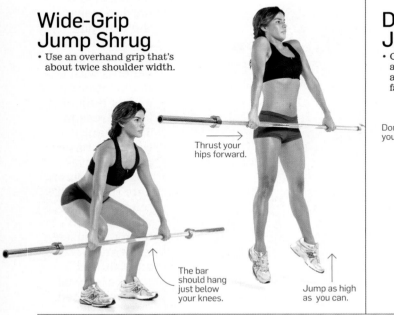

Thrust your hips forward.

The bar should hang just below your knees.

Jump as high as you can.

Dumbbell Jump Shrug

- Grab a pair of dumbbells and let them hang at arm's length, your palms facing your sides.

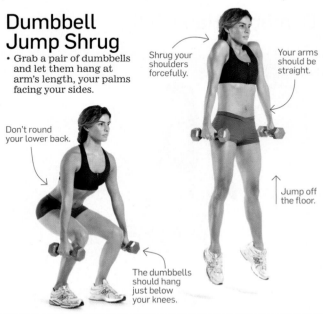

Shrug your shoulders forcefully.

Your arms should be straight.

Don't round your lower back.

Jump off the floor.

The dumbbells should hang just below your knees.

348

Single-Arm Dumbbell Snatch

A

- Grab a dumbbell with an overhand grip.
- Bend at your hips and knees to squat down until the weight is centered between your feet, your arm straight.

Your lower back should be slightly arched.

Drive your heels into the floor.

B

- In a single movement, try to throw the dumbbell at the ceiling—without letting go of it.

Keep the dumbbell as close to your body as possible at all times.

Your feet should be slightly wider than shoulder-width apart.

Bend your arm and raise your elbow as high as you can.

C

- Allow your forearm to rotate up and back from the momentum of the lift, until your arm is straight and your palm is facing forward.
- Pull your body under the weight.

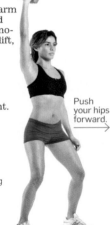

You should be thrusting the dumbbell upward so forcefully that you rise up on your toes.

Push your hips forward.

Single-Arm Hang Snatch
• Instead of starting from the floor, hold the dumbbell just below knee height.

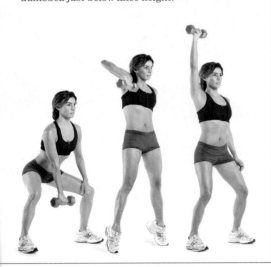

Single-Arm Kettlebell Snatch
• Substitute a kettlebell for a dumbbell.

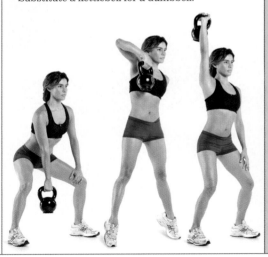

Power Up Your Workout

Try a doing a power move before a traditional strength exercise. For instance, perform a single-arm snatch or jump shrug before squats, or explosive pushups before standard pushups. In a study published in the *Journal of Strength and Conditioning Research*, people who did a squat after a power exercise performed better in the squat than those who skipped the explosive movement. The researchers speculate that performing a power exercise causes chemical changes within the muscle fiber, stimulating a greater number of nerves to be activated during the second exercise.

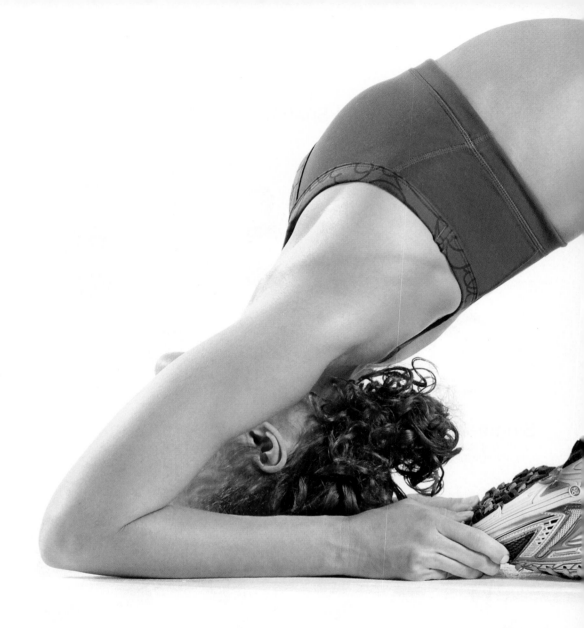

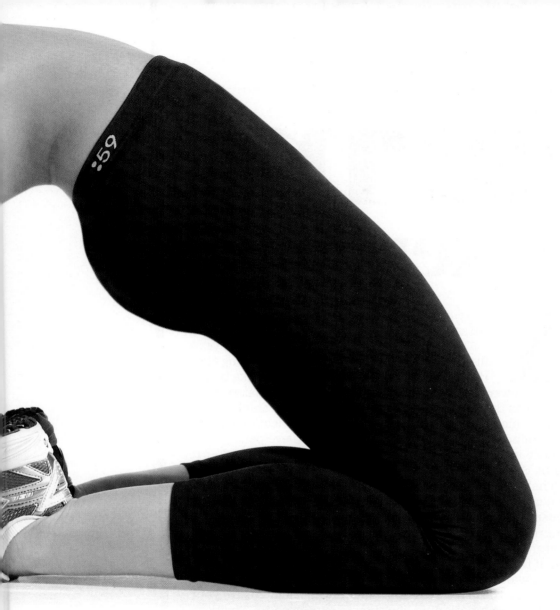

Chapter 12:
Warmup Exercises
MOVES THAT REALLY MATTER

Warmup Exercises

You're probably tempted to flip past this chapter. After all, who has time to warm up?

The answer is everyone. You see, over the years, fitness experts have discovered that doing the right movements before a workout is like turning on the power to your muscles. Scientists believe that exercises known as dynamic stretches—what you might think of as calisthenics—appear to enhance the communication between your mind and muscles, allowing you to achieve peak performance in the gym. Translation: faster fat loss and better results. Surely that isn't something you want to miss out on.

That's why this chapter provides a library of exercises that you can perform before any workout. Besides activating your muscles, the movements that have been chosen will also improve your flexibility, mobility, and posture—all critical factors for keeping your body both young and injury-free. All of this and it'll only require 5 to 10 minutes of your time.

But wait, there's more! You'll find a section on foam-roller exercises, too. These are movements that help ensure your muscles are functioning like they're supposed to. The best part: They can be done at any time—whether it's at the gym as part of your workout or after dinner on your living room floor. Just consider it the regular muscle maintenance you need to keep your body moving like a well-oiled machine.

Warmup Exercises

In this chapter, you'll find 49 exercises that help prepare your muscles for just about any activity, while also improving your flexibility and mobility.

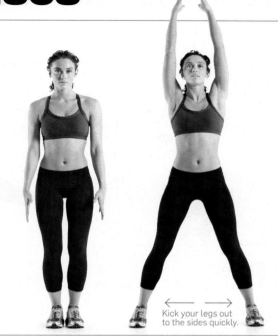

Jumping Jacks

- Stand with your feet together and your hands at your sides.
- Simultaneously raise your arms above your head and jump up just enough to spread your feet out wide.
- Without pausing, quickly reverse the movement and repeat.

Kick your legs out to the sides quickly.

Split Jacks

- Stand in a staggered stance, your right foot in front of your left.
- Simultaneously jump back with right foot and forward with your left as you swing your right arm forward and above your shoulder and swing your left arm back.
- Continue to quickly switch legs back and forth as you raise and lower your arms.
- Repeat as many times as you can in 30 seconds.

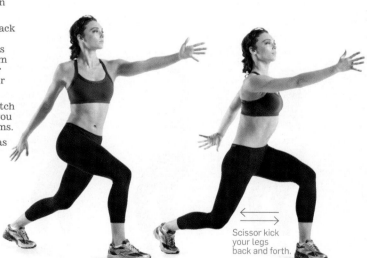

Scissor kick your legs back and forth.

Warmup Exercises

Squat Thrusts

- Stand with your feet shoulder-width apart and your arms at your sides.
- Push your hips back, bend your knees, and lower your body as deep as you can into a squat.
- Kick your legs backward, so that you're now in a pushup position.
- Then quickly bring your legs back to the squat position.
- Stand up quickly and repeat the entire movement.

If you want a greater challenge, do a pushup here.

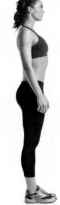

As you squat down, place your hands on the floor in front of you, shifting your weight onto them.

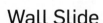

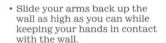

Wall Slide

- Lean your head, upper back, and butt against the wall.
- Place your hands and arms against the wall in the "high-five" position, your elbows bent 90 degrees and your upper arms at shoulder height.
- Keeping your elbows, wrists, and hands pressed into the wall, slide your elbows down toward your sides as far as you can. Squeeze your shoulder blades together.
- Slide your arms back up the wall as high as you can while keeping your hands in contact with the wall.
- Lower and repeat.

Don't allow your head, upper back, or butt to lose contact with the wall.

Hold for 1 second.

When your hands start to lose contact with the wall, slide your arms back down again.

THE BENEFIT *Enhances the function of your shoulder blades, which can help improve posture and shoulder health.*

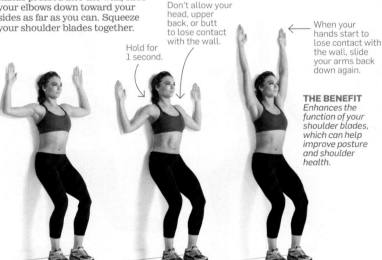

Hand Crossover

- Hold your arms so that, together, they form a straight line and a 45-degree angle with the floor.
- Your left arm should be raised, with your palm facing forward and your thumb pointing up.
- Your right arm should be held low, with your palm facing behind you and your thumb pointing down.
- Bring your arms across your body as if they were swapping positions, only keep the palm of each hand facing the same direction it was in the starting position.
- Alternate back and forth, gradually increasing the speed of the crossovers, so that you're loosely and quickly swinging your arms across your body. Do all your reps, then switch to the starting position and repeat.

Palm facing behind you, thumb up.

Palm facing forward, thumb up.

Palm facing behind you, thumb down.

Palm facing forward, thumb down.

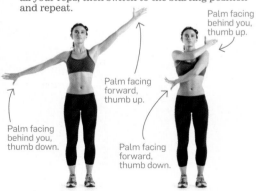

THE BENEFIT *Improves the mobility of your shoulders.*

Neck Rotations

- Stand tall with your feet shoulder-width apart.
- Roll your neck in a circular motion to the right 10 times (or as prescribed).
- Reverse directions, rolling in a circular motion to the left 10 times.

THE BENEFIT
Enhances the mobility of your neck.

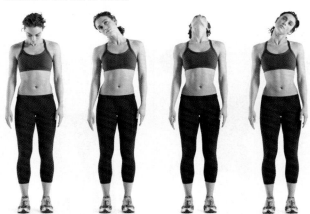

Side-Lying Thoracic Rotation

- Lie on your left side on the floor, with your hips and knees bent 90 degrees.
- Straighten both arms in front of you at shoulder height, palms pressed together.
- Keeping your left arm and both legs in position, rotate your right arm up and over your body and rotate your torso to the right, until your right hand and upper back are flat on the floor.
- Hold for 2 seconds, then bring your right arm back to the starting position.
- Complete the prescribed number of reps, then turn over and do the same number for your other side.

THE BENEFIT
Loosens the muscles of your middle and upper back.

Your arm and shoulder should touch the floor.

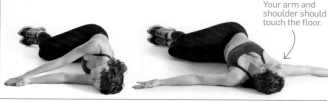

Thoracic Rotation

- Get down on on all fours.
- Place your right hand behind your head.
- Brace your core.
- Rotate your upper back downward so your elbow is pointed down and to your left.
- Raise your right elbow toward the ceiling by rotating your head and upper back up and to the right as far as possible.
- Complete the prescribed number of reps, then do the same number on your left.

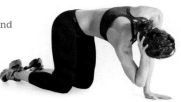

Bracing your abs—as if you were about to be punched in the gut—ensures that the rotation takes place at your upper back, and not your lower back.

THE BENEFIT
Enhances the mobility of your upper back, which can help improve posture.

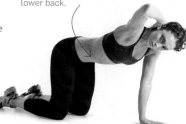

Reach, Roll, and Lift

- Kneel down and place your elbows on the floor, allowing your back to round.
- Your elbows should be bent 90 degrees.
- Your palms should be flat on the floor.
- Slide your right hand forward until your arm is straight.
- Rotate your right palm so that it's facing up.
- Raise your right arm as high as you can.
- Do all your reps, then repeat with your left arm.

THE BENEFIT
Enhances the mobility of your shoulders and upper back.

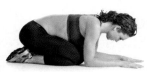

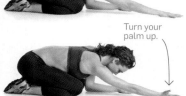

Turn your palm up.

Lift your arm.

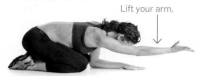

Warmup Exercises

Bent-Over Reach to Sky

- Keeping your lower back naturally arched, bend at your hips and knees and lower your torso until it's almost parallel to the floor.
- Let your arms hang straight down from your shoulders, palms facing each other.
- Brace your core.
- Rotate your torso the right as you reach as high as you can with your right arm.
- Pause, then return and reverse the movement to your left. That's one rep. (For even greater benefit, touch your toes between reps.)

THE BENEFIT
Enhances the mobility of your upper back.

Keep your arms straight for the entire movement.

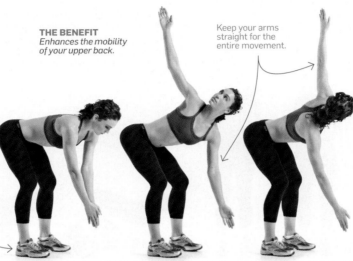

Set your feet shoulder-width apart.

Over-Under Shoulder Stretch

- Simultaneously reach behind your head with your right hand and behind your back with your left hand, and clasp your fingers together. Hold for 10 to 15 seconds.
- Release, and repeat with your left hand behind your head and your right hand behind your back

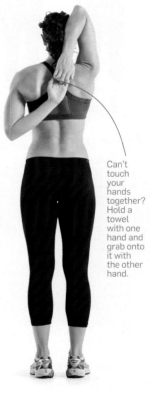

Can't touch your hands together? Hold a towel with one hand and grab onto it with the other hand.

THE BENEFIT
Loosens your rotator cuff and enhances shoulder mobility.

Shoulder Circles

- Stand tall with your feet placed shoulder-width apart.
- Without moving any other part of your body, roll your shoulders backward in a circular motion 10 times.

THE BENEFIT
Enhances the mobility of your shoulders.

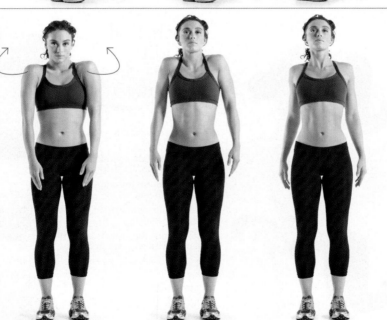

Arm Circles

- Stand tall, holding your arms straight out to your sides, so that they're parallel to the floor.
- Start by making small circles with your arm progressing to bigger circles. Do 10 reps forward, and 10 reps backward.

THE BENEFIT
Enhances the mobility of your shoulders.

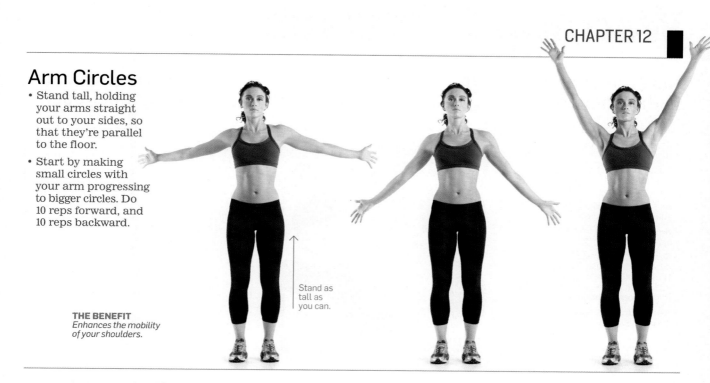

Stand as tall as you can.

Low Side-to-Side Lunge

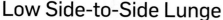

- Stand with your feet set about twice shoulder-width apart, your feet facing straight ahead.
- Clasp your hands in front of your chest.
- Shift your weight over to your right leg as you push your hips backward and lower your body by dropping your hips and bending your knees.
- Your lower right leg should remain nearly perpendicular to the floor.
- Your left foot should remain flat on the floor.
- Without raising yourself back up to a standing position, reverse the movement to the left. Alternate back and forth.

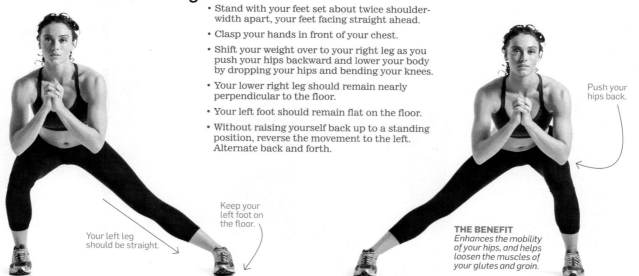

Your left leg should be straight.

Keep your left foot on the floor.

Push your hips back.

THE BENEFIT
Enhances the mobility of your hips, and helps loosen the muscles of your glutes and groin.

Warmup Exercises

Reverse Lunge with Reach Back

- Stand tall with your arms hanging at your sides.
- Brace your core and hold it that way.
- Lunge back with your right leg, lowering your body until your left knee is bent at least 90 degrees.
- As you lunge, reach back over your shoulders and to the left.
- Reverse the movement back to the starting position.
- Complete the prescribed number of repetitions with your left leg, then step back with your left leg and reach over your right shoulder for the same number of reps.
- Keep your torso upright for the entire movement.

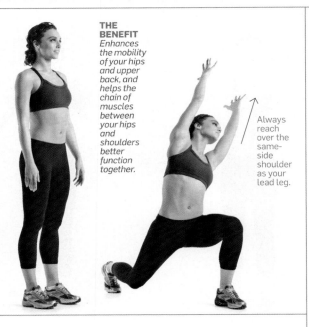

THE BENEFIT
Enhances the mobility of your hips and upper back, and helps the chain of muscles between your hips and shoulders better function together.

Always reach over the same-side shoulder as your lead leg.

Lunge with Diagonal Reach

- Grab a light dumbbell in your left hand and hold it in the "high-five" position—your upper arm perpendicular to your body and your elbow bent 90 degrees.
- Lunge forward with your right leg, lowering your body until your right knee is bent at least 90 degrees.
- As you lunge, rotate your torso to the right and reach across your body with your left arm, almost as if you were trying to put the dumbbell in your right back pocket.
- Reverse the movement back to the starting position.
- Do all your reps and repeat with your right arm, lunging with your left leg.

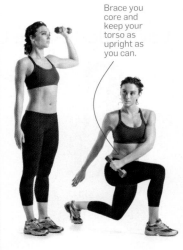

Brace you core and keep your torso as upright as you can.

THE BENEFIT
Enhances the mobility of your hips, and helps the chain of muscles between your hips and shoulders function better together.

Reverse Lunge with Twist and Overhead Reach

- Stand tall with your arms hanging at your sides and your palms facing the sides of your thighs.
- Brace your core.
- Step backward with your left leg, and lower your body until your right knee is bent at least 90 degrees.
- As you lunge, rotate your torso to your right as you reach high with both hands.
- Return to the starting position.
- Complete the prescribed number of repetitions with your left leg stepping back and your torso rotating right, then step back with your right leg and rotate left for the same number of reps.

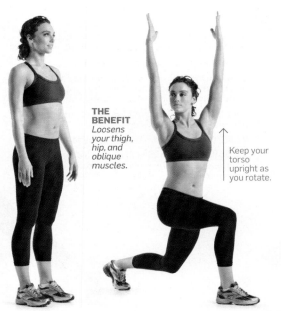

THE BENEFIT
Loosens your thigh, hip, and oblique muscles.

Keep your torso upright as you rotate.

358

Lunge with Side Bend

- Stand tall with your arms hanging at your sides.
- Step forward with your right leg, and lower your body until your right knee is bent at least 90 degrees.
- As you lunge, reach over your head with your left arm as you bend your torso to your right.
- Reach for the floor with your right hand.
- Return to the starting position.
- Complete the prescribed number of reps, then lunge with your left leg and bend to your left for the same number of reps.

Overhead Lunge with Rotation

- Hold a broomstick above your head with your hands about twice shoulder-width apart.
- Your arms should be completely straight.
- Step forward with your right leg and lower your body until your right knee is bent at least 90 degrees.
- As you lunge, rotate your upper body to the right.
- Reverse the movement back to the starting position.
- Complete the prescribed number of reps, then do the same number with your left leg, rotating to your left.

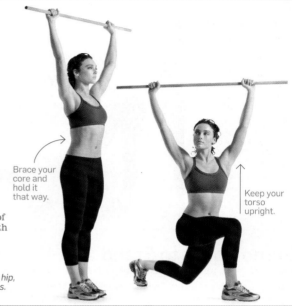

Brace your core and hold it that way.

Keep your torso upright.

THE BENEFIT
Loosens your thigh, hip, and oblique muscles.

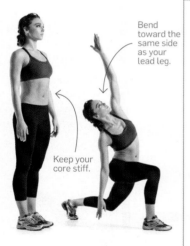

Bend toward the same side as your lead leg.

Keep your core stiff.

THE BENEFIT
Loosens your thigh, hip, and oblique muscles.

Elbow-to-Foot Lunge

- Stand tall with your arms at your sides.

- Brace your core, and lunge forward with your right leg.
- As you lunge, lean forward at your hips and place your left hand on the floor so that it's even with your right foot.
- Place your right elbow next to the instep of your right foot (or as close as you can), and hold for 2 seconds.

- Next, rotate your torso up and to the right and reach as high as you can with your right hand.

- Now, rotate back and place your right hand on the floor outside your right foot, then push your hips upward. That's one rep.
- Step forward with your left leg and repeat.

THE WORLD'S GREATEST STRETCH? *That's what Mark Verstegen, the famed strength coach who popularized this movement, calls the elbow-to-foot lunge.*

THE BENEFIT
Loosens your quadriceps, hamstrings, glutes, and groin.

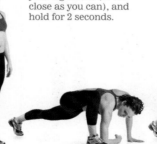

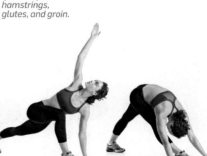

Warmup Exercises

Inchworm

- Stand tall with your legs straight and bend over and touch the floor.

- Keeping your legs straight, walk your hands forward.

- Then take tiny steps to walk your feet back to your hands. That's one repetition.

If you can't reach the floor with your legs straight, bend your knees just enough so you can. As your flexibility improves, try to straighten them a little more.

THE BENEFIT
Loosens your thigh, hip, and oblique muscles.

Walk your hands out as far as you can without allowing your hips to sag.

Keep your core braced.

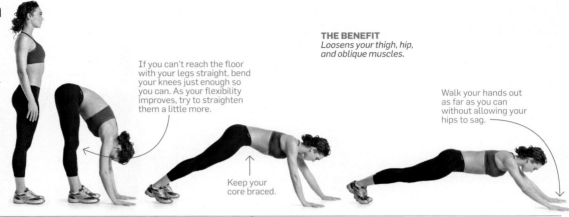

Sumo Squat to Stand

- Stand tall with your legs straight and your feet shoulder-width apart.

- Keeping your legs straight, bend over and grab your toes. (If you need to bend your knees you can, but bend them only as much as necessary.)

- Without letting go of your toes, lower your body into a squat as you raise your chest and shoulders up.

- Staying in the squat position, raise your right arm up high and wide. Then raise your left arm.

- Now stand up.

THE BENEFIT
Loosens your quadriceps, hamstrings, glutes, groin, and lower back.

Your arms should be straight.

Keep your chest and head up.

Raise one arm straight above your shoulder, and then the other.

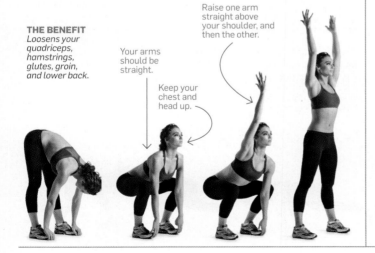

Inverted Hamstring

- Stand on your left leg, your knee bent slightly.

- Raise your right foot slightly off the floor.

- Without changing the bend in your left knee, bend at your hips and lower your torso until it's parallel to the floor.

- As you bend over, raise your arms straight out from your sides until they're in line with your torso, your palms facing down.

- Your right leg should stay in line with your body as you lower your torso.

- Return to the start. Complete the prescribed number of reps on your left leg, then do the same number on your right.

Keep your lower back naturally arched.

Your arms should form a T with your body.

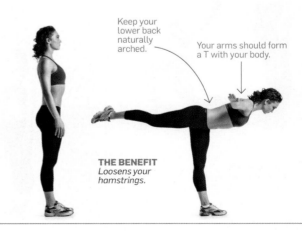

THE BENEFIT
Loosens your hamstrings.

Lateral Slide

- Stand with your feet just beyond shoulder width.
- Push your hips back, bend your knees, and lower your body until your hips are just slightly higher than your knees.
- Shuffle to your left by taking a step to your left with your right foot and then one with your left foot. Slide about 10 feet.
- Slide back to your right.
- Repeat for 30 seconds, or as prescribed.

Walking High Knees

- Stand tall with your feet shoulder-width apart.
- Without changing your posture, raise your left knee as high as you can and step forward.
- Repeat with your right leg. Continue to alternate back and forth.

THE BENEFIT
Loosens your glutes and hamstrings.

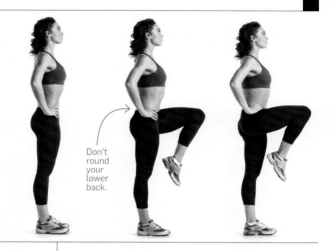

Don't round your lower back.

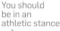
You should be in an athletic stance.

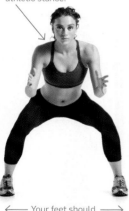

← Your feet should be just beyond shoulder width. →

THE BENEFIT
Improves the rotational and side-to-side mobility of your hips.

Walking Leg Cradles

- Stand with your feet shoulder-width apart and your arms at your sides.
- Step forward with your left leg as you lift your right knee and grasp it with your right hand and grasp your right ankle in your left hand.
- Stand up as tall as you can while you gently pull your right leg toward your chest.
- Release your leg, take three steps forward, and repeat by raising your left knee. Continue to alternate back and forth.

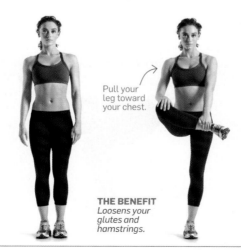

Pull your leg toward your chest.

THE BENEFIT
Loosens your glutes and hamstrings.

Walking Knee Hugs

- Stand with your feet shoulder-width apart and your arms at your sides.
- Step forward with your left leg, bend your knee, and lean forward slightly at your hips.
- Lift your right knee toward your chest, grasping it with both hands just below your kneecap. Then pull it as close to the middle of your chest as you can, while you stand up tall.
- Release your leg, take three steps forward, and repeat by raising your left knee. Continue to alternate back and forth.

THE BENEFIT
Loosens your glutes and hamstrings.

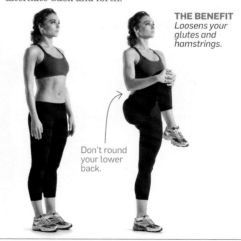

Don't round your lower back.

Warmup Exercises

Lateral Stepover

- Stand with your right side facing a bench.
- Lift your right knee in front of you, then rotate your thigh to step over the bench.
- Follow with your left leg.
- As soon as your left leg touches the floor, reverse the movement, back to the other side. That's one rep.

THE BENEFIT
Enhances the mobility of your thighs and hips.

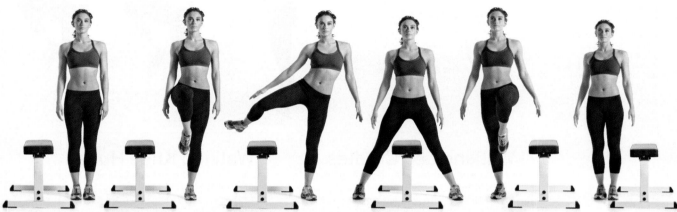

Lateral Duck Under

- Set a barbell in a squat rack or Smith machine a little higher than waist level.
- Stand with your right side next to the bar.
- Take a long stride under the bar, and shift your weight toward your right leg as you squat low to duck under the bar in one movement.
- Rise to a standing position on the other side of the bar.
- Reverse the movement to return to the starting position.

THE BENEFIT
Enhances the mobility of your thighs and hips.

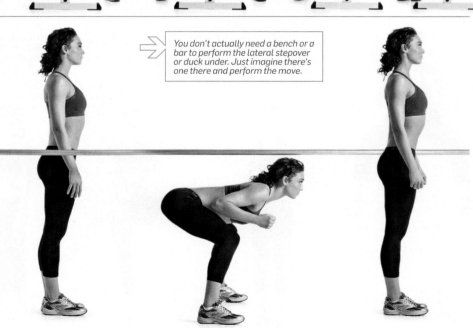

You don't actually need a bench or a bar to perform the lateral stepover or duck under. Just imagine there's one there and perform the move.

Lying Side Leg Raise

- Lie on your left side with your legs straight, your right leg on top of your left. Brace your left upper arm on the floor, and support your head with your left hand.
- Keeping your knee straight, raise your right leg as high as possible in a straight line.
- Lower your leg back to the starting position.

THE BENEFIT
Loosens your hip adductors, or groin.

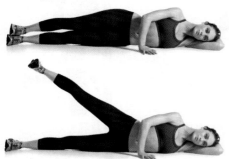

Walking Heel to Butt

- Stand tall with your arms at your sides.
- Step forward with your left leg, then lift your right ankle toward your butt, grasping it with your right hand.
- Pull your ankle as close to your butt as you can.
- Release your ankle, take three steps forward, and repeat by raising your left ankle.

THE BENEFIT
Loosens your quadriceps.

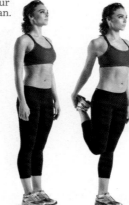

MUSCLE MISTAKE
You Only Do Slow, Static Stretches

That's so 20th century. Here's why: Static stretches—the kind you learned in grade school—boost your flexibility in a specific posture at a slow speed. So they're beneficial for improving your general range of motion and for loosening tight muscles that can contribute to poor posture. (Static stretches appear throughout the book, one for each muscle group.)

Dynamic stretches, on the other hand, give you the flexibility you need when your muscles stretch at fast speeds and in various body positions, such as during weight training and when you play sports. Dynamic stretches also excite your central nervous system and increase blood-flow and strength and power production. So they're the ideal warmup for any physical activity. That's why they constitute most of the movements in this chapter. And it's also why you should regularly do *both* dynamic and static stretches. That way, your body will benefit from the best of both modes.

Lying Straight Leg Raise

- Lie faceup on the floor with your legs straight.
- Keeping both knees straight, raise your left leg upward as far as possible. (Imagine that you're trying to kick a ball that's hanging over your body.)
- Complete the prescribed number of reps with your left leg, then do the same number with your right leg.

THE BENEFIT
Loosens your hamstrings.

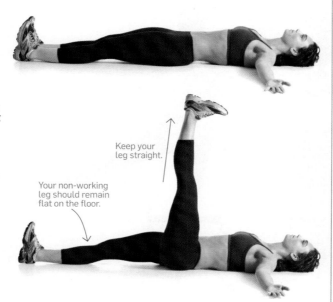

Keep your leg straight.

Your non-working leg should remain flat on the floor.

Warmup Exercises

Forward-and-Back Leg Swings

- Stand tall and hold on to a sturdy object with your left hand.

- Brace your core.

- Keeping your right knee nearly straight, swing your right leg forward as high as you comfortably can.

- Swing your right leg backward as far as you can. That's one rep.

- Swing back and forth continuously. Complete all your reps, then do the same with your left leg.

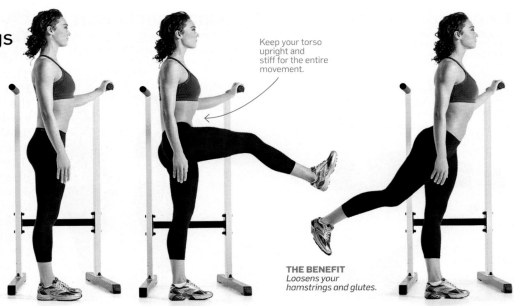

Keep your torso upright and stiff for the entire movement.

THE BENEFIT
Loosens your hamstrings and glutes.

Side-to-Side Leg Swings

- Stand tall and hold on to a sturdy object with both hands.

- Keeping your right knee straight, swing your right leg as high out to the side as you comfortably can.

- Swing your leg back toward your body so that it crosses in front of your left leg. That's one rep.

- Swing back and forth continuously until you complete the pre-scribed number of reps, then do the same with your left leg.

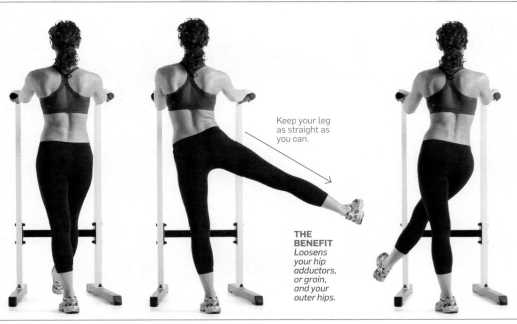

Keep your leg as straight as you can.

THE BENEFIT
Loosens your hip adductors, or groin, and your outer hips.

364

Walking High Kicks

- Stand tall with arms hanging at your sides.
- Keeping your knee straight, kick your left leg up—reaching with your right arm out to meet it—as you simultaneously take a step forward. (Just imagine that you're a Russian soldier.)
- As soon as your left foot touches the floor, repeat the movement with your right leg and left arm. Alternate back and forth.

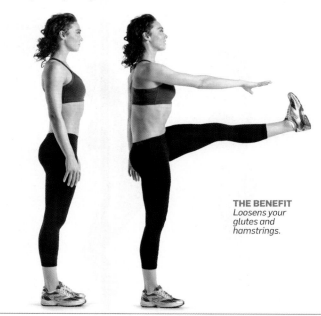

THE BENEFIT
Loosens your glutes and hamstrings.

Prone Hip Internal Rotation

- Lie facedown on the floor with your knees together and bent 90 degrees.
- Without allowing your hips to rise off the floor, lower your feet straight out to the sides as far as you comfortably can. Hold for 1 or 2 seconds, then return to the starting position.

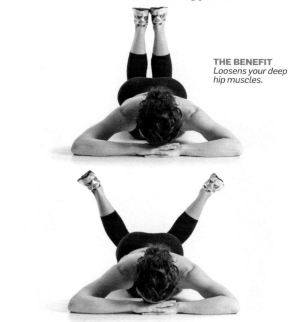

THE BENEFIT
Loosens your deep hip muscles.

Groiners

- Get into pushup position.

THE BENEFIT
Loosens your hip adductors, or groin, and enhances hip mobility.

- Bring your right foot forward, place it next to your right hand (or as close as you can), and lower your hips for a brief moment.

- Return to the start, and repeat with your left leg.

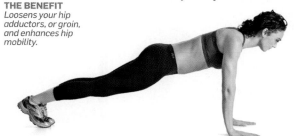

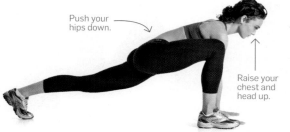

Push your hips down.

Raise your chest and head up.

Warmup Exercises

Ankle Circles

- Stand tall on one foot, and raise your left thigh until it's parallel to the floor. Clasp your hands under your left knee to support your leg.

- Without moving your lower leg, rotate your ankle clockwise. Each circle is one repetition.

- Complete all your reps, then do the same number in a counterclockwise direction. Repeat with your right leg.

THE BENEFIT
Enhances the mobility of your ankles.

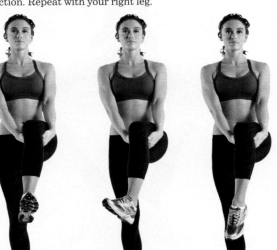

Ankle Flexion

- Place the balls of your feet on a surface that's about 2 inches high, with your heels on the floor.

- Stand tall with your legs nearly straight.

- Bend your knees and shift your weight forward until you feel a stretch in the backs of your heels. Hold for 2 or 3 seconds, then return to the starting position. That's one repetition.

THE BENEFIT
Enhances the mobility of your ankles.

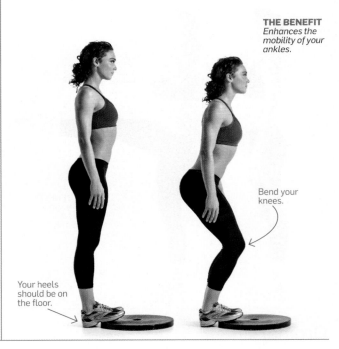

Bend your knees.

Your heels should be on the floor.

Supine Hip Internal Rotation

- Lie faceup on the floor with your knees bent 90 degrees.

- Your feet should be flat on the floor and about twice shoulder-width apart.

- Without allowing your feet to move, lower your knees inward as far as you comfortably can. Hold for 1 or 2 seconds, then return to the starting position.

THE BENEFIT
Loosens the muscles of your inner thighs and hips.

Your feet should remain stationary.

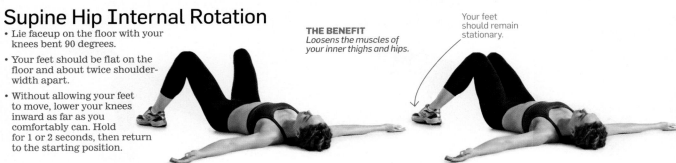

FOAM-ROLL EXERCISES

You might liken these foam-roller exercises to a deep massage. By rolling the hard foam over your thighs, calves, and back, you'll loosen tough connective tissue and decrease the stiffness of your muscles. This helps enhance your flexibility and mobility and keeps your muscles functioning properly. As a result, foam-rolling exercises are valuable both before and after a hard workout, and really, anytime you have the opportunity. Want to multi-task? Pull out the foam roller while you're watching TV.

At first, you may find foam rolling to be uncomfortable. This will be especially true for the muscles that need it most. The more it hurts; the more you need to roll. The good news: Roll regularly, and you'll notice that your muscles will become a little less tender with every subsequent session. For each muscle that you work, slowly move the roller back and forth over it for 30 seconds. If you hit a point that's particularly tender, pause on it for 5 to 10 seconds.

Your main objective: Focus on foam rolling the muscles that need it the most. Trust me, you'll know which ones those are as soon as you start experimenting with the exercises that follow. You can buy your own 36-inch foam roll at most fitness-equipment stores. But in a pinch, you can substitute a basketball, tennis ball, or a section of PVC pipe.

Hamstrings Roll

- Place a foam roller under your right knee, with your leg straight.
- Cross your left leg over your right ankle.
- Put your hands flat on the floor for support.
- Keep your back naturally arched.
- Roll your body forward until the roller reaches your glutes. Then roll back and forth.
- Repeat with the roller under your left thigh.

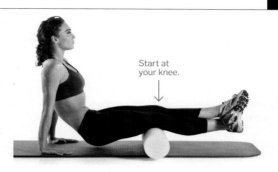

Start at your knee.

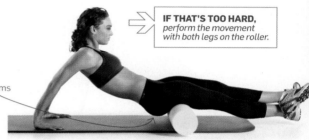

Roll to the bottoms of your glutes.

IF THAT'S TOO HARD, perform the movement with both legs on the roller.

Glutes Roll

- Sit on a foam roller, with it positioned on the back of your right thigh, just below your glutes.
- Cross your right leg over the front of your left thigh.
- Put your hands flat on the floor for support.
- Roll your body forward until the roller reaches your lower back. Then roll back and forth.
- Repeat with the roller under your left glutes.

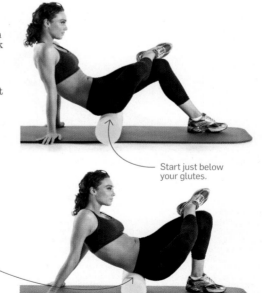

Start just below your glutes.

Roll to your lower back.

Warmup Exercises

Iliotibial-Band Roll

- Lie on your left side and place your left hip on a foam roller.
- Put your hands on the floor for support.
- Cross your right leg over your left, and place your right foot flat on the floor.
- Roll your body forward until the roller reaches your knee. Then roll back and forth.
- Lie on your right side and repeat with the roller under your right hip.

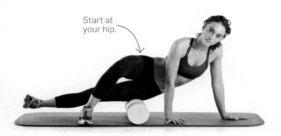

Start at your hip.

WHEN THAT BECOMES TOO EASY, *place your right leg on top of your left instead of bracing it on the floor.*

Roll to your knee.

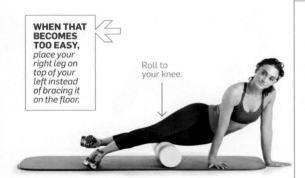

ROLL AWAY TENSION
Your iliotibial band—commonly called the IT band—is a tough strip of connective tissue that runs down the side of your thigh, starting on your hip bone and connecting just below your knee. When it comes to foam rolling, you'll probably find this tissue is one of the most sensitive areas that you can roll over, perhaps due to high tension in the band. You should make it a priority, though: Over time, an overly tense IT band can lead to knee pain.

Calf Roll

- Place a foam roller under your right ankle, with your right leg straight.
- Cross your left leg over your right ankle.
- Put your hands flat on the floor for support.
- Keep your back naturally arched.
- Roll your body forward until the roller reaches the back of your right knee. Then roll back and forth.
- Repeat with the roller under your left calf.

IF THAT'S TOO HARD, *perform the movement with both legs on the roller.*

Start at your ankle.

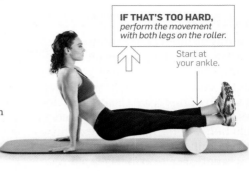

Roll to your knee.

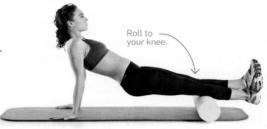

Quadriceps-and-Hip-Flexors Roll

- Lie facedown on the floor with a foam roller positioned above your right knee.
- Cross your left leg over your right ankle and place your elbows on the floor for support.
- Roll your body backward until the roller reaches the top of your right thigh.
- Then roll back and forth.
- Repeat with the roller under your left thigh.

IF THAT'S TOO HARD, *perform the movement with both thighs on the roller.*

Start at your knee.

Roll to the top of your thigh.

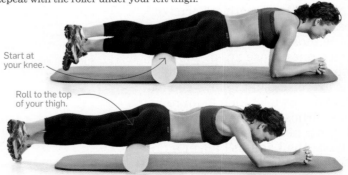
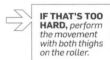

368

Groin Roll

- Lie facedown on the floor.
- Place a foam roller parallel to your body.
- Put your elbows on the floor for support.
- Position your right thigh nearly perpendicular to your body, with the inner portion of your thigh, just above the level of your knee, resting on top of the roller.
- Roll your body toward the right until the roller reaches your pelvis. Then roll back and forth.
- Repeat with the roller under your left thigh.

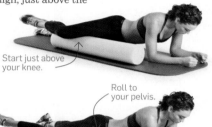

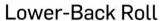
Start just above your knee.

Roll to your pelvis.

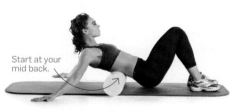

Upper-Back Roll

- Lie faceup with a foam roller under your mid back, at the bottoms of your shoulder blades.
- Clasp your hands behind your head and pull your elbows toward each other.
- Raise your hips off the floor slightly.
- Slowly lower your head and upper back downward, so that your upper back bends over the foam roller.
- Raise back to the start and roll forward a couple of inches—so that the roller sits higher under your upper back—and repeat.
- Roll forward one more time and do it again. That's one rep.

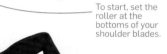

To start, set the roller at the bottoms of your shoulder blades.

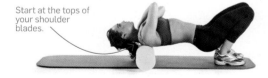

Lower-Back Roll

- Lie faceup with a foam roller under your mid back.
- Your knees should be bent, with your feet flat on the floor.
- Raise your hips off the floor slightly.
- Roll back and forth over your lower back.

Start at your mid back.

Roll to the top of your glutes.

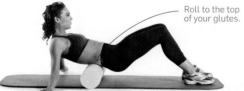

Shoulder-Blades Roll

- Lie faceup with a foam roller under your upper back, at the tops of your shoulder blades.
- Cross your arms over your chest.
- Your knees should be bent, with your feet flat on the floor.
- Raise your hips so they're slightly elevated off the floor.
- Roll back and forth over your shoulder blades and your mid and upper back.

Start at the tops of your shoulder blades.

Roll to the bottoms of your shoulder blades.

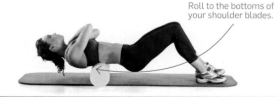

369

Warmup Exercises

CREATE YOUR OWN WARMUP

Besides the movements shown in this chapter, many of the exercises that appear elsewhere in this book also double as great warmup moves. They've been included here in order to give you a full roster of exercises to choose from. (For convenience, the appropriate page number follows the exercise.) To create your own 5-minute warmup, use these guidelines from Mike Wunsch, CSCS, director of fitness programs at Results Fitness in Santa Clarita, California. Simply choose your moves from the categories that follow, using the accompanying

CATEGORY 1
Choose one movement from this list exercises.

Hand crossover (page 354)

Wall slide (page 354)

Reach, roll, and lift (page 355)

Pushup plus (page 64)

CATEGORY 2
Choose one movement from this list exercises.

Floor Y raise (page 87)

Floor T raise (page 88)

Incline Y raise* (page 86)

Incline T raise* (page 88)

Incline W raise* (page 90)

Incline L raise* (page 89)

Swiss-ball Y raise* (page 87)

Swiss-ball T raise* (page 88)

Swiss-ball W raise* (page 90)

Swiss-ball L raise* (page 89)

CATEGORY 3
Choose one movement from this list of exercises.

Side-lying thoracic rotation (page 355)

Thoracic rotation (page 355)

Bent-over reach to sky (page 356)

CATEGORY 4
Choose three movements from this list of exercises—one from each category.

QUADRICEPS AND HIP ADDUCTORS (GROIN)

Walking heel to butt (page 363)

Supine hip internal rotation (page 366)

Groiners (page 365)

Side-to-side leg swings (page 364)

HAMSTRINGS

Walking high knees, (page 361)

Walking knee hugs, (page 361)

Walking high kicks, (page 365)

Lying straight leg raise (page 363)

Forward-and-back leg swings (page 364)

GLUTES AND HIP ABDUCTORS (OUTER HIPS)

Hip raises (page 236)

Single-leg hip raise with knee hold (page 241)

Lateral band walks (page 267)

Walking leg cradles (page 361)

Prone hip internal rotation (page 365)

Clamshell (page 267)

Lying side leg raise (page 361)

For these exercises, use the form shown, but perform the movement without the dumbbells.

directions. You can either do 5 to 10 reps of each exercise or perform each one for 30 seconds. Do the movements in a circuit, completing one set of each exercise without resting. *One additional option:* If you can't get to the gym or don't have time for your regular workout, do this warmup as a quickie bodyweight routine. Use the same directions for each category, only choose three exercises—instead of just one—from Category 6, and do as many sets of the three exercises in Category 7 as you have time for.

CATEGORY 5

Choose any Core exercise in Chapter 10, from the section labeled "Stability Exercises." For example, any version of the plank, side plank, or mountain climber.

CATEGORY 6

Choose one to three movements—as time allows—from this list of exercises.

Jumping jacks (page 353)

Split jacks (page 353)

Squat thrusts (page 354)

CATEGORY 7

Choose three movements—one of each movement type—from this list of exercises. So you'll select one side-to-side movement, one forward and back movement, and one rotational movement.

SIDE-TO-SIDE MOVEMENTS

Low side-to-side lunge (page 357)

Lateral slide (page 361)

Lateral stepover (page 362)

Lateral duck under (page 362)

Dumbbell side lunge* (page 221)

FORWARD AND BACK MOVEMENTS

Prisoner squat (page 192)

Body-weight squat (page 190)

Dumbbell lunge* (page 218)

Reverse dumbbell lunge* (page 217)

Dumbbell crossover lunge* (page 219)

Reverse dumbbell crossover lunge* (page 219)

Inverted hamstring (page 360)

Inchworm (page 360)

Elbow-to-foot lunge (page 359)

Sumo squat to stand (page 360)

ROTATIONAL MOVEMENTS

Reverse lunge with reach back (page 358)

Lunge with diagonal reach (page 358)

Lunge with side bend (page 359)

Reverse lunge with twist and overhead reach (page 358)

Overhead lunge with rotation (page 359)

Chapter 13:
The Best Workouts for Everything
YOUR COMPLETE GUIDE
TO TRANSFORMING YOUR BODY

Here are the blueprints for the body you want.

Whether your goal is to tone your arms, shrink your hips, or to lose the last 10 pounds, there's a workout for you. In fact, there are lots of workouts. That's because I've enlisted the world's top fitness experts to create cutting-edge plans for just about everything—a bikini-ready body, a smaller jeans size, even your wedding day. There's also a workout for every lifestyle. Too busy for the gym? Try an intense 15-minute routine. Always on the road? There's a bodyweight workout you can do in your room. Never picked up a weight before? The Get-Your-Body-Back Workout on page 376 is what you need.

Simply choose one of the plans that follow, then use the instructions on page 375 to make sure you do it right. (And for even more routines, downloaded straight to your iPhone, check out the *Women's Health Workouts* app from the iTunes store.) If you have additional questions, you're likely to find the answers in Chapter 2.

Now get to work. Your new body is waiting.

Best Workouts for Everything

Before You Start: What You Need to Know

Use these instructions to ensure you understand how to do each workout in this chapter.

How to Do These Workouts

• Always perform the exercises in the order shown.

• When you see a number without a letter next to it—such as "1" or "4"—perform the exercise as a straight set. That is, do one set of the exercise, rest for the prescribed amount of time, and then do another set. Complete all sets of this exercise before moving on to the next.

• When you see a number with a letter next to it—such as "2A"—it indicates that the exercise is to be performed as part of a group of exercises. (A group of exercises all share the same number, but will each have a different letter; for example, 1A, 1B, and 1C.) Do one set of the exercise, rest for the prescribed amount of time, and then do one set of the next exercise in the group. For instance, if you see 2A and 2B in a workout, complete one set of Exercise 2A, rest for the prescribed amount of time, then do one set of Exercise 2B, and rest again. Repeat until you've completed all of your sets for each exercise. Follow this procedure regardless of how many exercises are in a group.

• You'll notice that sometimes the prescribed rest period is actually "0"— zero seconds. That means you're not to rest between movements; move directly to the next exercise.

• When a duration (for example, 30 seconds) is given for the number of reps, simply perform the exercise for the prescribed time. So if it's a plank or side plank, hold the position for the duration of the set. If it's an exercise in which you normally do repetitions, complete as many reps as you can in the given time period.

• The acronym AMAP stands for *as many as possible*. So when AMAP is indicating the number of repetitions you should do, it means that you're to complete as many repetitions as you can. When it's indicating the number of sets you do, complete as many sets as you can in the given time frame.

• The acronym ALAP stands for *as little as possible*. So when ALAP is indicating your rest period, it means that you're to rest only as long as you feel you need. Basically, catch your breath and get back to work.

Best Workouts

The Get-Your-Body-Back Workout
Phase 1: Weeks 1 to 4

Whether you've never lifted weights before or you just haven't made time for exercise lately, this 12-week plan, from Joe Dowdell, CSCS, was created with you in mind. It's designed to blast fat and tone your muscles, while taking into account that you're not yet in peak condition. And it does all of this while targeting the weaknesses brought on by a sedentary lifestyle— the kind that often slow your results and lead to frustration. So you'll not only transform your body, you'll do it faster than ever.

About the Expert
Joe Dowdell, CSCS, is co-owner of Peak Performance in New York City. He makes his living training models, athletes, and celebrities, and has worked with such names as Anne Hathaway, Claire Danes, Molly Sims, and Kate Hudson, as well as Victoria's Secret and Sports Illustrated swimsuit models. He's widely recognized as one of the best strength coaches in the world. (Search for his new book at www.amazon.com.)

How to Do This Workout

• Do the Weight Workout 3 days a week, resting for at least a day after each session. So you might lift weights on Monday, Wednesday, and Friday.
• Do the Cardio Workout twice a week, on the days in between your Weight Workouts. So you might do your cardio sessions on Tuesday and Thursday. (If you can't find time to exercise 5 days a week, just do the Cardio Workout immediately following two of your weight workouts.)
• Prior to each Weight Workout, complete the warmup.
• Questions? Flip back to page 375, where you'll find complete instructions for performing all of the workouts.

Warmup

EXERCISE	SETS	REPS	REST
1A. Side-lying thoracic rotation (page 355)	1	5	0
1B. Body-weight lunge (page 217)	1	4	0
1C. Low side-to-side lunge (page 357)	1	4	0
1D. Hip raise with knee press-out (page 238)	1	10–12	0
1E. Plank (page 278)	1	4–6	0
1F. Swiss-ball W raise (page 90)	1	8–10	0

For the plank and the prone cobra, hold the position for 1 second, then relax momentarily and repeat. That's one repetition.

Weight Workout

If the barbell or dumbbell squat is too hard, substitute a body-weight squat.

EXERCISE	SETS	REPS	REST
1A. Barbell or dumbbell squat (page 198 or 203)	2–3	10–12	1 min
1B. Pushup (page 34)	2–3	10–12	1 min
2A. Hip raise with feet on a Swiss ball (page 239)	2–3	10–12	1 min
2B. Cable row to neck with external rotation (page 95)	2–3	10–12	1 min
3A. Reverse crunch (page 322)	2–3	10–12	1 min
3B. Prone cobra (page 295)	2–3	10–12	1 min

If you have difficulty with the pushup, choose a variation that's easier—such as the modified pushup or incline pushup—but still challenging.

Cardio Workout

THE PLAN

Warm up by walking on a treadmill at an easy pace—about 30 to 50 percent of your best effort—for 3 to 5 minutes. Then do this interval workout:

- Raise the incline on the treadmill until you're exercising at an intensity that's 40 to 60 percent of your best effort. Go for 2 minutes.
- Lower the incline back to 0 percent and go for 2 more minutes. That's one set.
- Do a total of three sets, then cool down for 3 to 5 minutes, walking at an easy pace.
- During the course of this 4-week phase, try to work up to a total of five sets.

Best Workouts

The Get-Your-Body-Back Workout
Phase 2: Weeks 5 to 8

How to Do This Workout
• Do the Weight Workout three days a week, resting for at least a day after each session. So you might lift weights on Monday, Wednesday, and Friday.
• Do the Cardio Workout three times a week, on the days in between each Weight Workout. For your first two workouts, perform the Interval Workout. For the last workout, do the Aerobic Workout. So you might do the Interval Workout on Tuesday and Thursday, and the Aerobic Workout on Saturday.
• Prior to each Weight Workout, complete the warmup.
• Questions? Flip back to page 375, where you'll find complete instructions for performing all of the workouts.

Warmup

EXERCISE	SETS	REPS	REST
1A. Hip crossover (page 303)	1	5	0
1B. Elbow-to-foot lunge (page 359)	1	4	0
1C. Body-weight side lunge (page 221)	1	4	0
1D. Clamshell (page 267)	1	8–10	0
1E. Side plank (page 284)	1	4–6	0
1F. Swiss-ball T raise (page 88)	1	8–10	0

Weight Workout

EXERCISE	SETS	REPS	REST
1A. Dumbbell split squat (page 209)	2–3	10–12	1 min
1B. Dumbbell bench press (page 52)	2–3	10–12	1 min
2A. Swiss-ball hip raise and leg curl (page 243)	2–3	10–12	1 min
2B. Band-assisted chinup (page 98)	2–3	10–12	1 min
3A. Side crunch (page 332)	2–3	8–10	1 min
3B. Bird dog (page 283)	2–3	8–10	1 min

For the side crunch, hold the up position of each crunch for 2 seconds.

For the side plank (in the warmup) and bird dog, hold the position for 1 second, then relax momentarily and repeat. That's one repetition.

Cardio Workout

THE PLAN

Warm up by walking on a treadmill at an easy pace—about 30 to 50 percent of your best effort—for 3 to 5 minutes. Then do one of these workouts, performing the Interval Workout on your first and second cardio day each week, and do the Aerobic Workout on your third cardio day.

INTERVAL WORKOUT

- Increase the treadmill speed to an intensity that's 65 to 75 percent of your best effort. Go for 60 seconds.
- Lower the speed to 3.5 miles per hour and go for 2 minutes. That's one set.
- Do a total of four sets, then cool down for 3 to 5 minutes, walking at an easy pace.
- Try to work up to a total of six sets during the course of this 4-week phase.

AEROBIC WORKOUT

- Increase the treadmill speed or incline until you're exercising at an intensity that's 40 to 60 percent of your best effort. Go at that pace for 15 minutes.
- During the course of this 4-week phase, try to work up to 25 minutes.

Best Workouts

The Get-Your-Body-Back Workout
Phase 3: Weeks 9 to 12

How to Do This Workout

• Alternate between Workout A and Workout B three days a week, resting for at least a day between each session. So if you plan to lift on Monday, Wednesday, and Friday, you'd do Workout A on Monday, Workout B on Wednesday, and Workout A again on Friday. The next week, you'd do Workout B on Monday and Friday, and Workout A on Wednesday.

• Do the Cardio Workout three times a week, on the days in between Weight Workouts. For your first two workouts, perform the Interval Workout. For the last workout, do the Aerobic Workout. So you might do the Interval Workout on Tuesday and Thursday, and the Aerobic Workout on Saturday. Note that you do Interval Workout A for the first 2 weeks (weeks 9 and 10), then transition to Interval Workout B for the last 2 weeks (weeks 11 and 12).

• Prior to each workout, complete the warmup.

• Questions? Flip back to page 375, where you'll find complete instructions for performing all of the workouts.

Warmup

EXERCISE	SETS	REPS	REST
1A. Cat camel (page 283)	1	5–6	0
1B. Elbow-to-foot lunge (page 359)	1	4	0
1C. Walking knee hugs (page 361)	1	5	0
1D. Lateral band walks (page 267)	1	10–12	0
1E. Inchworm (page 360)	1	3–5	0
1F. Swiss-ball Y raise (page 87)	1	8–10	0

Workout A

EXERCISE	SETS	REPS	REST
1A. Barbell deadlift (page 248)	3	8–10	1 min
1B. Incline dumbbell bench press (page 54)	3	8–10	1 min
2A. Partial single-leg squat (page 197)	3	8–10	1 min
2B. Kneeling supported neutral-grip dumbbell row (page 80)	3	8–10	1 min
3A. Hammer curl to press (page 159)	3	8–10	1 min
3B. Swiss-ball crunch (page 318)	3	8–10	1 min

Workout B

EXERCISE	SETS	REPS	REST
1A. Dumbbell stepup (page 262)	3	10–12	1 min
1B. Dumbbell bench press (page 52)	3	10–12	1 min
2A. Barbell straight-leg deadlift (page 252)	3	8–10	1 min
2B. Rear lateral raise (page 83)	3	10–12	1 min
3A. Dumbbell lying triceps extension (page 166)	3	8–10	1 min
3B. Back extension (page 258)	3	8–10	1 min

Cardio Workout

THE PLAN

Perform the appropriate Interval Workout on your first and second cardio day each week, and do the Aerobic Workout on your third cardio day.

INTERVAL WORKOUT A

- Increase the treadmill speed you're exercising at to an intensity that's 70 to 80 percent of your best effort. Go for 45 seconds.
- Lower the speed to 3.5 miles per hour and go for 2 minutes. That's one set.
- Do a total of five sets, then cool down for 3 to 5 minutes, walking at an easy pace.
- Try to work up to a total of seven sets during the course of this 4-week phase.

INTERVAL WORKOUT B

- Increase the treadmill speed you're exercising at to an intensity that's 70 to 80 percent of your best effort. Go for 30 seconds.
- Lower the speed to 3.5 miles per hour and go for 90 seconds. That's one set.
- Do a total of six sets, then cool down for 3 to 5 minutes, walking at an easy pace.
- Try to work up to a total of eight sets during the course of this 4-week phase.

AEROBIC WORKOUT

- Increase the treadmill speed or incline until you're exercising at an intensity that's 40 to 60 percent of your best effort. Go at that pace for 25 minutes.
- During the course of this 4-week phase, try to work up to 30 minutes at an effort of 60 percent.

Best Workouts

The Best Workouts for a Crowded Gym

You should never have to wait in line at the gym. And these three workout plans—all designed to burn fat fast—ensure you won't have to.

About the Expert
Craig Ballantyne, MS, CSCS, has been a fitness advisor to *Men's Health* for nearly a decade. Based in Toronto, Craig is the owner of TurbulenceTraining.com, one of the most popular and effective online training programs.

Workout Plan 1

How to Do This Workout
• The only equipment you need: one pair of dumbbells. This routine is designed so that you won't have to even change the amount of weight you use from one move to the next.
• Do each workout (Workout A, Workout B, and Workout C) once a week, resting for at least a day after each session.
• Questions? Flip back to page 375, where you'll find complete instructions for performing all of the workouts.

Workout A

EXERCISE	SETS	REPS	REST
1A. Dumbbell bench press (page 52)	4	8	1 min
1B. Kneeling supported neutral-grip dumbbell row (page 80)	4	8–12	1 min
2A. Incline dumbbell bench press (page 54)	3	5	0
2B. Dumbbell squat (page 202)	3	12	1 min

Workout B

EXERCISE	SETS	REPS	REST
1A. Dumbbell split squat (page 209)	4	8	1 min
1B. Single-arm dumbbell shoulder press (page 122)	4	12	1 min
2A. Dumbbell straight-leg deadlift (page 256)	3	10	0
2B. Single-arm dumbbell swing (page 268)	3	15–20	1 min

Workout C

EXERCISE	SETS	REPS	REST
1A. Dumbbell stepup (page 262)	4	8	1 min
1B. Lying supported neutral-grip dumbbell row (page 80)	4	12	1 min
2A. Standing dumbbell curl (page 154)	4	10	0
2B. Lying dumbbell triceps extension (page 179)	4	12	1 min

Best Workouts

The Best Workouts for a Crowded Gym

Workout Plan 2

How to Do This Workout

• This unique 45-minute workout is designed so that you stay at each station for 10 minutes, using the same weight the entire time. This keeps you in one place and working hard for the whole session, with no need to change exercises or weights.

• Do each Weight Workout (Workout A, Workout B, and Workout C) once a week, resting for at least a day after each session. So you might do Workout A on Monday, Workout B on Wednesday, and Workout C on Friday. Follow these guidelines:

• For Exercise 1 in each workout, choose the heaviest weight that allows you to complete 10 to 12 repetitions. This is the weight you'll use for each set that you perform.

• Set a timer for 10 minutes.

• Do three repetitions, rest for 10 seconds, and repeat. Continue in this manner until you can't complete all three reps. Then increase your rest by 10 seconds, so that you're resting for

20 seconds after each three-repetition set. When you're once again unable to complete three reps, increase your rest to 30 seconds, and so on. Follow this procedure until your 10 minutes are up. That's your cue to move on to the next exercise.

• Use these same guidelines for Exercise 2 and Exercise 3.

• Each week, increase the weight you use for each exercise by 5 to 10 pounds.

• For Exercises 4 and 5, simply choose one core exercise (Chapter 10) and one arm exercise (Chapter 7). Do two sets of 10 to 12 reps of each, using the heaviest weight that allows you to complete all of your repetitions. Rest for 60 seconds between sets. One caveat: If you choose a core exercise such as the plank or side plank, hold the position for 30 seconds.

• Do the Cardio Workout immediately after each Weight Workout.

• Questions? Flip back to page 375, where you'll find complete instructions for performing all of the workouts.

About the Expert
Nick Nilsson is the vice president of BetterU, Inc., an online personal-training company. Nick has a degree in kinesiology and has been a personal trainer for more than a decade.

Workout A

EXERCISE
1. Dumbbell bench press (page 52)
2. Chinup (page 96)
3. Barbell squat (page 198)
4. Core exercise: your choice (Chapter 10)
5. Arm exercise: your choice (Chapter 7)

Workout B

EXERCISE
1. Dumbbell split squat (page 209)
2. Barbell bench press (page 46)
3. Barbell row (page 76)
4. Core exercise: your choice (Chapter 10)
5. Arm exercise: your choice (Chapter 7)

Workout C

EXERCISE
1. Barbell deadlift (page 248)
2. Pushup (page 34)
3. Barbell front squat (page 199)
4. Core exercise: your choice (Chapter 10)
5. Arm exercise: your choice (Chapter 7)

Cardio Workout

THE PLAN

- You can perform this workout on a treadmill, on a stationary bike, or outside on the sidewalk or a track. Do it for a total of 10 minutes.
- Exercise at an intensity that's about 90 percent of your best effort. Go for 30 seconds.
- Rest for 30 seconds. Then repeat until your 10 minutes are up.

Best Workouts

The Skinny Jeans Workout
Phase 1: Weeks 1 to 4

Want a look sexier in pair of jeans? Then this is the workout for you, courtesy of Rachel Cosgrove, CSCS. It's based entirely on the Skinny Jeans Challenge she conducted at her gym, in which 20 women dropped two jeans sizes in 8 weeks. (The ladies' reward: new designer jeans, purchased by Rachel.) If you're up for the challenge—and a reason to go shopping—get ready to slim down and tone up. It's the perfect routine for any woman, since it's designed to allow you to start at the pace that's right for your body—whether you're a beginner or a long-time exerciser.

How to Do This Workout

• Alternate between Workout A and Workout B three days a week, resting at least a day between each session. So if you plan to exercise on Monday, Wednesday, and Friday, you'd do Workout A on Monday, Workout B on Wednesday, and Workout A again on Friday. The next week, you'd do Workout B on Monday and Friday, and Workout A on Wednesday.

• If you're a beginner or you haven't exercised in some time, perform the number of sets on the low end of the recommended range. So if you're to do one to three sets of an exercise, just do one set the first week. Then increase the number of sets you do weekly so that you're performing three sets by week 4.

When you start a new phase, drop back down to the beginner-level sets. That is, in Phase 2, you'll start with one set again and work your way back up to three.

• For each exercise in which you raise and lower a weight, take 2 seconds to lower the weight or your body, pause in the down position, and then take 2 seconds to lift the weight, keeping tension on your muscles the entire time.

• If you already regularly exercise, you can start with two or three sets per exercise.

• Prior to each workout, complete the warmup.

• Questions? Flip back to page 375, where you'll find complete instructions for performing all of the workouts.

About the Expert
Rachel Cosgrove, CSCS, is the owner of Results Fitness in Santa Clarita, California, and a fitness columnist for *Women's Health*. You can find more workouts and advice from Rachel in her terrific new book, *The Female Body Breakthrough*, available everywhere books are sold.

Warmup

EXERCISE	SETS	REPS	REST
1A. Upper-back roll (page 369)	1	10	0
1B. Reach, roll, and lift (page 355)	1	10	0
1C. Sumo squat to stand (page 360)	1	10	0
1D. Bent-over reach to sky (page 356)	1	10	0
1E. Inchworm (page 360)	1	10	0
1F. Lateral band walk (page 267)	1	10	0

Workout A

EXERCISE	SETS	REPS	REST
1A. Body-weight lunge (page 217)	1–3	10	60 sec
1B. Incline Y-T-W-L raises (page 86)	1–3	10	60 sec
2A. Single-leg hip raise (page 240)	1–3	10	60 sec
2B. Swiss-ball dumbbell shoulder press (page 122)	1–3	10	60 sec
3A. Bird dog (page 283)	1–2	10	60 sec
3B. Prone cobra (page 295)	1–2	60 sec	60 sec

For the bird dog, raise your arm and leg and hold for 2 seconds, then slowly lower and repeat with your other arm and leg. That's one rep.

Workout B

EXERCISE	SETS	REPS	REST
1A. Body-weight overhead squat (page 202)	1–3	10	60 sec
1B. Incline pushup (page 36)	1–3	10	60 sec
2A. Single-leg dumbbell straight-leg deadlift (page 257)	1–3	10	60 sec
2B. Standing-supported neutral-grip row (page 81)	1–3	10	60 sec
3A. Hip raise with feet on a Swiss ball (page 239)	1–2	10	60 sec
3B. Swiss-ball rollout (page 292)	1–3	10	60 sec
4. Swiss-ball crunch (page 318)	1–2	10	60 sec

For the body-weight overhead squat, perform an overhead barbell squat, but while holding a broomstick or light pole instead of a barbell. Each time you lower your body, pause for 2 seconds in the down position.

Best Workouts

The Skinny Jeans Workout
Phase 2: Weeks 5 to 8

Workout A

EXERCISE	SETS	REPS	REST
1A. Dumbbell box lunge (page 218)	1–3	8	60 sec
1B. Underhand-grip rear lateral raise (page 84)	1–3	8	60 sec
1C. Swiss-ball Russian twist (page 302)	1–2	10	60 sec
2A. Alternating dumbbell shoulder press (page 121)	1–3	5	60 sec
2B. Plank (page 278)	1–2	60 sec hold	60 sec
2C. Swiss-ball hip raise and leg curl (page 243)	1–3	8	60 sec
3. Prone cobra (page 295)	1–2	90 sec hold	60 sec

Workout B

If the single-leg deadlift is too hard, simply allow the toes of your back foot to touch the floor as you lower your body, providing you with extra support.

EXERCISE	SETS	REPS	REST
1A. Single-leg deadlift (page 251)	1–3	8	60 sec
1B. Pushup (page 34)	1–3	8	60 sec
1C. Dumbbell row (page 78)	1–3	8	60 sec
2A. Wide-grip lat pulldown (page 104)	1–3	8	60 sec
2B. Dumbbell stepup (page 262)	1–3	8	60 sec
2C. Single-leg hip raise (page 240)	1–2	8	60 sec
3. T-stabilization (page 287)	1–2	6–8	60 sec

The Skinny Jeans Workout
Phase 3: Weeks 9 to 12

Workout A

EXERCISE	SETS	REPS	REST
1A. Body-weight or dumbbell side lunge (pages 217 or 221)	1–3	15	60 sec
1B. Inverted row (page 72)	1–3	12–15	60 sec
1C. Single-leg Swiss-ball hip raise and leg curl (page 244)	1–3	15	60 sec
1D. Dumbbell alternating shoulder press and twist (page 123)	1–3	15	60 sec
2A. Swiss-ball plank (page 281)	1–2	60 sec hold	60 sec
2B. Core stabilization (page 334)	1–3	15	60 sec
3. Side plank (page 284)	1–2	30 sec hold	60 sec

For core stabilization, take 2 seconds to rotate to the left, pause for 2 seconds, and then take 2 seconds to return to the starting position.

Workout B

EXERCISE	SETS	REPS	REST
1A. Reverse dumbbell lunge (page 217)	1–3	15	60 sec
1B. Standing cable row (page 95)	1–3	15	60 sec
1C. Partial single-leg squat (page 197)	1–3	15	60 sec
1D. Close-grip lat pulldown (page 105)	1–3	15	60 sec
2A. T-pushup (page 41)	1–3	15	60 sec
2B. Dumbbell straight-leg deadlift (page 256)	1–2	15	60 sec
3. Swiss-ball jackknife (page 290)	1–2	15	60 sec

Best Workouts

The Bikini-Ready Workout
Phase 1: Weeks 1 to 3

From a flat stomach to a tight butt, this 6-week plan will ensure that you look your very best in a bikini—and in the bedroom. It's designed by celebrity trainer Valerie Waters, who's perfected the body-shaping workouts you see here on dozens of Hollywood stars, including Jennifer Garner, Rachel Nichols, Kate Beckinsale, and Jessica Biel. Add your name to Valerie's client list to tone your total body and feel more confident than ever.

How to Do This Workout

• Alternate between Workout A and Workout B three days a week, resting at least a day between each session. So if you plan to exercise on Monday, Wednesday, and Friday, you'd do Workout A on Monday, Workout B on Wednesday, and Workout A again on Friday. The next week, you'd do Workout B on Monday and Friday, and Workout A on Wednesday.

• For each circuit, do one set of each exercise in succession. Rest for the prescribed amount of time, and repeat until you've completed all sets of each exercise. Then move on to the next circuit.

• Prior to each workout, complete the warmup.

• Questions? Flip back to page 375, where you'll find complete instructions for performing all of the workouts.

About the Expert
Valerie Waters is one of Hollywood's most sought after trainers. She's the creator of the Red Carpet Ready program, where she shares all of her body transformation secrets. You can read more about the plan at www.redcarpetready.com and learn more about Valerie at www.valeriewaters.com.

Warmup

EXERCISE	SETS	REPS	REST
1A. Forward-and-back leg swings (page 364)	1	10	0
1B. Side-to-side leg swings (page 364)	1	10	0
1C. Sumo squat to stand (page 360)	1	10	0
1D. Reverse lunge with reach back (page 358)	1	8	0
1E. Low side-to-side lunge (page 357)	1	8	0

Workout A
Circuit 1

EXERCISE	SETS	REPS	REST
1A. Single-leg hip raise (page 240)	2–3	12	0
1B. Side plank (page 284)	2–3	30 sec hold	0
1C. Plank (page 278)	2–3	30–40 sec hold	0
1D. Situp (page 310)	2–3	12	1–2 min

← If the situp is too hard, perform the negative situp instead.

Circuit 2

EXERCISE	SETS	REPS	REST
2A. Body-weight squat (page 190), dumbbell squat (page 203), or goblet squat (page 204)	3	15	0
2B. Single-arm cable row (page 95)	3	12	0
2C. Dumbbell straight-leg deadlift (page 256)	3	12	0
2D. Dumbbell bench press (page 52)	3	15	1–2 min

Circuit 3

EXERCISE	SETS	REPS	REST
3A. Valslide reverse dumbbell lunge (page 217)	3	12	0
3B. Dumbbell shoulder press (page 120)	3	12	0
3C. Dumbbell lunge (page 218)	3	10	0
3D. Triceps pressdown (page 171)	3	12	0
3E. Dumbbell curl (page 154)	3	12	1–2 min

← For the Valslide reverse dumbbell lunge, perform a reverse dumbbell lunge, but with one foot on a Valslide. So instead of stepping back into a lunge, slide back into a lunge. No Valslide? Just perform the reverse dumbbell lunge as shown.

Best Workouts

The Bikini-Ready Workout
Phase 1: Weeks 1 to 3

Workout B
Circuit 1

EXERCISE	SETS	REPS	REST
1A. Lateral band walks (page 267)	2–3	20	0
1B. Body-weight squat with knee press-out (page 192)	2–3	20	0
1C. Dumbbell stepup (page 262)	2–3	15	0
1D. Mountain climber with feet on Valslides (page 289)	2–3	20	0
1E. Alternating slide out (page 293)	2–3	12	1–2 min

For the mountain climber with feet on Valslides, slide one foot forward as you slide the other one back.

Circuit 2

EXERCISE	SETS	REPS	REST
2A. Dumbbell side lunge (page 221)	3	15	0
2B. Dumbbell row (page 78)	3	15	0
2C. Pushup (page 34)	3	10–12	0
2D. Crunch (page 318)	3	20	0
2E. Reverse crunch (page 322)	3	20	1–2 min

If the standard pushup is too hard, choose an easier variation, such as the modified pushup or incline pushup.

Circuit 3

EXERCISE	SETS	REPS	REST
3A. Lateral raise (page 126)	2–3	15	0
3B. Twisting dumbbell curl (page 155)	2–3	15	0
3C. Dumbbell kickback (page 173)	2–3	15	0
3D. Half-kneeling rotational chop (page 307)	2–3	12–15	1–2 min

For the lateral raise, use 5-pound dumbbells. (If that's too hard, use a lighter weight or no weight at all.)

For the twisting dumbbell curl and the dumbbell kickback, use 8-pound dumbbells. (If that's too hard, use a lighter weight.)

The Bikini-Ready Workout
Phase 2: Weeks 4 to 6

Workout A
Circuit 1

EXERCISE	SETS	REPS	REST
1A. Single-leg hip raise with foot on a foam roller (page 241)	3	12	0
1B. Side plank with reach under (page 286)	3	30–40 sec	0
1C. Wide-stance plank with leg lift (page 280)	3	30–40 sec hold	0
1D. Swiss-ball rollout (page 292)	3	15	1-2 min

For the single-leg hip raise with foot on a foam roller, place your foot on a short step if you don't have a foam roller.

Circuit 2

EXERCISE	SETS	REPS	REST
2A. Single-leg squat (page 196)	3	12	0
2B. Single-arm cable row and rotation (page 95)	3	12	0
2C. Single-leg, dumbbell straight-leg deadlift (page 257)	3	10	0
2D. Dumbbell bench press (page 52)	3	12–15	1–2 min

If the single-leg squat is too hard, perform the partial single-leg squat instead.

Circuit 3

EXERCISE	SETS	REPS	REST
3A. Single-arm reverse lunge and press (page 344)	3	10	0
3B. Walking dumbbell lunge (page 217)	3	12	0
3C. Triceps pressdown (page 171)	3	12	0
3D. Dumbbell curl (page 154)	3	12	1–2 min

Best Workouts

The Bikini-Ready Workout
Phase 2: Weeks 4 to 6

Workout B
Circuit 1

EXERCISE	SETS	REPS	REST
1A. Lateral band walks (page 267)	2–3	20	0
1B. Body-weight squat with knee press-out (page 192)	2–3	20	0
1C. Lateral slide (page 361)	2–3	12	0
1D. Single-arm stepup and press (page 344)	2–3	12	0
1E. Swiss-ball pike (page 328)	2–3	15	0
1F. Alternating slide out (page 293)	2–3	15	1–2 min

For the single-arm stepup and press, use a 5-pound dumbbell.

Circuit 2

EXERCISE	SETS	REPS	REST
2A. Valslide reverse dumbbell lunge (page 217)	3	20	0
2B. Dumbbell side lunge (page 221)	3	20	0
2C. Dumbbell row (page 78)	3	15	0
2D. T-pushup (page 41)	3	10	0
2E. Elevated-feet Russian twist (page 301)	3	15	1–2 min

For the Valslide reverse dumbbell lunge, perform a reverse dumbbell lunge, but with one foot on a Valslide. So instead of stepping back into a lunge, slide back into a lunge. No Valslide? Just perform the reverse dumbbell lunge as shown.

If the T-pushup is too hard, choose an easier variation, such as the pushup or incline pushup.

Circuit 3

EXERCISE	SETS	REPS	REST
3A. Swiss-ball L raise (page 89)	2–3	12	0
3B. Twisting standing dumbbell curl (page 155)	2–3	15	0
3C. Lying dumbbell triceps extension (page 179)	2–3	12	0
3D. Half-kneeling rotational reverse chop (page 309)	2–3	15	1–2 min

For the twisting dumbbell curl, use 8-pound dumbbells. (If that's too hard, use a lighter weight.)

For the lying dumbbell triceps extension, use 8- to 10-pound dumbbells. (If that's too hard, use a lighter weight.)

Best Workouts

The Wedding Workout
Phase 1: Weeks 1 to 4

What's a "Wedding Workout"? It's the workout you do to get in shape for your wedding day. And that's what this 8-week plan, courtesy of Charlotte Ord, is all about. It's designed to tone your legs and butt, narrow your waist, and sculpt your shoulders. All so that you'll not only look great walking down the aisle, but on your honeymoon, too.

About the Expert
Charlotte Ord is a UK-based fitness expert who specializes in fat loss and what she calls "feel-good fitness." Charlotte has competed internationally in five different sports, including lacrosse and equestrian sports.

How to Do This Workout
• Alternate between Workout A and Workout B three days a week, resting at least a day between each session. So if you plan to exercise on Monday, Wednesday, and Friday, you'd do Workout A on Monday, Workout B on Wednesday, and Workout A again on Friday. The next week, you'd do Workout B on Monday and Friday, and Workout A on Wednesday.
• Prior to each workout, warm up for 10 minutes by exercising at an easy pace on a treadmill or stationary bike for 10 minutes.
• Questions? Flip back to page 375, where you'll find complete instructions for performing all of the workouts.

Workout A

EXERCISE	SETS	REPS	REST
1A. Body-weight side lunge (page 221)	1	5	0
1B. Inchworm (page 360)	1	5	0
2. Dumbbell lunge (page 218)	2	8	60 sec
3A. Wide-grip lat pulldown (page 104)	2	12	60 sec
3B. Dumbbell shoulder press (page 120)	2	12	60 sec
4A. Plank (page 278)	2	30 sec hold	60 sec
4B. Standing rotational chop (page 307)	2	10	60 sec
5A. Jump rope	2–3	30 sec	0
5B. Medicine ball slam (page 320)	2–3	15	0
5C. Mountain climber (page 288)	2–3	20	30 sec

Perform the mountain climber as directed in the book, with one tweak: Do the movement quickly, switching your leg positions simultaneously, as if you were performing a split jack (page 351) in a pushup position.

Workout B

EXERCISE	SETS	REPS	REST
1A. Prisoner squat (page 192)	1	10	0
1B. Inchworm (page 360)	1	6–8	0
2. Prone cobra (page 295)	2	15	60 sec
3A. Inverted row (page 72)	2	8–10	60 sec
3B. Dumbbell bench press (page 52)	2	15	60 sec
4A. Hip crossover (page 303)	2	5	0
4B. Reverse dumbbell curl (page 156)	2	10	0
4C. Swiss-ball rollout (page 292)	2	30 sec	60 sec
5A. Body-weight jump squat (for fat loss) (page 194)	2–3	15	0
5B. Pushup (page 34)	2–3	10	0
5C. Squat thrusts (page 354)	2–3	10	30 sec

For the prone cobra, perform as instructed, only hold the up position for 2 seconds, then lower back down. That's one rep.

Best Workouts

The Wedding Workout
Phase 2: Weeks 5 to 8

Workout A

EXERCISE	SETS	REPS	REST
1A. Low side-to-side squat (page 357)	1	10	0
1B. Inchworm (page 360)	1	8	0
1C. Single-leg hip raise (page 240)	1	5	0
2. Single-leg squat (page 196)	2	5	60 sec
3A. Close-grip chinup (page 99)	2	5	60 sec
3B. Dumbbell push press (page 121)	2	12	0
4A. Side plank with reach under (page 286)	2	20	60 sec
4B. Reverse crunch (page 322)	2	6	60 sec
5A. Jump rope	2–3	30 sec	0
5B. Elbow-to-knee crunch (page 315)	2–3	20 sec	0
5C. Thrusters (page 343)	2–3	10	60 sec

If the single-leg squat is too hard, perform a partial single-leg squat.

If the close-grip chinup is too hard, perform a negative chinup or a band-assisted chinup.

Workout B

EXERCISE	SETS	REPS	REST
1A. Sumo squat to stand (page 360)	1	10	0
1B. Inchworm (page 360)	1	8	0
2. Barbell deadlift (page 248) or dumbbell deadlift (page 250)	2	12	60 sec
3A. Incline dumbbell bench press (page 54)	2	12	60 sec
3B. Dumbbell row (page 78)	2	12	60 sec
4A. Plank (page 278)	2	30 sec hold	60 sec
4B. Incline Y-T-W-L raises (page 86)	2	6 reps of each	60 sec
5A. Box jump (page 195)	2	10	0
5B. Dumbbell chop (page 304)	2	12	0
5C. Dumbbell split squat (page 209)	2	12	30 sec

Best Workouts

The Hard-Body Workout

If you want a tight, toned body, try this 6-week workout from personal trainer Jen Heath. It uses mini-circuits to keep your heart rate high as you sculpt your hips, legs, and abs. So once you start moving, you keep moving—until you've worked every inch of your body, from every direction. The result: a complete total-body workout that'll have you beach-ready in no time.

About the Expert
Jen Heath is certified as a personal trainer by the American College of Sports Medicine. Along with helping her clients transform their bodies, Jen also works as both a commercial and fitness model, and is a frequent expert contributor to FigureAthlete.com.

How to Do This Workout

• Do each workout (Workout A, Workout B, and Workout C) once a week, resting at least a day between each session. So you might do Workout A on Monday, Workout B on Wednesday, and Workout C on Friday.
• Questions? Flip back to page 375, where you'll find complete instructions for performing all of the workouts.

Workout A

EXERCISE	SETS	REPS	REST
1A. Overhead barbell or dumbbell squat (page 202 or page 205)	2	12	0
1B. Pushup (page 34)	2	12	0
1C. Dumbbell Bulgarian split squat (page 210)	2	12	0
1D. Incline dumbbell bench press (page 54)	2	12	0
1E. Hanging leg raise (page 329)	2	12	60 sec
2A. Goblet squat (page 204)	2	12	0
2B. Dumbbell bench press (page 52)	2	12	0
2C. Dumbbell lunge (page 218)	2	12	0
2D. Dumbbell chest fly (page 60)	2	12	0
2E. V-up (page 316)	2	12	60 sec

Workout B

EXERCISE	SETS	REPS	REST
1A. Single-leg dumbbell straight-leg deadlift (page 257)	2	12	0
1B. Pullup (or assisted pullup) (page 99)	2	12	0
1C. Cable pull through (page 259)	2	12	0
1D. Cable row (page 92)	2	12	0
1E. Single-leg side plank (page 285)	2	12	60 sec
2A. Barbell row (page 76)	2	12	0
2B. Underhand-grip lat pulldown (page 104)	2	12	0
2C. Swiss-ball hip raise and leg curl (page 243)	2	12	0
2D. Rear lateral raise (page 83)	2	12	0
2E. Cable crunch (page 321)	2	12	60 sec

Perform the single-leg side plank as directed with one tweak: Instead of keeping your top leg elevated the entire time, raise and lower it slowly as you hold the side plank. Each time you return to a standard side plank counts as one repetition. If that's too hard, brace the back of your body against a wall as you perform the movement.

If the Swiss-ball hip raise and leg curl is too easy, use the single-leg version of the exercise (page 244).

Workout C

EXERCISE	SETS	REPS	REST
1A. Single-leg dumbbell straight-leg deadlift (page 257)	2	12	0
1B. Close-hands pushup (page 38)	2	12	0
1C. Incline dumbbell bench press (page 54)	2	12	0
1D. Dumbbell stepup (page 262)	2	12	0
1E. Side plank and row (page 286)	2	12	60 sec
2A. Lateral raise (page 126)	2	12	0
2B. Lat pulldown (page 102)	2	12	0
2C. Dumbbell Bulgarian split squat (page 210)	2	12	0
2D. Pushup and row (page 43)	2	12	0
2E. Swiss-ball rollout (page 292)	2	12	60 sec

Best Workouts

The Lose-the-Last-10-Pounds Workout

Finish off the fat for good with this 8-week plan from North Carolina–based trainer Leigh Peele. It's designed to help you finally shed those last few hard-to-lose pounds.

How to Do This Workout
• Do the Weight Workout 3 days a week, resting at least a day between each session.
• Do the Cardio Workout immediately after each Weight Workout.
• Prior to each workout, do the warmup.
• Questions? Flip back to page 375, where you'll find complete instructions.

About the Expert
Leigh Peele is certified as a personal trainer by the National Academy of Sports Medicine. She's known by her clients as the "fat-loss troubleshooter," for her unique ability to help women break through longtime weight loss plateaus and achieve the bodies they want.

For the overhead triceps stretch, perform as directed, only hold the stretch for just 1 second, and release. Then repeat with your other arm. That's one rep.

If the plank is too hard, try the modified plank instead.

If the side plank is too hard, try the modified side plank instead.

Warmup

EXERCISE	SETS	REPS	REST
1A. Reverse lunge with twist and overhead reach (page 358)	1	12	15 sec
1B. Walking leg cradles (page 361)	1	12	15 sec
1C. Overhead triceps stretch (page 181)	1	10	15 sec
1D. Swiss-ball Y-T-W-L raises (pages 87–91)	1	8	15 sec

Weight Workout: Weeks 1–4

EXERCISE	SETS	REPS	REST
1A. Single-leg hip raise with foot on bench (page 241)	3	15	15–30 sec
1B. Cable row (page 92)	3	15	15–30 sec
1C. Cable hip adduction (page 222)	3	12	15–30 sec
1D. Incline chest fly (page 81)	3	12	15–30 sec
1E. Dumbbell shoulder press (page 120)	3	12	15–30 sec
1F. Dumbbell lying triceps extension (page 166)	3	15	15–30 sec
1G. Plank (page 278)	3	30 sec hold	15–30 sec
1H. Side plank (page 284)	3	30 sec hold	2–3 min

Weight Workout: Weeks 5–8

EXERCISE	SETS	REPS	REST
1A. Single-leg dumbbell straight-leg deadlift (page 257)	4	15	15–30 sec
1B. Cable face pull (page 108)	4	15	15–30 sec
1C. Cable pull-through (page 259)	4	12	15–30 sec
1D. Dumbbell bench press (page 52)	4	12	15–30 sec
1E. Rear lateral raise (page 83)	4	12	15–30 sec
1F. Triceps pressdown (page 171)	4	15	15–30 sec
1G. Single-leg side plank (page 285)	4	30 sec hold	15–30 sec
1H. T-stabilization (page 287)	4	30 sec	2–3 min

For the single-leg side plank, perform the exercise as instructed, but instead of keeping your top leg elevated for the duration, raise and lower it slowly as you hold your position.

Cardio Workout

EXERCISE

You can perform this workout on a treadmill, stationary bike, or outside on the sidewalk. Before each workout, warm up for 5 minutes by walking or cycling. The workout is divided into three parts.

Part 1: Exercise for 5 minutes at an intensity that's about 75 percent of your best effort.

Part 2: Exercise for 2 minutes at an intensity that's about 85 percent of your best effort.

Part 3: Exercise for 3 minutes at an intensity that's about 65 percent of your best effort.

• Perform each part in succession without stopping to rest. Once you've completed each part one time, start over again with Part 1. Repeat the entire process two times, so that you've done each part of the workout three times. On your final round, add an extra 5 minutes to Part 3. That is, instead of going for 3 minutes, go for 8 minutes.

Best Workouts

The Best Sports Workout

There's a popular notion that if you train like an athlete, you'll look like an athlete. And it's true. That's why I asked Mike Boyle, CSCS, one of the world's top sports performance coaches, to create a workout that'll enhance your game *and* your figure. The end result: You'll look as fit as a tennis pro—even if you never step foot on a court.

How to Do This Workout

• Do Workout A and Workout B once a week, on consecutive days. Then rest for a day or two, and do Workout C and Workout D on consecutive days. Rest for a day or two again, and start over the following week. So you might do Workout A on Monday, Workout B on Tuesday, Workout C on Thursday, and Workout D on Friday.

• Questions? Flip back to page 375, where you'll find complete instructions for performing all of the workouts.

About the Expert
Mike Boyle, CSCS, is the owner of Mike Boyle Strength and Conditioning, with locations in both Winchester and North Andover, Massachusetts. Over the years, he's trained numerous NBA, NFL, and NHL athletes. Mike also owns Strength coach.com, one of the best sources of training information on the Web.

Workout A

EXERCISE	WEEK 1			WEEK 2			WEEK 3		
	SETS	REPS	REST	SETS	REPS	REST	SETS	REPS	REST
1A. Single-arm kettlebell swing (page 268)	3	10	1 min	3	10	1 min	3	10	1 min
1B. Cable core press (page 295)	2	12	1 min	2	14	1 min	2	16	1 min
2A. Chinup (page 96)	2	8	1 min	3	8	1 min	3	8	1 min
2B. Single-leg squat (page 196)	2	8	1 min	3	8	1 min	3	8	1 min
2C. Side plank (page 284)	2	30-sec hold	30 sec	2	40-sec hold	30 sec	2	50-sec hold	30 sec
3A. Dumbbell row (page 78)	2	8	30 sec	2	8	30 sec	2	8	30 sec
3B. Single-leg barbell straight-leg deadlift (page 254)	2	8	30 sec	2	8	30 sec	2	8	30 sec
3C. Cable face pull with external rotation (page 108)	2	8	30 sec	2	8	30 sec	2	8	30 sec
3D. Half-kneeling stability reverse chop (page 299)	2	8	30 sec	2	8	30 sec	2	8	30 sec

Workout B

EXERCISE	WEEK 1			WEEK 2			WEEK 3		
	SETS	REPS	REST	SETS	REPS	REST	SETS	REPS	REST
1A. Dumbbell bench press (page 52)	2	8	1 min	3	8	1 min	3	8	1 min
1B. Swiss-ball rollout (page 292)	2	20	1 min	2	30	1 min	2	40	1 min
2A. Hammer curl to press (page 159)	2	8	1 min	2	8	1 min	2	8	1 min
2B. Wall slide (page 354)	2	10	0	2	12	0	2	14	0
2C. Plank (page 278)	2	30-sec hold	30 sec	2	40-sec hold	30 sec	2	50-sec hold	30 sec
3A. Mountain climber (page 288)	2	10	1 min	2	12	1 min	2	14	1 min
3B. Incline Y-T-W-L raises (page 86)	2	8	1 min	2	10	1 min	2	12	1 min
3C. Standing cable hip adduction (page 222)	2	10	1 min	2	12	1 min	2	14	1 min

Best Workouts

The Best Sports Workout

Workout C

EXERCISE	WEEK 1			WEEK 2			WEEK 3		
	SETS	REPS	REST	SETS	REPS	REST	SETS	REPS	REST
1A. Single-arm kettlebell swing (page 268)	3	5	1 min	3	5	1 min	3	5	1 min
1B. Cable core press (page 295)	2	12	1 min	2	14	1 min	2	16	1 min
2A. Single-leg squat (page 196)	2	8	1 min	3	8	1 min	3	8	1 min
2B. Inverted row (page 72)	2	15	1 min	3	15	1 min	3	15	1 min
2C. Side plank (page 284)	2	30-sec hold	30 sec	2	40-sec hold	30 sec	2	50-sec hold	30 sec
3A. Lat pulldown (page 102)	2	15	30 sec	2	15	30 sec	2	15	30 sec
3B. Dumbbell lunge (page 218)	2	8	30 sec	2	12	30 sec	2	15	30 sec
3C. Swiss-ball hip raise and leg curl (page 243)	2	8	30 sec	2	10	30 sec	2	12	30 sec
3D. Half-kneeling stability chop (page 297)	2	8	30 sec	2	8	30 sec	2	8	30 sec

Workout D

EXERCISE	WEEK 1			WEEK 2			WEEK 3		
	SETS	REPS	REST	SETS	REPS	REST	SETS	REPS	REST
1A. Close-grip bench press (page 47)	2	8	1 min	3	8	1 min	3	8	1 min
1B. Swiss-ball rollout (page 292)	2	20	1 min	2	30	1 min	2	40	1 min
2A. Combo shoulder raise (page 129)	2	10	1 min	2	10	1 min	2	10	1 min
2B. Wall slide (page 354)	2	10	0	2	12	0	2	14	0
2C. Plank (page 278)	2	30-sec hold	30 sec	2	40-sec hold	30 sec	2	50-sec hold	30 sec
3A. Mountain climber (page 288)	2	10	1 min	2	12	1 min	2	14	1 min
3B. Incline Y-T-W-L raises (page 86)	2	8	1 min	2	10	1 min	2	12	1 min
3C. Standing cable hip adduction (page 222)	2	10	1 min	2	12	1 min	2	14	1 min
3D. Cable core press (page 295)	2	8	1 min	2	8	1 min	2	8	1 min

The Best Three-Exercise Workouts

Flatten your belly and shrink your hips with just three moves, courtesy of fitness coach Galya Talkington, CPT. You even have a choice of routines. That's because Galya has create three separate fat-burning workouts, each of which will help you tone your total body—with less hassle than ever before.

How to Do These Workouts

• Choose one of the three workouts that follow, and do it 3 days a week for 4 weeks. Then simply switch to one of the other workouts for another 4 weeks.
• Do the exercises as a circuit, performing one set of each exercise in succession, resting as prescribed. Complete a total of three circuits. To keep your body challenged, work your way up to four or five circuits, and eliminate the rest periods. So as you progress, you should move from exercise to exercise without taking a break.

Workout 1

EXERCISE	SETS	REPS	REST
1A. T-pushup (page 41)	3	8–10	30 sec
1B. Dumbbell lunge and rotation (page 219)	3	6–8	30 sec
1C. Dumbbell straight-leg deadlift (page 256)	3	10–12	30 sec

If the T-pushup is too hard, choose from any pushup in Chapter 4, including the incline pushup and modified pushup.

Workout 2

EXERCISE	SETS	REPS	REST
1A. Swiss-ball chest press (page 56)	3	8–10	30 sec
1B. Swiss-ball Y raise (page 87)	3	10–12	30 sec
1C. Swiss-ball hip raise and leg curl (page 243)	3	6–8	30 sec

Workout 3

EXERCISE	SETS	REPS	REST
1A. Alternating dumbbell row (page 78)	3	6–8	30 sec
1B. Dumbbell sumo squat (page 204)	3	10–12	30 sec
1C. Mountain climber (page 288)	3	10	30 sec

Best Workouts

The Prenatal Workout
Phase 1: Months 1 to 3

This 9-month plan, from Galya Talkington, CPT, is designed to give you the strength, stability, and overall fitness you need to make your pregnancy easier. As always, make sure you consult your obstetrician before you engage in any physical activity.

How to Do This Workout

• Do the Weight Workout 3 days a week, resting at least a day between each session. So you might lift weights on Monday, Wednesday, and Friday.
• Do the Cardio Workout three times a week, on the days in between your Weight Workouts. So you might do your cardio sessions on Tuesday, Thursday, and Saturday.
• Prior to each Weight Workout, complete the warmup.
• Questions? Flip back to page 375, where you'll find complete instructions for performing all of the workouts.

Warmup

EXERCISE	SETS	REPS	REST
1A. Wall slide (page 354)	1	12	0
1B. Body-weight squat (page 190)	1	10	0
1C. Cat camel (page 283)	1	10	0
1D. Clamshell (page 267)	1	15	0
1E. Hip raises (page 236)	1	12	0
1F. Pelvic tilt	1	10	0
1G. Lying tummy pull	1	10	0
1H. Kegels	1	30	0

For the body-weight squat, perform as instructed, only set your feet about twice shoulder-width apart, as you would for a dumbbell sumo squat (page 204).

For each rep of the hip raise, hold the up position for 1 second.

For the pelvic tilt, assume an all-fours position, as if you were performing a quadruped (page 282). Draw your stomach in toward your spine and hold while breathing deeply. Then without moving your thighs, push your hips forward so that only your pelvis moves and your lower back flattens. Hold for a moment, then release. That's one rep.

For kegels, sit comfortably on a chair or bench, squeeze your pelvic floor muscle, and hold for 3 seconds. To locate this muscle, imagine you are trying to stop yourself from peeing. (It's that simple.)

For the lying tummy pulls, lie on your back as if you're about to perform a situp (page 310). Now inhale like you have lungs in your stomach. Exhale as you use your abdominal muscles to pull your belly button toward your spine. Hold for 2 or 3 seconds and release. (You should be able to talk while you hold the position.) That's one rep.

408

Weight Workout

EXERCISE	SETS	REPS	REST
1A. Bent-over Y raise	2	8	0
1B. Underhand-grip rear lateral raise (page 84)	2	8	60 sec
1C. Modified pushup (page 36)	2	AMAP	60 sec
1D. Braced Squat (page 194)	2	12	60 sec
1E. Side plank (page 284)	2	ALAP	60 sec
1F. Reverse dumbbell lunge (page 217)	2	8	60 sec
1G. Dumbbell row (page 78)	2	12	60 sec
1H. Bird dog (page 283)	2	10	60 sec
1I. Alternating dumbbell shoulder press (page 121)	2	10	60 sec
2. Glute stretch (page 270)	1	30 sec	0
3. Doorway stretch (page 66)	1	30 sec	0

For the bent-over Y raise, use the instructions for the incline Y raise (page 86), but instead of lying down, perform the movement in a bent-over position, as you would the underhand-grip rear lateral raise (page 84; also known as a bent-over T raise).

For the bird dog, apply these tweaks to the instructions: Start by drawing your stomach in as if you were trying to pull your belly button to your spine. Then raise one arm and one leg as directed, but hold only for a moment, and without allowing your lower back posture to change, bring your elbow to your knee. That's one rep. Raise them up again and repeat. Do all your reps and then switch arms and legs.

Cardio Workout

Perform a low-intensity aerobic workout at least three times a week. If you are already involved in cardio activity, just lower the intensity to match the goals in this workout and stay away from any group classes and recreational sports that might cause you to trip or fall. While specific workouts for walking outside and riding a stationary bike have been provided, you can use similar guidelines when swimming, or when using an elliptical trainer or treadmill. Just choose whichever workout best suits you.

About the Expert
Galya Talkington, CPT, is a fitness coach and nutrition counselor from Sofia, Bulgaria. She splits her time training clients in Sofia and Los Angeles, and is certified as a personal trainer by the National Strength and Conditioning Association. You can find her online at www.eatloveandtrain.com.

Best Workouts

The Prenatal Workout
Phase 1: Months 1 to 3

The Walking Workout
• Walk at a speed so that you're exercising at an intensity that's about 50 percent of your best effort. Go for 5 minutes.
• Next, increase your intensity so that you're walking at about 60 percent of your best effort and go for 10 minutes.
• Slow down slightly, so that you're walking at about 50 percent of your best effort for the last 5 minutes.
• 5-minute break and then repeat the 20-minute walk.
• After walking perform the stretching routine below.

EXERCISE	SETS	REPS	REST
1A. Bulgarian split squat stretch	1	30 sec	0
1B. Straight-leg calf stretch (page 229)	1	30 sec	0

For the Bulgarian squat stretch, perform a body-weight Bulgarian split squat (no dumbbell; page 210), but instead of pushing yourself back up to the starting position, hold the down position for the prescribed time. Then repeat with your other leg.

THE STATIONARY BIKE WORKOUT

• Warm up for 5 minutes by pedaling at a pace that's about 50 percent of your best effort.
• Increase your speed until you're exercising at an intensity that's about 60 percent of your best effort. Go for 3 minutes.
• Lower your intensity so that you're exercising at 30 percent of your best effort for 3 minutes. That's one set.
• Do a total of four to six sets, then cool down for 5 minutes, pedaling at about 40 percent of your best effort.

Turn the page to start
PHASE 2 OF THE PRENATAL WORKOUT

Best Workouts

The Prenatal Workout
Phase 2: Months 4 to 7

Warmup

For the pelvic tilt, assume an all-fours position, as if you were performing a bird dog (page 283). Draw your stomach in toward your spine and hold while breathing deeply. Then without moving your thighs, push your hips forward so that only your pelvis moves and your lower back flattens. Hold for a moment, then release. That's one rep.

EXERCISE	SETS	REPS	REST
1A. Wall slide (page 354)	1	12	0
1B. Thoracic rotation (page 355)	1	10	0
1C. Cat camel (page 283)	1	10	0
1D. Clamshell (page 267)	1	15	0
1E. Pelvic tilt	1	10	0
1F. Quadruped tummy pull	1	10	0
1G. Kegels	1	30	0

For quadruped tummy pulls, use the directions for the quadruped (page 282), with one tweak: Start by drawing your stomach in as if you were trying to pull your belly button to your spine. Then hold for 5 seconds while breathing deeply. Relax for a moment and repeat. That's one rep.

For kegels, sit comfortably on a chair or bench, squeeze your pelvic floor muscle, and hold for 3 seconds. To locate this muscle, imagine you are trying to stop yourself from peeing. (It's that simple.)

Weight Workout

For the bent-over Y raise, use the instructions for the incline Y raise (page 86), but instead of lying down, perform the movement in a bent-over position, as you would the rear lateral raise (page 83; also known as a bent-over T raise).

EXERCISE	SETS	REPS	REST
1A. Bent-over Y raise	3	8	0
1B. Underhand-grip rear lateral raise (page 84)	3	10	60 sec
1C. Braced squat (page 194)	3	10	60 sec
1D. Modified side plank (page 285)	3	ALAP	60 sec
1E. Incline pushup (page 36)	3	AMAP	60 sec
1F. Dumbbell stepup (page 262)	3	8	60 sec
1G. Bird dog (page 283)	3	30 sec	60 sec
2. Glute stretch (page 270)	1	30 sec	0
3. Doorway stretch (page 66)	1	30 sec	0

If the incline pushup is too hard, simply do the same movement, but with your hands placed on a wall, so that your body is even more vertical. (Think of it as a "standing pushup.")

Perform the bird dog as in Phase 1.

Cardio Workout

Perform a low-intensity aerobic workout at least three times a week. If you are already involved in cardio activity, just lower the intensity to match the goals in this workout and stay away from any group classes and recreational sports that might cause you to trip or fall. While specific workouts for walking outside and riding a stationary bike have been provided, you can use similar guidelines when swimming, or when using an elliptical trainer or treadmill. Just choose whichever workout best suits you.

The Walking Workout

• Walk on a fairly flat route at a speed so that you're exercising at an intensity that's about 50 percent of your best effort. Go for 10 minutes.
• Next, find a hill that's no steeper than what looks like 45 degrees (compared to a flat surface). For 10 minutes walk up the hill and back down at a speed that is 60 percent of your maximum speed on the way up and 30 percent of your maximum speed on the way down.
• Slow down slightly and return to the flat route, so that you're walking at about 50 percent of your best effort for the last 10 minutes.
• After walking perform the stretching routine below.

EXERCISE	SETS	REPS	REST
1A. Kneeling hip flexor stretch (page 228)	1	30 sec	0
1B. Straight-leg calf stretch (page 229)	1	30 sec	0

THE STATIONARY BIKE WORKOUT

• Warm up for 5 minutes by pedaling at a pace that's about 50 percent of your best effort.
• Increase your speed until you're exercising at an intensity that's about 60 percent of your best effort. Go for 2 minutes.
• Lower your intensity so that you're exercising at 30 percent of your best effort for 2 minutes. That's one set.
• Do a total of four to six sets, then cool down for 5 minutes, pedaling at about 40 percent of your best effort.

Best Workouts

The Prenatal Workout
Phase 3: Months 8 to 9

For quadruped tummy pulls, use the directions for the quadruped, with one tweak: Start by drawing your stomach in as if you were trying to pull your belly button to your spine. Then hold for 5 seconds while breathing deeply. Relax for a moment and repeat. That's one rep.

For kegels, sit comfortably on a chair or bench, squeeze your pelvic floor muscle, and hold for 3 seconds. To locate this muscle, imagine you are trying to stop yourself from peeing. (It's that simple.)

Warmup

EXERCISE	SETS	REPS	REST
1A. Wall slide (page 354)	1	12	0
1B. Thoracic rotation (page 355)	1	10	0
1C. Cat camel (page 283)	1	15	0
1D. Clamshell (page 267)	1	15	0
1E. Quadruped tummy pull	1	10	0
1F. Kegels	1	40	0

Weight Workout

EXERCISE	SETS	REPS	REST
1A. Bent-over Y raise (page 409)	2	10	0
1B. Rear lateral raise (page 83)	2	10	60 sec
1C. Swiss-ball wall squat (page 193)	2	10	60 sec
1D. Modified side plank (page 285)	2	ALAP	60 sec
1E. Single-arm dumbbell shoulder press (page 122)	2	8	60 sec
1F. Crossover dumbbell stepup (page 263)	2	10	60 sec
1G. Bird dog (page 283)	2	20 sec	60 sec
1H. Glute stretch (page 270)	2	30 sec	0
1I. Doorway stretch (page 66)	2	30 sec	0
1J. Neck rotations (page 355)	2	30 sec	0
1K. Kneeling hip flexor stretch (page 228)	2	30 sec	0

The Walking Workout

• Choose an enjoyable path and walk for 5 minutes, at 40 percent of your best effort.
• Increase your speed slightly, so that you're walking at 50 percent of your best effort. Go for 5 minutes.
• Take a break for as long as you need to feel ready to go again. Repeat for two more bouts of walking for 10 minutes.
• After walking perform the stretching routine below.

EXERCISE	SETS	REPS	REST
1A. Kneeling hip flexor stretch (page 228)	2	30 sec	0
1B. Straight-leg calf stretch (page 229)	2	30 sec	0
1C. Glute stretch (page 270)	2	30 sec	0

THE STATIONARY BIKE WORKOUT

• Warm up for 5 minutes by pedaling at a pace that's about 40 percent of your best effort.
• Increase your speed until you're exercising at intensity that's about 50 percent of your best effort. Go for 3 minutes.
• Lower your intensity so that you're exercising at 30 percent of your best effort for 3 minutes. That's one set.
• Do a total of two to four sets, then cool down for 5 minutes, pedaling at about 30 percent of your best effort.

Best Workouts

The Time-Saving Couples Workout

This fat-burning plan is designed so that you can work out with your spouse but still ensure that you get the results you want. The weight workouts are performed in a circuit. You can do them simultaneously, or if you're sharing the same equipment, perform them follow-the-leader style, with one of you completing the first exercise before the other starts. After you've finished the main workout, you can then choose an optional workout that allows you to customize your routine for the body you want.

How to Do This Workout

• Do each Weight Workout (Workout A, Workout B, and Workout C) once a week, resting for at least a day after each session. So you might do Workout A on Monday, Workout B on Wednesday, and Workout C on Friday.

• Prior to each Weight Workout, complete the warmup.

• Each Weight Workout is designed to last 10 minutes. Simply do as many sets of each exercise as you can in that time frame. Note that you'll be performing the exercises in a circuit. So complete one set of the first exercise, then move immediately to the second exercise, and so on. Stop your workout when you run out of time.

• After each Weight Workout, you can also choose one of the 4-Minute Add-

On Workouts. These are optional, so do them only if you have time. They're designed to both burn fat and give a little extra attention to the muscles that you may want to show off. As a result, you'll find there are different routines for men and women (although you can choose from any of them).

• Do the Cardio Workout twice a week, on the days in between your Weight Workouts. So you might do your cardio sessions on Tuesday and Thursday. (If you can't find time to exercise 5 days a week, just do the Cardio Workout immediately following two of your Weight Workouts.)

• Questions? Flip back to page 375, where you'll find complete instructions for performing all of the workouts.

About the Expert
Ed Scow, CPT, is the owner of ELS Massage and Personal Training in Lincoln, Nebraska. Ed specializes in helping busy men and women lose fat and get fit fast.

Weight Workouts
Warmup

EXERCISE	SETS	REPS	REST
1A. Jumping jacks (page 353)	1	15	0
1B. Prisoner squat (page 192)	1	10	0
1C. Pushup (page 34)	1	8	0

Workout A

EXERCISE	SETS	REPS	REST	DURATION
1A. Incline dumbbell bench press (page 54)	AMAP	8	0	8 min
1B. Dumbbell row (page 78)	AMAP	8	0	8 min
1C. Single-arm dumbbell swing (page 268)	AMAP	8	0	8 min
2. Squat thrusts (page 354)	AMAP	20 sec	10 sec	2 min

• This workout is split into two separate routines. One routine lasts 8 minutes and the other is to be performed for 2 minutes. Simply do as many sets of each exercise as you can in the given time frame.
• For the 8-minute routine, you'll be performing the three exercises in an 8-minute circuit. So complete one set of the first exercise, then move immediately to the second exercise, and so on. When time is up, move on to the 2-minute routine.
• For the 2-minute routine, you'll simply do one exercise. Do as many reps as you can in 20 seconds, rest for 10 seconds, then repeat until you run out of time.

Best Workouts

The Time-Saving Couples Workout

Workout B

EXERCISE	SETS	REPS	REST	DURATION
1A. Thrusters (page 343)	AMAP	8	0	
1B. Rear lateral raise (page 83)	AMAP	8	0	
1C. Pushup (page 34)	AMAP	12	0	10 min
1D. Reverse dumbbell lunge (page 217)	AMAP	8	0	
1E. Mountain climber (page 288)	AMAP	30 sec	0	

Workout C

EXERCISE	SETS	REPS	REST	DURATION
1A. Elbows-out dumbbell row (page 80)	AMAP	10	0	
1B. Incline dumbbell bench press (page 54)	AMAP	10	0	
1C. Squat thrusts (page 354)	AMAP	8	0	10 min
1D. Dumbbell push press (page 121)	AMAP	10	0	
1E. Single-arm dumbbell swing (page 268)	AMAP	12	0	

4-Minute Add-On Workouts for Women
Option 1: Hips, Triceps, and Core

EXERCISE	SETS	REPS	REST	DURATION
1A. Hip raise with feet on a Swiss ball (page 239)	AMAP	20 sec	10 sec	
1B. Mountain climber (page 288)	AMAP	20 sec	10 sec	4 min
1C. Dumbbell lying triceps extension (page 166)	AMAP	20 sec	10 sec	
1D. Mountain climber (page 288)	AMAP	20 sec	10 sec	

Option 2: Hips, Thighs, and Core

EXERCISE	SETS	REPS	REST	DURATION
1A. Swiss-ball jackknife (page 290)	AMAP	20 sec	10 sec	
1B. Swiss-ball hip raise and leg curl (page 243)	AMAP	20 sec	10 sec	4 min
1C. Swiss-ball jackknife (page 290)	AMAP	20 sec	10 sec	
1D. Split jump (page 211)	AMAP	20 sec	10 sec	

Option 3: Hips, Thighs, Shoulders, and Arms

EXERCISE	SETS	REPS	REST	DURATION
1A. Dumbbell squat (page 203)	AMAP	20 sec	10 sec	
1B. Single-arm dumbbell swing (page 268)	AMAP	20 sec	10 sec	4 min
1C. Hammer curl to press (page 159)	AMAP	20 sec	10 sec	
1D. Single-arm dumbbell swing (page 268)	AMAP	20 sec	10 sec	

Best Workouts

The Time-Saving Couples Workout

4-Minute Add-On Workouts for Men
Option 1: Arms and Core

EXERCISE	SETS	REPS	REST	DURATION
1A. Standing dumbbell curl (page 154)	AMAP	20 sec	10 sec	
1B. Squat thrusts (page 354)	AMAP	20 sec	10 sec	4 min
1C. Dumbbell lying triceps extension (page 166)	AMAP	20 sec	10 sec	
1D. Squat thrusts (page 354)	AMAP	20 sec	10 sec	

Option 2: Hips, Arms, and Core

EXERCISE	SETS	REPS	REST	DURATION
1A. Close-hands pushup (page 38)	AMAP	20 sec	10 sec	
1B. Single-arm dumbbell swing (page 268)	AMAP	20 sec	10 sec	4 min
1C. Hammer curl to press (page 159)	AMAP	20 sec	10 sec	
1D. Single-arm dumbbell swing (page 268)	AMAP	20 sec	10 sec	

Option 3: Arms and Core

EXERCISE	SETS	REPS	REST	DURATION
1A. Swiss-ball jackknife (page 290)	AMAP	20 sec	10 sec	
1B. Hammer curl (page 156)	AMAP	20 sec	10 sec	4 min
1C. Swiss-ball jackknife (page 290)	AMAP	20 sec	10 sec	
1D. Dumbbell lying triceps extension (page 166)	AMAP	20 sec	10 sec	

The 16-Minute Cardio Workout

THE PLAN

- You can perform this workout on a treadmill, on a stationary bike, or outside on the sidewalk or a track.
- Start by going at an easy pace—about 30 percent of your best effort—for 4 minutes. Then do this interval workout:
- Exercise at an intensity that's about 80 percent of your best effort. Go for 30 seconds.
- Slow down until your intensity is about 40 percent of your best effort and go for 60 seconds. That's one set. Do six sets.
- Once you've completed all of your sets, slow down to 30 percent of your best effort and go for 3 minutes.

Best Workouts

The Best Body-Weight Workouts

You don't need a gym membership to sculpt a great body. In fact, you don't even need equipment. Tone your arms, legs, and abs and burn fat anywhere with these super-simple body-weight workouts.

Workout 1

EXERCISE	SETS	REPS	REST
1. Body-weight Bulgarian split squat (page 210)	3	10–12	1 min
2A. Pushup (page 34)	3	12–15	1 min
2B. Hip raises (page 236)	3	12–15	1 min
3A. Side plank (page 284)	3	30-sec hold	30 sec
3B. Floor Y-T-I raises (pages 87, 88, and 91)	3	10	30 sec

If any of the first four exercises are too hard, feel free to substitute the variation of the movement that allows you to perform the prescribed number of reps. Likewise, if you find an exercise is too easy, use a harder variation instead.

For the floor Y-T-I raises, do 10 repetitions of each letter. That is, do 10 reps of the floor Y raise, followed by 10 reps of the floor T raise and 10 reps of the floor I raise.

Workout 2

EXERCISE	SETS	REPS	REST
1. Iso-explosive jump squat (page 194)	4	6–8	1 min
2A. Iso-explosive pushup (page 42)	3	6–8	1 min
2B. Single-leg hip raise (page 240)	3	12–15	1 min
3A. Inverted shoulder press (page 123)	3	AMAP	1 min
3B. Prone cobra (page 295)	2	1-min hold	1 min

For the iso-explosive jump squat and the iso-explosive pushup, make sure to hold the down position for 5 seconds each repetition.

If the iso-explosive pushup is too hard, use an easier variation of the exercise.

Workout 3

EXERCISE	SETS	REPS	REST
1A. Jumping jacks (page 353)	2–5	30 sec	0
1B. Prisoner squat (page 192)	2–5	20	0
1C. Close-hands pushup (page 38)	2–5	20	0
1D. Walking dumbbell lunge (page 217)	2–5	12	0
1E. Mountain climber (page 288)	2–5	10	0
1F. Inverted hamstring (page 360)	2–5	8	0
1G. T-pushup (page 41)	2–5	8	0
1H. Run in place	2–5	30 sec	0

The first time you try this routine, do two sets of each exercise. In future workouts, work your way up to five sets for each.

← If the T-pushup is too hard, use an easier version of the exercise.

Best Workouts

The Best 15-Minute Workouts

Ready to start sculpting a leaner, stronger body? It won't take you long. Just three 15-minute weight workouts a week can double a beginner's strength, report scientists at the University of Kansas. What's more, unlike the average person, who quits a new weight-training program within a month, 96 percent of the participants in the study easily fit the quickie workouts into their lives. You can do the same, with the 10 workouts that follow—all of which are designed to shape your muscles while melting fat.

Workout 1

EXERCISE	SETS	REPS	REST
1A. Goblet squat (page 204)	3	15	0
1B. Pushup (page 34)	3	AMAP	0
1C. Hip raises (page 236)	3	12–15	0
1D. Dumbbell row (page 78)	3	10–12	0
1E. Plank (page 278)	3	30-sec hold	0

Workout 2

EXERCISE	SETS	REPS	REST
1A. Swiss-ball hip raise and leg curl (page 243)	3	AMAP	0
1B. Pushup plus (page 64)	3	AMAP	0
1C. Swiss-ball jackknife (page 290)	3	AMAP	30 sec
2A. Chinup (page 96)	2–3	AMAP	30 sec
2B. Dumbbell shoulder press (page 120)	2–3	8–10	30 sec

Before You Start

If any of the body-weight exercises in these workouts are too hard or too easy, feel free to substitute the variation of the movement that allows you to perform the prescribed number of reps. Remember, each set should challenge your muscles to the point where you start to struggle but don't quite reach complete failure. (See Chapter 2 for a more detailed explanation of this concept.)

And make no mistake: These workouts aren't easy. They're fast paced and intense. So if they're too hard when you first start, go ahead and take longer rest between sets, and finish as much of the workout as you can in the 15 minutes. In each subsequent workout, try to do a little more, until you're able to complete the entire routine.

How to Do These Workouts

• Option 1: Choose a workout and do it three times a week, resting for at least a day after each session. After 2 or 3 weeks, switch to a new workout.

• Option 2: Choose two workouts and alternate between them 3 days a week. Always rest for at least a day after each session. So you might do Workout 1 on Monday and Friday, and Workout 2 on Wednesday. The following week, you'd do Workout 2 on Monday and Friday, and Workout 1 on Wednesday. After 4 weeks, it's time to choose two new workouts.

Workout 3

EXERCISE	SETS	REPS	REST
1. Single-arm reverse lunge and press (page 344)	3	10–12	1 min
2A. Chinup (page 96)	3	AMAP	0
2B. Side plank (page 284)	3	30-sec hold	0
2C. Pushup (page 34)	3	AMAP	45 sec

Workout 4

EXERCISE	SETS	REPS	REST
1A. Single-arm dumbbell swing (page 268)	3	12	30 sec
1B. Pushup and row (page 43)	3	12	30 sec
2A. Thrusters (page 343)	2	12	30 sec
2B. Swiss-ball jackknife (page 290)	2	12–15	30 sec

Best Workouts

The Best 15-Minute Workouts

Workout 5

EXERCISE	SETS	REPS	REST
1. Side lunge and press (page 345)	3	10–12	1 min
2A. Single-leg dumbbell row (page 79)	3	12–15	0
2B. Single-leg hip raise (page 240)	3	AMAP	0
2C. T-pushup (page 41)	3	AMAP	30 sec

Workout 6

EXERCISE	SETS	REPS	REST
1A. Overhead dumbbell lunge (page 219)	3	10–12	0
1B. Single-arm neutral-grip dumbbell row and rotation (page 82)	3	10–12	0
1C. Single-arm stepup and press (page 344)	3	10–12	0
1D. Pushup (page 34)	3	AMAP	0
1E. Prone cobra (page 295)	3	30-sec hold	60

Workout 7

EXERCISE	SETS	REPS	REST
1. Wide-grip barbell deadlift (page 248)	4	5	90 sec
2A. Incline dumbbell bench press (page 54)	2	10–12	0 sec
2B. Swiss-ball Russian twist (page 302)	2	10–12	0 sec
2C. Dumbbell lunge (page 218)	2	10–12	1 min

Workout 8

EXERCISE	SETS	REPS	REST
1A. Barbell good morning (page 254) or back extension (page 258)	3	8	0
1B. Dumbbell bench press (page 52)	3	8	0
1C. Body-weight squat (page 190)	3	30 sec	0
1D. Dumbbell row (page 78)	3	10	0
1E. Mountain climber (page 288)	3	30 sec	15–30 sec

Workout 9

EXERCISE	SETS	REPS	REST
1A. Dumbbell deadlift (page 250)	4	6	0
1B. Jump rope	4	45 sec	0
1C. Dumbbell push press (page 121)	4	6	0
1D. Jump rope	4	45 sec	1 min

Workout 10

EXERCISE	SETS	REPS	REST
1. Goblet squat (page 204)	3	6–8	1 min
2A. Barbell row (page 76)	3	6–8	0
2B. Core stabilization (page 334)	3	30 sec	0
2C. Single-arm dumbbell swing (page 268)	3	10–12	0
2D. Decline pushup (page 36)	3	AMAP	30 sec

Best Workouts

The Spartacus Workout

Ever wonder how Hollywood actors get in such incredible shape? It's not rocket science. But it is exercise science. So when executives at Starz asked me to create a training plan inspired by the network's new show, *Spartacus*—in preparation for the program's January 2010 premiere—I knew exactly who to consult: Rachel Cosgrove, one of the world's top fitness experts who's known industry-wide for her ability to meld the latest in muscle and fat loss science to achieve stunning results.

To create the Spartacus workout, we chose 10 exercises that collectively work every part of your body, and then placed each at a 60-second station—in order to challenge your heart and lungs as well as your muscles. The final product: A cutting-edge circuit routine that will strip away fat; shape your shoulders, arms, and legs; and send your fitness levels soaring. So you'll sculpt a lean, athletic-looking body—while getting in the best shape of your life.

How to Do This Workout

• Do this workout three days a week. You can do it as your primary weight workout, or as a "cardio" workout on the days between your regular weight workouts. This approach will help you speed fat loss even more.

• Perform the workout as a circuit, doing one set of each exercise—or "station"—in succession. Each station in the circuit lasts for 60 seconds. Do as many repetitions as you can in that duration, then move on to the next station in the circuit. Give yourself 15 seconds to transition between stations, and rest for 2 minutes after you've done one circuit of all 10 exercises. Then repeat two times. If you can't go for the entire minute on the body-weight exercises, go as long as you can, rest for a few seconds, then go again until your time at that station is up.

• Prior to each workout, complete a 5- to 10-minute warmup. Use the "Create Your Own Warmup" guide in Chapter 12 to design your routine.

STATION 1

Goblet squat (page 204)

STATION 2

Mountain climber (page 288)

STATION 3

Single-arm dumbbell swing (page 268)

STATION 4

T-pushup (page 41)

← If the T-pushup is too hard, use an easier version of the pushup.

STATION 5

Split jump (page 211)

STATION 6

Dumbbell row (page 78)

STATION 7

Dumbbell side lunge and touch (page 221)

STATION 8

Pushup position row (page 43)

For the pushup position row, refer to the pushup and row on page 43. Simply do the row portion of the exercise, without the pushup.

STATION 9

Dumbbell lunge and rotation (page 219)

STATION 10

Dumbbell push press (page 121)

Chapter 14:
The Best Cardio Workouts
FINISH STRONG, EVERY TIME

Let's clear something up:

The term *cardio* doesn't just mean "aerobic exercise." After all, *cardio* is really short for *cardiovascular conditioning*. And the fact is, weight training and sprints are highly beneficial to your heart and lungs, too. So you'll see plenty of great cardio routines throughout this entire book.

But in the pages that follow, you'll find a dozen more fast, unique workouts that may forever change the way you think about cardio. Whether you want to bust out of your rut, train for a 10-K, or just finish in a flurry, you'll find there's a cutting-edge plan for you.

8 World-Class Ways to Run Faster

If you're tired of long, boring runs, try these short speed workouts from Ed Eyestone, MS, a two-time Olympic marathoner and head coach of the Brigham Young University men's cross-country team. These routines not only help break up the monotony, they'll boost your speed and endurance to an all-time high. A great way to mix them up: Do one of the first three workouts early in the week, then choose a second from numbers 4 through 7 later in the week, at the track. Do the last run on the weekend.

1. Tempo Run

What: A fuel-injected version of your 4-mile jog, run at a "comfortably hard" pace.

Why: Tempo runs train your body to clear the waste products that cause your muscles to "burn" and thereby force you to slow down. As a result, you can go harder, longer.

How: Estimate your fastest 3-mile time (think back to your best recent 5-K). Calculate the pace per mile and add 30 seconds to it. So if you think the fastest you can run 3 miles is 24 minutes—that's an 8-minute pace—try for a tempo pace of 8 minutes, 30 seconds per mile for your 4-mile run.

Tip: Be precise. Wear a watch.

2. Tempo 1,000s

What: A series of 1,000-meter runs at your tempo pace, with rest in between.

Why: Short tempo runs help you maintain a strict pace, and the brief recoveries keep your effort level high.

How: Run at your 4-mile tempo pace (determined in #1, tempo run) for 1,000 meters—that's about $2\frac{1}{2}$ times around a track—then rest for 60 seconds before repeating. Start with a total of six 1,000-meter intervals and progress to 10, adding one each time you perform the workout.

Tip: If you'd prefer, measure in time instead of distance. Perform each interval for $3\frac{1}{2}$ minutes before resting.

3. Step-Down Fartlek

What: *Fartlek* is Swedish for "speed play," meaning you accelerate and slow down according to how you feel. (How European!)

Why: In a step-down fartlek, the intervals are more structured (how American!) and become harder at the end of your run. Working hard when you're tired will make you faster when you're fresh.

How: Start at a pace that's about 75 percent of your full effort and go for 5 minutes. Then slow down to about 40 percent effort for 5 minutes. Continue this fast-then-slow pattern, but shorten the hard-running segment by a minute each time, while increasing your speed. By the last 1-minute burst, you should be almost sprinting.

Tip: Each week, add 1 minute to your

first segment—but keep doing the same step-down sequence—until your first interval is 10 minutes.

4. Mile Repeats

What: Hard 1-mile runs with rest in between. The ultimate training tool for the serious runner.

Why: The length and intensity of mile repeats force you to work at the edge of your aerobic limit, giving you the endurance and mental toughness you need to run hard for long periods of time.

How: Run three or four 1-mile intervals at your 5-K race pace. After each mile, rest for 4 minutes.

Tip: Budget your effort so that you run each quarter mile at the same pace.

5. 800 Repeats

What: Hard runs with jogging recoveries.

Why: Running at your maximum aerobic capacity is a great way to improve it.

How: Warm up till you're sweating. Subtract 10 seconds from your mile-repeat pace and maintain that speed for 800 meters (twice around the track). After each 800-meter run, jog once around the track before repeating.

Tip: Start with only four intervals per session and add one each workout until you can comfortably do eight.

6. 400 Repeats

What: Hard runs with jogging recoveries.

Why: You'll be training to finish strong.

How: Run at your fastest 1-mile pace. (So if your personal record, or PR, for

the mile is 7 minutes, you'll want to perform each 400-meter interval in 105 seconds, or 1:45.) After each 400-meter run, jog for 1 or 2 minutes, then repeat. Start with a six-interval workout and add one interval each time you go to the track, until you reach 10.

Tip: Do the math before you start. And warm up first!

7. In-and-Outs

What: Fast 200-meter runs alternating with not-so-fast 200-meter runs for 2 miles total.

Why: This workout forces you to recover on the go, allowing you to train at higher overall intensity for a longer distance than you otherwise could.

How: At your mile PR pace, run 200 meters, then slow down so it takes you 10 seconds longer to complete the next 200 meters. Continue to alternate between these speeds until you've run 2 miles.

Tip: If you slow by more than 2 seconds in either your fast or slow segment, run at a light pace until you finish the entire 2 miles.

8. Fast-Finish Long Run

What: A long run with a speed surge in the second half.

Why: You'll train your body to go long and finish hard.

How: Double your regular easy run. Do the first half at your normal pace, and at the midway point, pick up the pace by 5 to 10 seconds per mile.

Tip: Stash or carry water to help you in that second half.

The Ultimate 10-K Plan

Kick tail in your next 10-K with this 8-week speed plan from Len Kravitz, PhD, associate professor of exercise science at the University of New Mexico. It uses the Pledge of Allegiance—that's right, the Pledge you recited in grade school—to help you run faster than ever before. In a University of Wisconsin-Lacrosse study, researchers found that a person's ability to recite the Pledge of Allegiance—all 31 words—while running is a highly accurate gauge of intensity. Learn how to use it strategically, and you'll ensure that you run at the ideal pace every single workout, whether it's a long, easy run or high-intensity intervals. The end result: You'll turn in your best 10-K time ever.

The Science of Speed

Before we get to the Pledge, a lesson in lactate threshold. Lactate is your body's buffering agent for the acid that builds up in your legs and causes them to burn during a run. (This "acid" is commonly thought of as lactic acid, but scientists no longer think that's true.) The faster you run, the faster your acid levels rise. At a certain point, there's too much acid to neutralize, and you have to slow down. This is when you've crossed your lactate threshold.

You can also think of your lactate threshold as the fastest pace you can run that allows you to start and finish at the same speed without feeling any burn. So by pushing your lactate threshold higher, you'll be able to run faster, longer. That's where the Pledge of Allegiance comes in: It's the tool that will help you raise your threshold.

Training Days

In this program, you'll run 3 or 4 days a week and vary the distance and intensity of the workouts. Follow the guidelines below for performing each workout at the ideal intensity.

Volume training. On volume days, you have just one goal: Log the miles. Volume training is designed to develop your ability to perform prolonged exercise, as well as to prepare your muscles and joints for the repeated impact of running. Run at a pace that allows you to recite the Pledge of Allegiance easily.

Maximal steady-state training. Do these runs as close to your lactate threshold as possible. Maximal steady-state training simulates race pace and improves your body's ability to clear speed-limiting acid from your blood and muscles. Run at a pace that allows you to recite the Pledge of Allegiance with difficulty, in spurts of only three or four words at a time.

Interval training: You'll intersperse short bouts of running that are above your lactate threshold with longer periods of running that fall below it. Intervals train your body to tolerate high amounts of acid. Start by running at your volume-training intensity for 5 minutes. Then increase your speed until you can't recite a single word of the Pledge. Maintain this pace for 30 seconds, then slow down to your starting pace for the next 3 minutes, before beginning another 30-second high-intensity stint. Start with five intervals and try to do more each workout, while shortening the recovery periods.

The Multi-Level 10-K Plan

Determine which program is appropriate for your level of fitness, then use the chart below as a guide for your day-by-day workout calendar. Next to each mileage amount is a corresponding letter that indicates whether you perform volume training (V), maximal steady-state training (M), or interval training (I) that day. Complete the entire plan, then repeat it to continue to push your fitness level higher.

Beginner: Follow the Beginner program if you perform aerobic exercise or sports up to 2 or 3 days a week.

Advanced: Do the Advanced plan if, on 3 or more days each week, you run for at least 20 minutes or 2 miles.

WEEK		Monday	Tuesday	Wednesday	Thursday	Friday	Saturday	Sunday
Week 1	Beginner	2 miles (V)	Rest	2.5 miles (V)	Rest	3 miles (V)	Rest	3.5 miles (V)
	Advanced	3 miles (V)	Rest	3.5 miles (V)	Rest	4 miles (V)	Rest	4.5 miles (V)
Week 2	Beginner	Rest	4 miles (V)	Rest	4 miles (V)	Rest	4 miles (V)	Rest
	Advanced	Rest	5 miles (V)	Rest	5 miles (V)	Rest	5 miles (V)	Rest
Week 3	Beginner	4.5 miles (V)	Rest	4.5 miles (V)	Rest	4.5 miles (V)	Rest	5 miles (V)
	Advanced	5.5 miles (V)	Rest	5.5 miles (M)	Rest	5.5 miles (V)	Rest	6 miles (V)
Week 4	Beginner	Rest	5 miles (M)	Rest	5 miles (V)	Rest	5.5 miles (V)	Rest
	Advanced	Rest	6 miles (V)	Rest	5 miles (M)	Rest	6 miles (V)	5 miles (I)
Week 5	Beginner	4 miles (V)	Rest	4.5 miles (M)	Rest	4.5 miles (V)	Rest	4.5 miles (V)
	Advanced	Rest	6.5 miles (V)	Rest	5 miles (M)	Rest	6 miles (V)	5 miles (I)
Week 6	Beginner	Rest	5 miles (I)	Rest	6 miles (V)	Rest	5 miles (M)	6 miles (V)
	Advanced	Rest	7 miles (V)	Rest	5 miles (M)	Rest	6 miles (V)	5 miles (I)
Week 7	Beginner	Rest	5 miles (I)	Rest	6 miles (V)	Rest	5 miles (M)	6 miles (V)
	Advanced	Rest	7 miles (M)	Rest	6 miles (V)	Rest	5 miles (I)	6 miles (V)
Week 8	Beginner	Rest	5 miles (V)	Rest	4 miles (V)	Rest	Rest	Race
	Advanced	Rest	6 miles (V)	Rest	5 miles (V)	Rest	Rest	Race

The Fastest Cardio Workouts of All Time

Strapped for time? Try these novel cardio workouts used by top strength coach Alwyn Cosgrove, CSCS, and his team at Results Fitness in Santa Clarita, California. They're actually called metabolic circuits, and they're designed to challenge your cardiovascular system and speed fat loss just like hard sprints do. The big difference: You can do these routines in your basement. What's more, they also improve your aerobic capacity, just like jogging a few miles at a moderate pace. These workouts, however, take a fraction of the time, since you exercise far more intensely.

Medley Conditioning

Do one set of each exercise below in the order shown. Perform each exercise for 15 seconds, then rest for 15 seconds. Perform as many circuits as you can in 5 minutes. One note: For the dumbbell jump squat, lower your body until your thighs are at least *parallel* to the floor each repetition, then jump as high as you can.

- **Sprints or stairclimbing**
  Rest
- **Dumbbell jump squat** (page 205)
  Rest
- **Dumbbell chop** (page 304)
  Rest
- **Single-arm dumbbell or kettlebell swing** (page 268)
  Rest

Finishers

These are quickie cardio routines that you can do at the end of each workout. They're called finishers not just because they're a great way to finish off an exercise session but also because they'll help you finish off your fat.

THE LEG MATRIX

Do one set of each exercise without resting, and keep track of how long it takes to complete the circuit. Then rest for twice that duration, and repeat once. When you can finish the circuit in 90 seconds, skip the rest.

- **Body-weight squat** (page 190): 24 reps
- **Body-weight alternating lunge** (page 217): 12 reps with each leg
- **Body-weight split jump** (page 211): 12 reps with each leg
- **Body-weight jump squat** (for fat loss) (page 194): 24 reps

SQUAT SERIES

Do one set of each exercise without resting. That's one round. Complete a total of three rounds.

- **Body-weight jump squat** (for fat loss) (page 194): Do as many reps as you can in 20 seconds.
- **Body-weight squat** (page 190): Do as many reps as you can in 20 seconds.
- **Isometric squat:** Lower your body until your thighs are parallel to the floor. Hold that position for 30 seconds.

COUNTDOWNS

Alternate back and forth between two exercises (choose either option 1 or option 2), without resting. In your first round, do 10 repetitions of each exercise. In your second round, do 9 reps. Then do 8 reps in your third round. Work your way down as far as you can go. (If you get to zero, you're done.) Each week, raise the number of reps you start with by one—so in your second week, you'll begin your "countdown" with 11 reps.

Option 1
- Single-arm dumbbell swing (page 268)
- Squat thrusts (page 354)

Option 2
- Body-weight jump squat (for fat loss) (page 194)
- Explosive pushup (page 42)

Chapter 15:
The Big Chapter of Nutrition Secrets

UNLOCK THE POWER OF FOOD

Food is power.

In fact, it has too much power over so many of us. But that's why it's liberating to know the rules of good nutrition. The first lesson: Denial won't get you lean. Instead, think about making smart food choices—ones that will allow you to enjoy great-tasting, nutrient-rich meals that fill you up *without* filling you out. Once you learn to eat smart, you take control over your body and gain the power to flatten your belly and improve your health with every bite you take. So dive into the nutrition secrets that follow, and harness the power of food to improve your whole life.

The Simplest Diet Ever

There's one law of weight loss that can't be avoided: You have to burn more calories than you eat. Of course, there are dozens of ways to achieve this deficit. But it doesn't need to be complicated. Case in point: The eating plan that follows. It's designed to reduce your daily intake by trading empty-calorie fare that you're likely to binge on for nutritious whole foods that fill you up. The end result is that you'll lose your gut without feeling like you're on a diet. All you have to do is take it one step at a time—it's as easy as 1-2-3.

Your Three-Step Plan

Follow these three guidelines and you'll quickly find that everything else is just details when it comes to eating for a healthy, lean body. Start with step 1 and adhere to it for 2 weeks. You're likely to find that fat starts melting off you. If it doesn't, combine the advice in step 1 with the guidelines in step 2. Still having problems? Move on to step 3 to guarantee the results you want.

Step 1: Eliminate Added Sugars

This one step is the simplest way to quickly clean up any diet. According to a USDA survey, an average American eats 82 grams of added sugars every day. That's almost 20 teaspoons, contributing an empty 317 calories. The researchers report that 91 percent of these added sugars can be attributed to intake of regular soda (33 percent), baked goods and breakfast cereals (23 percent), candy (16 percent), fruit drinks (10 percent), and sweetened milk products (9 percent), such as chocolate milk, ice cream, and flavored yogurt.

What's not on the list? Meat, vegetables, whole fruit, and eggs, along with whole-grain and dairy products that haven't been sweetened. There's your menu; now eat accordingly. Also, go ahead and have whatever you want at one meal a week—great results don't depend on being perfect 100 percent of the time.

The key message here: Don't overanalyze your diet or worry too much about the details. By simply avoiding foods that contain added sugar, you'll automatically eliminate most junk food. So your diet will instantly become healthier. And for most people, this strategy also dramatically reduces calorie intake. So you start losing weight, without counting calories or restricting entire food groups. Try it for 2 weeks. If this doesn't kickstart fat loss, move on to step 2.

Step 2: Cut Back on Starch

Starches are the main carbs in bread, pasta, and rice. And not just in the processed versions—such as white bread—but also in the 100 percent whole-grain kind. Of course, you've probably been told you actually need more of these foods. You don't. Why? For starters, too much starch messes with your blood sugar.

Here's a more in-depth explanation:

Your blood sugar can fall too low after just 4 hours of not eating. You know when this happens; you become cranky, tired, and maybe even shaky. As a result, you start craving carbohydrates, particularly in the forms of starch and sugar, both of which quickly raise blood sugar. (Protein and fat have little effect on blood sugar.)

Now, chances are, you won't just eat a small amount of starch or sugar. You'll be more likely to binge, spiking your blood sugar high and fast. This fast-rising blood sugar triggers your pancreas to release a flood of insulin, a hormone that lowers blood sugar back to normal. Unfortunately, in nearly half the population, insulin tends to "overshoot," a dysfunction that sends blood sugar crashing. This reinforces the binge, because it makes you crave sugar and starch again. See the problem?

A review from the USDA Human Nutrition Research Center at Tufts University found that consuming carbohydrates such as bread, pasta, and rice, as well as sugar, promotes an increase in total calorie consumption. But by reducing your starch and cutting out foods with added sugars, you'll better control your blood sugar and be less likely to experience the intense carb cravings that tend to derail diets.

So how much starch can you eat? It depends. As a general guideline, limit yourself to two servings a day. Consider one serving to be about 20 grams of carbohydrates—equal to about one slice of bread, one cup of hot or cold cereal,

CARBOHYDRATES... EXPLAINED

Simple Carbohydrates (aka Sugar)

There are many types of sugar, but the two main ones in our diet are glucose and fructose. These are known as single sugars, and they combine with each other to create double sugars, such as sucrose (better known as table sugar). Typically, most foods with sugar contain a combination of glucose and fructose. This is true whether you're eating an apple or drinking a soda.

• *Glucose:* This is your body's primary energy source. It's also the "sugar" in blood sugar. And because it's already in the form your body needs, it's quickly absorbed into your blood. As a result, glucose is the type of carbohydrate that raises blood sugar the fastest.

• *Fructose:* Unlike glucose, fructose doesn't spike blood sugar. That's because to use fructose, your body must first send it from your intestines to your liver. From there, your body converts it to glucose and stores it. However, if your liver glucose stores are already full, then the fructose is converted to fat. This is why an excess can lead to weight gain, even though it has little impact on blood sugar.

Complex Carbohydrates

The definition of these is simple: any carbohydrate that's composed of more than two sugar molecules.

• *Starch:* This is the stored form of glucose in plant foods. There's an abundance of starch in grains, legumes, and root vegetables, such as potatoes. Essentially, starch is a bunch of glucose molecules that are held together by a weak chemical bond. So when you eat it, it breaks down easily, and you're left with pure glucose. The upshot: It raises blood sugar quickly when eaten without fat or fiber.

• *Fiber:* Also called a nondigestible carbohydrate, fiber is the structural material in the leaves, stems, and roots of plants. So it's found in vegetables, fruits, and grains. Fiber is composed of bundles of sugar molecules, but unlike starch, it has no effect on blood sugar. That's because human digestive enzymes can't break the bonds that hold those bundles together. What's more, fiber slows the absorption of starch into your bloodstream and is thought to help you feel full longer after a meal.

■

half of a large potato, or ½ cup cooked pasta, rice, or beans. (For a more accurate measure of the starch and sugar in a food, subtract the amount of fiber from the total carbohydrates.) As a rule, emphasize the highest-fiber, least-processed versions of these foods—breads, pastas, and cereals that are made with "100 percent whole wheat"; brown rice instead of white; and whole potatoes, including the skin.

To troubleshoot even further, reduce your starches to zero to one serving on days you don't work out; ramp back up to two servings on days when you exercise intensely. The reason: You burn more carbs on the days you work out. So give your body more fuel on the days you need it, and less on the days you don't.

As for the rest of your diet, follow these guidelines.

Never restrict your produce intake.
There's a popular saying in the diet industry: "No one ever got fat from eating produce." And it's true. Most whole fruits and vegetables contain very few calories, very little starch, and a wealth of belly-filling fiber. Don't worry about needing a list to double-check which ones meet these criteria. You can just consider potatoes, beans, corn, and peas to be your starchy exceptions, and enjoy the rest as desired. Sure, other root vegetables such as squash and parsnips could also fall under your starch limitations. But chances are, you won't be eating these foods every day anyway—much less *overeating* them.

Have some protein with every meal.
Eating protein ensures that your body always has the raw material to build and maintain your muscle, even while you lose fat. What's more, University of Illinois researchers determined that dieters who eat higher amounts of protein lose more fat and feel more satisfied than those who eat the lowest amounts of the nutrient. So at every meal and snack, make a conscious effort to have a serving or two of protein in the form of yogurt, cheese, milk, beef, turkey, chicken, fish, pork, eggs, nuts, or a protein shake.

If you want a number to shoot for, the ideal amount is about 1 gram of protein per pound of your target body weight. For example, if you want to weigh 120 pounds, eat 120 grams of protein a day. Of course, that much protein can be hard for some women to swallow—or even just inconvenient. If either is the case for you, consider your minimum requirement to be about 125 grams a day. Use the following chart to guide your selections.

FOOD	PROTEIN (G)
1 EGG	6
3 OZ BEEF, PORK, CHICKEN, OR FISH	25 TO 30
8 OZ MILK OR YOGURT	9
1 OZ (1 SLICE) CHEESE	7
1 OZ NUT BUTTER, NUTS, OR SEEDS	6

Don't be afraid of fat. You won't store it if you aren't eating too many total calories. For instance, research shows that diets containing upward of 60 percent fat are just as effective for weight loss as those in which fat provides only 20 percent of the calories. (Both approaches lower your risk of heart disease.) The fact is, fat is filling and it adds flavor to your meals, both of which help you avoid feeling deprived. And that means you can eat the natural fat in meat, cheese, milk, butter, avocados, nuts, and olive oil. Because you've already cut out foods with added sugar, you've also slashed many of the junk foods that provide the overload of fat and calories in the average person's diet.

Eat until you're satisfied, not stuffed. Focusing your diet on foods that provide healthy doses of protein, fiber, and fat fills you up, keeps you satisfied, and regulates your blood sugar. This combination of benefits helps diminish your appetite and often automatically reduces the number of calories you consume, speeding fat loss. However, if you eat mindlessly, you're not likely to lose fat. So pay attention to how you feel—and don't clean your plate out of habit. In a Cornell University nutrition survey, the heaviest people said they usually stopped eating when they thought they had consumed the "normal amount"—a typical restaurant entrée, say—instead of when they started to feel full.

Step 3: Watch Your Calories

If you've slashed sugar and starch for a month and your jeans haven't yet started fitting better, your problem is simple: You're still eating too much. It could be that you don't realize that you're satisfied *until* you're stuffed. Or maybe it's just hard to break old habits. The upshot? You need portion control.

Use this strategy from Alan Aragon, MS, *Men's Health* advisor and a nutritionist in Thousand Oaks, California. Simply multiply your desired body weight by 10 to 12. Then eat that many calories a day. One note: Choose your multiplier—10, 11, or 12—by how active you are. So if your desired weight is 180 pounds and you work out 5 days a week, you'd multiply 180 by 12—giving you a target of 2,160 calories a day. Just use your best judgment; you can always further adjust your intake if you're not achieving the results you want.

To ensure that you meet your calorie target, keep a food journal for 2 weeks. For each food you eat, estimate the serving size and write it down. (Be honest; otherwise, it doesn't work.) Then log each meal and snack into the free nutrient analysis tool like the one at www.nutritiondata.com or sparkpeople.com. This not only keeps you on track but also quickly teaches you how to eyeball meals to estimate their calorie counts. You'll begin to automatically realize what an appropriate portion is for your diet. Once you reach your desired weight, you can up your calorie intake to 14 to 16 calories per pound.

HOW SUGAR HIDES

Scanning a product's ingredients list to see if it contains sugar is smart—but you may need to expand your vocabulary. Here are 20 aliases that the sweet stuff goes by—none of which include the word *sugar*.

- **Barley malt**
- **Brown rice syrup**
- **Corn syrup**
- **Dextrose**
- **Evaporated cane juice invert syrup**
- **Fructose**
- **Fruit juice**
- **Galactose**
- **Glucose**
- **Granular fruit grape juice concentrate**
- **High-fructose corn syrup**
- **Honey**
- **Lactose**
- **Maltodextrin**
- **Maple syrup**
- **Molasses**
- **Organic cane juice**
- **Sorghum**
- **Sucrose**
- **Turbinado**

The Healthiest Foods You Aren't Eating

The real secret to eating better? Fill your diet with healthy fare that tastes good. Here are eight foods to make that task easier than ever.

Pork Chops

Taste isn't the only great thing about the pig meat in your butcher's case. Compared with other meats, pork chops contain relatively high amounts of selenium, a mineral that's linked to lower risk of cancer. Per gram of protein, pork chops pack almost five times the selenium of beef, and more than twice that of chicken. They're also loaded with riboflavin and thiamin, B vitamins that help your body more efficiently convert carbs to energy. But perhaps most important, Purdue researchers found that a 6-ounce daily serving helped people preserve their muscle as they lost weight on very low-calorie diets.

Mushrooms

Never mind that these edible fungi are more than 90 percent water—at least 700 different species are known to have a medicinal effect. Credit their metabolites, by-products that are created when mushrooms are broken down during the digestion process. Researchers in the Netherlands recently reported that metabolites have been shown to boost immunity and prevent cancer growth.

Red-Pepper Flakes

These hot little numbers may help extinguish your appetite. Dutch researchers have discovered that consuming a gram of red pepper—about $\frac{1}{2}$ teaspoon—30 minutes prior to a meal decreased total calorie intake by 14 percent. The scientists believe the appetite-reducing effect is due to capsaicin, the chemical compound that gives red peppers their heat. Emerging research suggests that capsaicin may also help kill cancer cells.

Full-Fat Cheese

Besides enhancing the flavor of broccoli, cheese is an excellent source of casein—a slow-digesting, high-quality protein that may be the best muscle-building nutrient you can eat. What's more, casein causes your body to utilize more of the bone-building calcium in cheese, according to a study in the *Journal of the American College of Nutrition*. Worried about your cholesterol? Don't be. Danish researchers found that even when men ate between seven and ten 1-ounce servings of full-fat cheese daily for 2 weeks, their LDL ("bad") cholesterol didn't budge.

Iceberg Lettuce

Conventional wisdom suggests this vegetable is nutritionally bankrupt. But that reputation is unfounded. As it turns out, $\frac{1}{2}$ head of iceberg lettuce has significantly more alpha-carotene, a powerful disease-fighting antioxidant, than either romaine lettuce or spinach. And at 10 calories per cup, you can consider it a nutritional freebie.

Scallops

These mollusks are composed almost entirely of protein. In fact, a 3-ounce serving provides 18 grams of the nutrient and just 93 calories. So it's a delicious and seemingly indulgent way to pack more protein into your diet. Clams and oysters provide a similar benefit.

Vinegar

Scientists in Sweden discovered that when people consumed 2 tablespoons of vinegar with a high-carb meal, their blood sugar was 23 percent lower than when they skipped the antioxidant-loaded liquid. They also felt fuller. Vinegar is packed with polyphenols, powerful chemicals that have been shown to improve cardiovascular health, report Arizona State University scientists. Besides combining it with olive oil for a salad dressing, you can use it to punch up your cooking: Add a splash of balsamic vinegar to mayonnaise before spreading it on a sandwich, drizzle a few tablespoons of red or white wine vinegar on a hot pan of sautéed vegetables (especially caramelized onions), or throw a shot of sherry vinegar into your next bowl of tomato soup.

Chicken Thighs

If you're bored with chicken breasts, try the thighs for a change. Sure, they have a little more fat, but that's why they taste so good. Nutritionally speaking, per ounce, thighs have just 1 more gram of fat and 11 more calories than breasts. Of course, if you judged all foods by calories per ounce, you'd end up on the celery diet. The key is portion size: If you like chicken thighs—or prime rib, for that matter—adjust the amount you eat so that it fits into your caloric budget. And don't forget that fat satisfies, so it may keep you full longer after your meal, causing you to eat less at your next.

TRACK YOUR LOSSES

Research shows that for every pound of weight you lose, you'll melt $1/4$ inch off your waist. See for yourself: Wrap a measuring tape around your abdomen—or have your significant other help—so that the bottom of the tape touches the tops of your hip bones. (Your navel moves as you lose weight, so targeting the hips ensures that you always take the measurement at precisely the same location.) The tape should be parallel to the floor and snug without compressing your skin.

NUTRITION SECRET #2

Fatty Foods You Can Eat Guilt-Free

As is true of other nutrients, the fat you eat shouldn't come from candy bars, cookies, and cake. Instead, it should be derived from whole, natural foods. And it's important to remember that calories still matter, too. But with that in mind, here are seven foods you can start eating again, as long as you keep the portions reasonable.

Meat with Flavor

I'm talking about beef (rib eye), poultry (dark meat), and pork (bacon and ham). The fat may add calories, but it also triggers your body to produce CCK, a satiety hormone that helps you feel full longer after you've eaten. And that can reduce your calorie intake at subsequent meals.

Whole Milk

While you've probably always been told to drink reduced-fat milk, the majority of scientific research shows that drinking whole milk actually improves cholesterol levels—just not as much as drinking skim. So choose milk based on your taste preference. A lower-fat option may save you a few calories, but you shouldn't consider it a necessity if your total calories are in check. Interestingly, scientists at the University of Texas Medical Branch, in Galveston, found that drinking whole milk after lifting weights boosted muscle protein synthesis—an indicator of muscle growth—2.8 times more than drinking skim.

Butter

Downing a basket of bread slathered in butter isn't healthy. But while many nutritionists object to the number of calories that butter adds to a meal, the reality is that one pat contains just 36 calories. And research shows the fat in butter improves your body's ability to absorb fat-soluble vitamins A, D, E, and K. Butter is also ideal for cooking, especially compared with polyunsaturated fats, such as those found in vegetable oils (corn or soybean). That's because under high heat, polyunsaturated fats are more susceptible to oxidation, an effect that may contribute to heart disease, according to Canadian researchers.

Sour Cream

For years, you've been told to avoid sour cream or to eat the light version. That's because 90 percent of the dairy product's calories are derived from fat, at least half of which is saturated. Sure, the percentage of fat is high, but the total amount isn't. Consider that a serving of sour cream is 2 tablespoons. That provides just 52 calories—half the amount that's in a single tablespoon of mayonnaise—and less saturated fat than you'd get from drinking a 12-ounce glass of 2% milk. Besides, full-fat tastes far better than the light or fat-free products, which also have added carbohydrates.

Coconut

Ounce for ounce, coconut contains even more saturated fat than butter does. As a result, health experts have warned that it will clog your arteries. But research shows that the saturated fat in coconut has a beneficial effect on heart disease risk factors. One reason: More than 50 percent of its saturated fat content is lauric acid. A recent analysis of 60 studies published in the *American Journal of Clinical Nutrition* reports that even though lauric acid raises LDL ("bad") cholesterol, it boosts HDL ("good") cholesterol even more. Overall, this means it decreases your risk of cardiovascular disease. The rest of the saturated fat in a coconut is believed to have little or no effect on cholesterol levels.

Chicken Skin

No, not the battered, fried kind. But leaving the skin on a roasted chicken breast makes the meat taste better and provides half your daily requirement of selenium.

Eggs

In a recent scientific review of dozens of studies, Wake Forest University researchers found no connection between egg consumption and heart disease. And more and more research suggests the nutrients in egg yolk are beneficial to your health.

Eggs may even be the perfect diet food: Saint Louis University scientists found that people who had eggs as part of their breakfast ate fewer calories the rest of the day than those who ate bagels instead. Even though both breakfasts contained the same number of calories, the egg eaters consumed 264 fewer calories for the entire day.

SPECIAL REPORT

The Saturated Fat Secret: Is Bad Fat Good for You?

You've probably come to believe that saturated fats are a high-fat health hazard. But do you really know the facts?

Turns out, there are more than 13 types of saturated fat. And though they've been damned as a whole by health experts for decades, some of them are actually *good* for your heart. You read right: Saturated fat is not a nutritional evil.

Take the saturated fat in beef, for example. Most of it actually decrease*s* your heart disease risk, either by lowering LDL ("bad") cholesterol or by reducing your ratio of total cholesterol to HDL ("good") cholesterol.

Let's dissect a sirloin into its various fatty acids, looking at the impact each has on your heart health. Although this analysis is specific to beef, it differs very little from in the results we'd get if we looked at chicken and turkey (think: dark meat and skin), pork (including ham and bacon), and eggs. That's because nearly all fat derived from animals is similar in composition. Dairy products, such as butter and cream, have a higher percentage of saturated fat than do beef, poultry, and pork. However, most of the saturated fat in dairy—about 70 percent—is from palmitic and stearic acids, neither of which raises heart disease risk.

MONOUNSATURATED FAT: 49%
Oleic acid: 45% [+]
Palmitoleic acid: 4% [+]

SATURATED FAT: 47%
Palmitic acid: 27% [+]
Stearic acid: 16% [0]
Myristic acid: 3% [-]
Lauric acid: 1% [+]

POLYUNSATURATED FAT: 4%
Linoleic acid: 4% [+]

+ = positive effect on cholesterol
− = negative effect on cholesterol
0 = no effect on cholesterol

So a simple analysis shows us that 97 percent of the fat in beef either has no effect on or lowers your risk for heart disease. You'll also notice, and perhaps be surprised by, the fact that the fat in beef isn't 100 percent saturated fat. That's because natural foods are typically made up of a combination of fats.

Consider lard: Because it's solid at room temperature—saturated fats are solid; unsaturated fats are liquid—it's often solely thought of as "saturated." Yet just as in beef, chicken, and pork, about 40 percent of lard's fat content is a monounsaturated fat called oleic acid. This is the very same heart-healthy fat that's found in olive oil, yet most people have never heard this fact.

But what about all the strong scientific evidence showing that saturated fat leads to heart disease? That case is actually pretty weak. The hypothesis that consuming saturated fat leads to heart disease was first proposed in the 1950s. Today, nearly 60 years later, that hypothesis has still never been proved. This despite the fact that billions of taxpayer dollars have been spent trying to prove it. For example, the Women's Health Initiative—the largest and most expensive diet study ever funded by the US government—showed that women who followed a diet low in total fat and saturated fat for an average of 8 years had the same heart disease and stroke rates as women who didn't change their eating habits. (The low-fat dieters ate 29 percent less saturated fat.)

What's more, your body is always making saturated fat. One reason: Saturated fats are part of every cell membrane in your body. They're also needed for production of hormones and serve as an important source of fuel. So even if you were to eat zero saturated fat, you'd make enough to serve these important functions. Bottom line: Saturated fat isn't poison to your body, despite what you may have been led to believe.

Of course, you don't want *too* much. Several studies indicate that higher levels of saturated fat in your blood are associated with increased risk for heart disease. Does that mean eating saturated fat boosts your chances of developing heart disease? Not likely, as long as you don't eat too many total calories overall.

In a recent study, University of Connecticut researchers compared people on a low-carb, high-fat diet—which didn't restrict saturated fat—to people following a low-fat, high-carb approach. The finding: Both groups ate fewer calories, lost weight, and lowered the amount of saturated fat in their bloodstreams. This shows the benefit of controlling your calories, regardless of the type of diet you're consuming. However, the low-carb dieters—who ate three times more saturated fat than the low-fat dieters—actually reduced their blood levels of saturated fat by twice as much. (The low-carb group also improved their HDL "good" cholesterol, and didn't raise their LDL "bad" cholesterol—a combination that lowered their risk of heart disease.)

Turns out, carbs are easily converted to saturated fat in your liver. In fact, eating carbs ramps up your liver's production of saturated fat, while consuming saturated fat itself lowers your internal production of the fat. So if you regularly *gorge* on carbs, your blood levels of the fat will likely skyrocket—even if you don't eat any saturated fat.

The take-home message: Eating too many calories is far worse for you than is consuming any specific fat or carb. And based on science, there's no good reason that whole foods containing saturated fat shouldn't be part of a healthy diet. So go ahead: Start enjoying fat again—just don't overindulge. Consider that your golden rule of eating for all foods.

PUMPKIN SEEDS: THE BEST SNACK YOU AREN'T EATING

These jack-o'-lantern waste products are the easiest way to consume more magnesium. That's important because French researchers have determined that people with the highest levels of magnesium in their blood have a 40 percent lower risk of early death than those with the lowest levels. On average, people consume 343 milligrams (mg) of the mineral daily, well under the 420 mg recommended by the Institute of Medicine.

How to eat them: Whole, shells and all. (The shells provide extra fiber.) Roasted pumpkin seeds contain 150 mg of magnesium per ounce, which will ensure you hit your daily target easily. Look for them in the snack section of your grocery store, next to the nuts and sunflower seeds.

Health Food Frauds

Just because the label says it's good for you doesn't mean that it is. Here's how to read beyond the marketing hype.

Yogurt with Fruit at the Bottom

The upside: Yogurt and fruit are two of the healthiest foods known to man.
The downside: Corn syrup is not. But that's exactly what's used to make these products super sweet. For example, a six-ounce carton of fruit-flavored yogurt contains 32 grams of sugar, only about half of which is found naturally in the yogurt and fruit. The rest comes from corn syrup, an "added"—or what we prefer to call "unnecessary"—sugar.
The healthier alternative: Mix ½ cup plain yogurt with ½ cup fresh fruit, such as blueberries or raspberries. You'll eliminate the excess sugar while more than doubling the amount of fruit you down.

Baked Beans

The upside: Beans are packed with fiber that helps keep you full and slows the absorption of sugar into your bloodstream.
The downside: The baked kind are typically covered in a sauce made with brown and white sugars. And because the fiber is located inside the bean, it doesn't have a chance to interfere with the speed at which the sugary glaze is digested. Consider that 1 cup of baked beans contains 24 grams of sugar: about the same amount that's in an 8-ounce soft drink. Not drinking regular soda? Then you should skip the baked beans, too.
The healthier alternative: Red kidney beans, packed in water. You get the nutritional benefits of legumes, without the extra sugar. They don't even need to be heated: Just open the can, rinse off the liquid and excess salt they're stored in, and serve. Try splashing some hot sauce on top for a spicy variation.

California Roll

The upside: The seaweed it's wrapped in contains essential nutrients, such as iodine, calcium, and omega-3 fats.
The downside: It's basically a Japanese sugar cube. That's because its two other major components are white rice and imitation crab, both of which are packed with fast-digesting carbohydrates and almost no protein.
The healthier alternative: Opt for real sushi, by choosing a roll that's made with tuna or salmon. This automatically reduces the number of blood sugar–boosting carbohydrates you're eating, while providing a hefty helping of high-quality protein. Or better yet, skip the rice, too, by ordering sashimi.

Fat-Free Salad Dressing

The upside: Cutting out the fat reduces the calories that a dressing contains.
The downside: Sugar is added to

provide flavor. Perhaps more important, the removal of fat reduces your body's ability to absorb many of the vitamins found in salad vegetables. In a recent study, Ohio State University researchers discovered that people who ate a salad dressing containing fat absorbed 15 times more beta-carotene and five times more lutein—both powerful antioxidants—than when they downed a salad topped with fat-free dressing.

The healthier alternative: Choose a full-fat dressing that is made with either olive oil or canola oil, and that provides less than 2 grams of carbohydrate per serving. Or keep it simple, tangy, and completely sugar-free by shaking liberal amounts of balsamic vinegar and olive oil over your salad.

Reduced-Fat Peanut Butter

The upside: Even the reduced-fat version is packed with healthy monounsaturated fat.

The downside: Many commercial brands are sweetened with "icing sugar"—the same finely ground sugar used to decorate cupcakes. And reduced-fat versions are the worst of all because they extract the healthy fat only to infuse more icing sugar. In fact, each tablespoon of reduced-fat Skippy contains $\frac{1}{2}$ teaspoon of the sweet stuff. So the label might as well read, "Stick a birthday candle in me."

The healthier alternative: An all-natural, full-fat peanut butter that contains no added sugar.

Corn Oil

The upside: It's considered good for you because it contains high levels of omega-6 fatty acid—an essential polyunsaturated fat that doesn't raise cholesterol.

The downside: Corn oil contains 60 times more omega-6 than omega-3, the type of healthy fat predominantly found in fish, walnuts, and flaxseed. This is a problem because research shows that a high intake of omega-6 fats relative to omega-3 fats is associated with increased inflammation that boosts your risk of cancer, arthritis, and obesity.

The healthier alternative: Olive or canola oils, which have a much better balance of omega-6 to omega-3 fats. They also have also a greater proportion of monounsaturated fat, which has been shown to lower LDL ("bad") cholesterol.

WHY DIETS WORK

Even lots of exercise is no match for bad eating habits, say University of Missouri researchers. In a recent study, a group of people lost their tummies with a strict diet and a vigorous, 5-day-a-week workout program. Then they were split into two groups: One that did no exercise, and another that continued the training regimen. However, they all ate an average of 500 additional calories a day. The result? The belly fat returned for everyone. The scientists point out that as long as you're taking in more calories than you're burning, abdominal fat will come back whether you exercise or not. The upshot: If you're starting to regain lost weight, it's likely that the solution is at the end of your fork.

NUTRITION SECRET #4

5 Food Rules You Should Break

Foolproof your diet for good with this nutrition-myth-busting guide from *Men's Health* nutrition advisor Alan Aragon, MS.

Myth #1: High Protein Intake Is Harmful to Your Kidneys

The origin: Back in 1983, researchers first discovered that eating more protein increases your glomerular filtration rate, or GFR. Think of GFR as the amount of blood your kidneys are filtering per minute. From this finding, many scientists made the leap that a higher GFR places your kidneys under greater stress.

What science really shows: Nearly 2 decades ago, Dutch researchers found that while a protein-rich meal did boost GFR, it didn't have an adverse effect on overall kidney function. In fact, there's zero published research showing that downing hefty amounts of protein—specifically, up to 1.27 grams per pound of body weight a day—damages healthy kidneys.

The bottom line: As a rule of thumb, shoot to eat your target body weight in grams of protein daily. For example, if you are a chubby 200 pounds and want to be a lean 180, then have 180 grams of protein a day.

Myth #2: Blueberries Are Better for You Than Bananas

The origin: Studies show that, per cup, blueberries have among the highest antioxidant content of almost any fruit. So they've been marketed as superior to other fruits—especially bananas.

What science really shows: They're both good for you, in different ways. For example, per calorie, bananas have about four times as much potassium and magnesium as blueberries have. So it's not as simple as one food being superior to another; it all has to do with your perspective—and it's likely that variety is best. For instance, Colorado State University scientists found that people who consume the widest array of fruits and vegetables experience more health benefits than those who eat just as much produce from among a smaller assortment.

The bottom line: Produce is good for you. And for the most benefits, you should eat a mix of the kinds you like the best—not limit yourself based on an antioxidant ranking.

Myth #3: Red Meat Causes Cancer

The origin: In a 1986 study, Japanese researchers discovered cancer in rats that were fed heterocyclic amines, compounds that are generated from overcooking meat via high heat. Since then, some studies of large populations have suggested a potential link between meat and cancer.

What science really shows: No study

has ever found a direct cause-and-effect relationship between red-meat consumption and cancer. As for the population studies, they're far from conclusive. They rely on broad surveys of people's eating habits and health afflictions, and the resulting numbers are crunched to find trends, not causes.

The bottom line: Don't stop grilling. Meat lovers who are worried about the supposed risks of grilled meat don't need to avoid burgers and steak; rather, they should just trim off the burned or overcooked sections of the meat.

Myth #4: High-Fructose Corn Syrup (HFCS) Is More Fattening Than Regular Sugar

The origin: In 2002, University of California at Davis researchers published a well-publicized paper noting that Americans' increasing consumption of fructose, including that in HFCS, paralleled our skyrocketing rates of obesity.

What science really shows: Both HFCS and sucrose—better known as table sugar—contain similar amounts of fructose. In fact, they're almost chemically identical in that they're both composed of about 50 percent fructose and 50 percent glucose. This is why the University of California at Davis scientists determined fructose intakes from *both* HFCS and sucrose. The truth is, there's no evidence to show any differences in these two types of sugar. Both will cause weight gain when consumed in excess.

The bottom line: HFCS and regular sugar are empty-calorie carbs that should be consumed in limited amounts.

Myth #5: Salt Causes High Blood Pressure and Should Be Avoided

The origin: In the 1940s, a Duke University researcher named Walter Kempner, MD, became famous for using salt restriction to treat people with hypertension. Later, studies confirmed that reducing salt could be helpful.

What science really shows: Large-scale scientific reviews have determined there's no reason for people with normal blood pressure to restrict sodium. Now, if you are already hypertensive, you may be "salt sensitive." As a result, reducing the amount of salt you eat could be helpful. However, it's been known for 20 years that people with high BP who don't want to lower their salt intake can simply consume more potassium-rich foods to achieve the same health benefits. Why? Because it's the balance of the two minerals that matters: Dutch scientists found that a low potassium intake has the same impact on blood pressure as high salt consumption does. And turns out, the average guy consumes 3,200 milligrams (mg) of potassium a day—1,500 mg less than recommended.

The bottom line: Strive for a diet rich in potassium by eating fruits, vegetables, and legumes. For instance, spinach (cooked), bananas, and most types of beans each contain more than 400 mg of potassium per serving.

THINK BEFORE YOU EAT

Before your next snack, review your previous meal. British researchers determined that people who used this strategy ate 30 percent fewer calories than those who didn't stop to think. The theory: Simply remembering what you've already eaten makes you less likely to overindulge.

Workout Nutrition Secrets

Whether you want to lose fat or build muscle, you'll achieve the best results by making sure your muscles are well fed. That means consuming a healthy dose of protein around your workout. This provides your body with the raw materials to repair and upgrade your muscles, enhancing your results.

What's more, after your workout is also the best time of the day to consume carbs. Why? Well, imagine that the carbs you eat go into a bucket. When the bucket is full, the carbs overflow and are converted to fat. This is what happens in your body, with the bucket representing your muscles. But when you exercise, you burn carbs, removing them from your bucket. As a result, you have more room in which to store the carbs you eat after your workout. That makes postworkout carbs less likely to end up stored as belly fat. Just as important, these carbs help speed the repair of your muscles.

The upshot: You can strategically eat most of your daily starch and sugar immediately before or after your workout, or you can stick with protein-only pre- and postworkout snacks to keep your carb bucket close to empty and your body burning fat at full blast. Simply choose the option you like best.

Protein-Only Workout Snacks

Option #1:

A convenient shake. Prepare a protein shake (mixed with water) that provides at least 20 grams of protein. (More is fine.) When choosing a product, look for one that contains only small amounts of carbs and fat. Here are three reputable products—they all have blends of whey and casein protein—but comparable protein powders work as well.

At Large Nutrition Nitrean
Available at: www.atlargenutrition.com
Per serving (make 2 servings): 24 grams (g) protein, 2 g carbohydrate, 1 g fat

Biotest Metabolic Drive Super Protein Shake
Available at: www.t-nation.com
and www.biotest.net
Per serving (make 2 servings): 20 g protein, 4 g carbohydrate, 1.5 g fat

MET-Rx Protein Plus Protein Powder (46-g Metamyosyn Protein Blend)
Available at: metrx.com
Per serving (make 1 serving): 46 g protein, 3 g carbohydrate, 1.5 g fat

Option #2:

Regular fare. Consume at least 20 grams of high-quality protein in the form of solid food.

- A small can (3.5 ounces) of tuna
- 3 to 4 ounces of lean deli meat
- A serving of any lean meat that's the size (length, width, thickness) of a deck of cards
- 3 eggs—an omelet, for instance

Protein-and-Carbs Workout Snacks

Option #1:

A convenient shake (with carbs). Prepare a shake (mixed with water or milk) that provides a blend of 40 to 80 grams of carbohydrates and at least 40 grams of whey and casein protein. When choosing a product, look for one that contains both types of protein. As for carbohydrates, this is the one time when sugar is perfectly acceptable. That's because it can be used immediately for energy during your workout, and it helps speed muscle growth after your workout. Three products that fit the criteria:

At Large Nutrition Opticen
Available at: www.atlargenutrition.com
Per serving (make 1 serving): 52 g protein, 25 g carbohydrate, 1.7 g fat

Biotest Surge Recovery
Available at: www.t-nation.com and www.biotest.net
Per serving (make 1 serving): 25 g protein, 46 g carbohydrate, 2.5 g fat

MET-Rx Xtreme Size Up
Available at: metrx.com
Per serving (make 1 serving): 59 g protein, 80 g carbohydrate, 6 g fat

Option #2:

Regular fare (that includes carbs). Take advantage of your half-empty carb bucket and enjoy a couple of servings of carbs without worrying about the impact on your waistline. Consume at least 20 grams of high-quality protein and up to 40 grams of carbohydrates from regular food. You can mix and match foods as desired, or use the general guidelines to figure out your own favorites. (Think: pizza!)

Foods that contain 20 grams of protein:
- A small can (3.5 ounces) of tuna
- 3 to 4 ounces of any kind of meat
- 3 eggs

Amounts and type of foods that contain 15 to 20 grams of carbs (you need two servings):
- 1 slice of bread
- ½ cup cooked pasta or rice
- ½ cup of cereal
- ½ medium potato
- 1 cup of berries or sliced fruit
- 1 whole apple, orange, or peach, or
- ½ large banana

Dairy foods that contain both protein and carbohydrates (per 8-ounce cup):

DAIRY FOOD	PROTEIN (G)	CARBS (G)
MILK	8	12
CHOCOLATE MILK	8	25
PLAIN YOGURT	8	12
FRUIT YOGURT	8	25
KEFIR	14	12
FLAVORED KEFIR	14	25
COTTAGE CHEESE	31	8

Surprising Fitness Foods

Meat, fish, and eggs are packed with protein—so they're great for your muscles. But here are four not-so-obvious foods that can help you tone your body, too.

Almonds

Crunch for crunch, almonds are one of the best sources of alpha-tocopherol vitamin E—the form that's best absorbed by your body. That matters to your muscles because vitamin E is a potent antioxidant that can help prevent free-radical damage after heavy workouts. And the fewer hits taken from free radicals, the faster your muscles will recover and start growing. How much to munch? Two handfuls a day. A Toronto University study found that people can eat that amount daily without gaining weight.

Almonds also double as brain insurance. A study published in the *Journal of the American Medical Association* found that those people who consumed the most vitamin E—from food sources, not supplements—had a 67 percent lower risk for Alzheimer's disease than those eating the least.

Olive Oil

The monounsaturated fat in olive oil appears to act as an anticatabolic nutrient. In other words, it prevents mus-cle breakdown by lowering levels of tumor necrosis factor, a cellular protein linked with muscle wasting. Monounsaturated fats have also been associated with lower rates of heart disease.

Spinach

Well, spinach and just about any other vegetable or fruit. Australian researchers found that people who reduced their antioxidant intake—eating just one serving of fruit and two of vegetables daily—for 2 weeks felt as if they were exerting more effort than when exercising on a diet rich in antioxidants. It seems that eating several servings of fruits and vegetables daily can make exercise seem easier—and help you finish those last reps.

Water

Whether they're in your shins or your shoulders, muscles are approximately 80 percent water. A reduction in body water of as little as 1 percent can impair exercise performance and adversely affect recovery. For example, a German study found that protein synthesis occurs at a higher rate in muscle cells that are well-hydrated, compared with dehydrated cells. English translation: The more parched you are, the slower your body uses protein to build muscle. Plus, researchers at Loma Linda University found that people who drank at least five 8-ounce glasses of water a day were 54 percent less likely to suffer a fatal heart attack than those who drank two or fewer.

The Protein-Powder Primer

Here's your guide to navigating the supplement aisle.

The Best Ingredients: Whey and Casein

What are they? The primary proteins found in milk. In fact, about 20 percent of the protein in milk is whey, and the other 80 percent is casein.

What's the diff? Both are high-quality proteins, meaning they contain all the essential amino acids that are needed by your body. However, whey is known as a "fast protein." That's because it's quickly broken down into amino acids and absorbed into your bloodstream. This makes it a very good protein to consume after your workout, as it can be delivered to your muscles right away. Casein, on the other hand, is digested more slowly, so it's ideal for providing your body with a steady supply of smaller amounts of protein for a longer period of time—such as between meals or while you sleep. Think of it as time-release protein.

Which one? Try a blend. Either will provide your muscles with the raw materials for growth, but combining them allows you to optimize your protein intake no matter when you down a shake.

The Label Decoder

To most people, the ingredients list of a protein powder may as well be written in Sanskrit. That's because it often contains several subtypes of whey and casein protein. Here's how to read the label like a chemist.

Concentrate: The cheapest form of most proteins. It contains slightly higher amounts of fat and carbohydrate than more pure versions and can be clumpy and hard to mix by hand; however, it provides the same basic muscle-building benefits. In the case of casein, it's referred to as caseinate.

Isolate: A protein that's more pure than concentrate—meaning it contains lower amounts of fat and carbohydrate—and is also easier to mix.

Hydrosylate, or hydrolyzed protein: A protein that's been broken down into smaller fractions than are in a concentrate or isolate, allowing it to be absorbed into your bloodstream more quickly. However, when it comes to casein hydrosylate, this defeats the purpose, since the benefit of casein is that it absorbs slowly.

Micellar casein, or isolated casein peptides: An expensive but easy-to-mix protein that's nearly pure casein, ensuring slow and steady absorption.

Milk protein: An ingredient that has the composition of natural milk protein—80 percent casein and 20 percent whey.

Egg-white protein: Like whey and casein, an excellent high-quality protein. It's sometimes called *instantized egg albumin* on the label.

BUILD A BETTER BREAKFAST

Skip the cold cereal: Eating eggs and bacon in the morning can help you control your hunger. In a recent study, Indiana University scientists found that dieters who consumed their biggest dose of daily protein at breakfast felt full longer than those who ate more of the nutrient at lunch or dinner, or who divided it equally across meals. Having greater amounts of protein at breakfast makes you less likely to overeat the rest of the day, say the researchers. The average woman consumes only a small portion of her daily protein intake at her morning meal. Shoot for at least 20 grams.

BONUS!

25 Fat-Fighting Snacks

End Mindless Eating with These Winning Combinations

Whenever you need a between-meals fix, just choose one item from each of the two categories below, mix-and-match style. Adhere to the suggested serving size, and you'll have 25 options for a balanced snack of approximately 200 calories. Each will provide you with a filling dose of protein, fat, and fiber, along with a shot of disease-fighting antioxidants.

EAT THIS ...	AMOUNT	WITH THAT ...	AMOUNT
ALMOND OR PEANUT BUTTER, NUTS, OR SEEDS	1 TBSP	**APPLE**	1 MEDIUM
PLAIN YOGURT	¾ CUP	**PEACH**	1 LARGE
HAM OR TURKEY SLICES	3 SLICES	**CELERY***	5 STALKS
HARD CHEESE (PARMESAN OR CHEDDAR)	1 OZ/1 SLICE	**BLUEBERRIES**	1 CUP
2% COTTAGE CHEESE	½ CUP	**BABY CARROTS***	1 CUP

*Because these are very low-calorie choices, you can double the serving size of the "Eat This" snack that you pair them with.

Index

Boldface page references indicate photographs. <u>Underscored</u> references indicate boxed text.

A

Abdominal muscles. *See also* Core
    muscles
  anatomy, **277**
  fast-tempo exercises, <u>321</u>
  workouts, 336–37
Airex Balance Pad, 21
Alcohol, 26
Almonds, 456
Alternating barbell lunge, 213
Alternating dumbbell bench press, 53,
  53
Alternating dumbbell lunge, 217
Alternating dumbbell lying triceps
  extension, 167, **167**
Alternating dumbbell shoulder press,
  121, **121**
Alternating incline dumbbell bench
  press, 54, **54**
Alternating lateral raise with static
  hold, 127, **127**
Alternating neutral-grip dumbbell
  bench press, 53, **53**
Alternating sets, 15
Alternating situp, 313, **313**
Alternating slide out, 293, **293**
Alternating Swiss-ball dumbbell chest
  press, 56, **56**
Alternating Swiss-ball dumbbell
  shoulder press, 122, **122**
Ankle circles, 366, **366**
Ankle flexion, 366, **366**
Arm circles, 357, **357**
Arm curls, 150–61, **150–61**, 178, **178**
Arm extensions, 162–73, **162–73**, 179, **179**
Arms
  benefits of strong, 148
  circumferences, measuring, <u>151</u>
  exercises
    arm curls, 150–61, **150–61**, 178, **178**
    arm extensions, 162–73, **162–73**, 179,
    179
    biceps, 150–61, **150–61**, 178, **178**
    forearms, 174–77, **174–77**

    triceps, 162–73, **162–73,** 179, **179**
    wrist and hand, 174–77, **174–77**
  muscles, **149**
  stretches, 180–81, **180–81**
  workouts, 182–84
At Large Nutrition Nitrean, 26, 454
At Large Nutrition Opticen, 455

B

Back
  benefits of strong, 70
  exercises, **72–109,** 72–111
    chinups and pullups, 96–101,
    96–101
    kneeling Swiss-ball lat stretch,
    109, **109**
    for latissimus dorsi, 96–107, **96–107**
    pulldowns and pullovers, 102–7,
    102–7
    rows and raises, 72–95, **72–95**
    for upper back, 72–95, **72–95**
  muscles, **71**
  pain, flossing away, <u>283</u>
  testing strength with scapular
    retraction, <u>101</u>
  workout, 110–11, 337
Back extension, 258, **258**
Back rest, for shoulder press, <u>117</u>
Baked beans, 450
Bananas, 452
Band-assisted chinup, 98, **98,** 110
Band side leg raise, 267, **267**
Barbell, 19
Barbell bench press, 46–47, **46–47**
  variations, 47–51, **47–51**
Barbell board press, 49, **49**
Barbell box lunge, 214, **214**
Barbell Bulgarian split squat, 208, **208**
Barbell crossover lunge, 215, **215**
Barbell deadlift, 248, **248**
Barbell floor press, 51, **51**
Barbell front split squat, 208, **208**
Barbell front squat, 199, **199**
  to push press, 341, **341**

Barbell good morning, 254, **254**
Barbell hack squat, 201, **201**
Barbell hang pull, 347, **347**
Barbell high pull, 346, **346**
Barbell jump shrug, 348, **348**
Barbell jump squat, 202, **202**
Barbell lateral stepup, 261, **261**
Barbell lunges, 212–13, **212–13**
  variations, 213–15, **214–15**
Barbell pin press, 49, **49**
Barbell push press, 118, **118**
Barbell quarter squat, 200, **200,** <u>201</u>
Barbell rollout, 292, **292**
Barbell row, 76–77, **76–77**
Barbell shoulder press, 116–17,
  116–17, <u>117</u>
  seated, 119, **119**
Barbell shrug, 130–31, **130–31**
  overhead, 132, **132**
  wide-grip, 132, **132**
Barbell side lunge, 215, **215**
Barbell split jerk, 119, **119**
Barbell split squats, 206–7, **206–7**
  variations, 208, **208,** 226, **226**
Barbell squats, 198, **198**
  variations, 199–202, **199–202**
Barbell stepover, 214, **214**
Barbell stepup, 260, **260**
Barbell stiff squat, 200, **200**
Barbell straight-leg deadlift, 252–53,
  252–53
  to row, 342, **342**
Barbell towel press, 48, **48**
Bar hold, 175, **175**
Beef, saturated fat in, 448
Bench, 18
Bent-arm lateral raise and external
  rotation, 128, **128**
Bent-knee reverse hip raise, 247, **247**
Bent-knee Swiss-ball reverse hip raise,
  247, **247**
Bent-leg calf stretch, 229, **229**
Bent-over reach to sky, 356, **356**
Beverages, 26

Core muscles
  exercises (cont.)
    side plank and row, 286, **286**
    side plank with feet on bench, 285, **285**
    side plank with feet on Swiss ball, 285, **285**
    side plank with knee tuck, 285, **285**
    side plank with reach under, 286, **286**
    single-leg elevated-feet plank, 280, **280**
    single-leg-lowering drill, 327, **327**
    single-leg side plank, 285, **285**
    single-leg Swiss-ball jackknife, 290, **290**
    situp, 310–11, **310–11**
    slide out, 293, **293**
    stability exercises, 278–99, **278–99,** 291, 334, **334**
    standing cable crunch, 321, **321**
    standing rotational chop, 307, **307**
    standing rotational reverse chop, 309, **309**
    standing split rotational chop, 307, **307**
    standing split rotational reverse chop, 309, **309**
    standing stability chop, 297, **297**
    standing stability reverse chop, 299, **299**
    static back extension, 294, **294**
    Swiss-ball crunch, 318, **318**
    Swiss-ball hip crossover, 304, **304**
    Swiss-ball jackknife, 290, **290**
    Swiss-ball opposite arm and leg lift, 283, **283**
    Swiss-ball pike, 328, **328**
    Swiss-ball plank, 281, **281**
    Swiss-ball plank with feet on bench, 281, **281**
    Swiss-ball reverse crunch, 323, **323**
    Swiss-ball rollout, 292, **292**
    Swiss-ball Russian twist, 302, **302**
    Swiss-ball side crunch, 333, **333**
    trunk flexion exercises, 310–21, **310–21**
    T-stabilization, 287, **287**
    V-up, 316, **316**
    weighted crunch, 315, **315**
    weighted Russian twist, 301, **301**
    weighted situp, 313, **313**
    weighted Swiss-ball crunch, 319, **319**

    wide-stance plank with diagonal arm lift, 281, **281**
    wide-stance plank with leg lift, 280, **280**
    wide-stance plank with opposite arm and leg lift, 281, **281**
    wrist-to-knee crunch, 315, **315**
  fast-tempo exercises, 321
  workouts, 336–37
Core stabilization, 334, **334**
Corn oil, 451
Corn syrup, 450, 453
Countdowns (cardio workout), 437
Couples, time-saving workout for, 416–21
Cross-body mountain climber, 289, **289** with feet on Swiss ball, 289, **289**
Crossed-arm barbell front squat, 200, **200**
Crossed-arms crunch, 315, **315**
Crossed-arms situp, 312, **312**
Crossover dumbbell stepup, 263, **263**
Crossover pullup, 100, **100**
Crossover rear lateral raise, 85, **85**
Crowded Gym Workouts, 382–85
Crunch, 314, **314**
  crossed-arms, 315, **315**
  fat burned by, 279
  foam-roller reverse on bench, 324, **324**
  foam-roller reverse with dumbbell, 325, **325**
  foam-roller reverse with medicine ball, 325, **325**
  incline reverse, 323, **323**
  kneeling cable, 321, **321**
  raised-legs, 315, **315**
  reverse, 322, **322**
  side, 332, **332**
  standing cable, 321, **321**
  Swiss-ball, 318, **318**
    reverse, 323, **323**
    side, 333, **333**
  weighted, 315, **315**
    Swiss-ball, 319, **319**
  wrist-to-knee, 315, **315**
Curls, arm, 150–61, **150–61,** 178, **178**
Curlup with raised elbows, 291, **291**
Cycling Russian twist, 302, **302**

D

Deadlift
  back extension, 258, **258**
  barbell, 248, **248**
  barbell good morning, 254, **254**

  barbell straight-leg, 252–53, **252–53**
  barbell straight-leg to row, 342, **342**
  cable pull through, 259, **259**
  dumbbell, 250, **250**
  dumbbell straight-leg, 256, **256**
  dumbbell straight-leg to row, 342, **342**
  rotational dumbbell straight-leg, 257, **257**
  seated barbell good morning, 255, **255**
  single-arm, 251, **251**
  single-leg, 251, **251**
  single-leg back extension, 258, **258**
  single-leg barbell, 249, **249**
  single-leg barbell good morning, 255, **255**
  single-leg barbell straight-leg, 254, **254**
  single-leg dumbbell straight-leg, 257, **257**
  split barbell good morning, 254, **254**
  sumo, 249, **249**
  wide-grip barbell, 249, **249**
  Zercher good morning, 255, **255**
Decline barbell bench press, 50, **50,** 51
Decline dumbbell bench press, 55, **55**
Decline dumbbell fly, 61, **61**
Decline hammer curl, 156, **156**
Decline pushup, 36, **36**
Decline situp, 313, **313**
Deltoids, **71, 115**
Depression, symptom reduction with weight lifting, 8
Depth jump, 195, **195**
Diabetes, decreasing risk by weight lifting, 6
Diagonal raise
  cable, 139, **139**
  dumbbell, 138, **138**
Diet. *See also* Food
  4-week plan, 24–26
  improvement by lifting weights, 7
  three-step plan, 440–43
  why diets work, 451
Dip, 44, **44**
  incline, 45, **45**
  weighted, 45
Doorway stretch, 66, **66**
Dumbbell alternating shoulder press and twist, 123, **123**
Dumbbell bench press, 52, **52**
  variations, 53–55, **53–55**
Dumbbell box lunge, 218, **218**
Dumbbell Bulgarian split squat, 210, **210**
Dumbbell chop, 304, **304**